The Backcountry Classroom:
Lessons, Tools, and Activities for Teaching Outdoor Leaders

Second Edition

Jack K. Drury

Bruce F. Bonney

Dene Berman

Mark C. Wagstaff

Edited by
Jack K. Drury

Illustrations by
John A. Drury

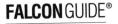

FALCON GUIDE®

GUILFORD, CONNECTICUT
HELENA, MONTANA
AN IMPRINT OF THE GLOBE PEQUOT PRESS

Falcon is a registered trademark of The Globe Pequot Press.

SPEC is a trademark of Leading Edge LLC.

Information on Leave No Trace in chapter 11 "Environmental Ethics" used with permission by Leave No Trace Center for Outdoor Ethics.

The Situational Leadership® Model on page 357 was reprinted from *Management of Organizational Behavior* by Hersey and Blanchard (1982) published by Prentice Hall, a Pearson Education Company, and is used by permission of the Center for Leadership Studies, Inc., © 2002. Situational Leadership® is a registered trademark of the Center for Leadership Studies, Inc.

Illustrations © by John A. Drury
Photos courtesy of the authors
Text design by Nancy Freeborn
Maps on pages 380, 413, and 414 by Zachary Parks © Globe Pequot Press; map illustrations on pages 416 and 417 by Mary Ballachino © Globe Pequot Press.

Library of Congress Cataloging-in-Publication Data
The backcountry classroom: lessons, tools, and activities for teaching outdoor leaders /
  Jack K. Drury . . . [et al.]; edited by Jack K. Drury; illustrations by John A. Drury. — 2nd ed.
      p. cm.
  Rev. ed. of: The backcountry classroom / by Bruce F. Bonney and Jack K. Drury. © 1992.
  Includes bibliographical references and index.
  ISBN 0-7627-2820-5
  1. Outdoor education. I. Drury, Jack K. II. Bonney, Bruce F. Backcountry classroom.

LB1047.B55 2005
371.3'8—dc22   2005040074

Manufactured in the United States of America
Second Edition/First Printing

To buy books in quantity for corporate use or incentives, call **(800) 962–0973, ext. 4551,** or e-mail **premiums@GlobePequot.com.**

Dedicated to the memory of Paul K. Petzoldt,
our teacher, our mentor, and our friend

Paper for this book donated by International Paper. Printed on Accent Opaque paper proudly produced at the Ticonderoga, New York Mill from trees harvested in working Adirondack forests that are managed responsibly in accordance with the principles of the *Sustainable Forestry Initiative*®, (SFI®), providing recreation, open space, and economic benefits for generations and the future.

Contents

Preface to the Second Edition

An education isn't how much you have committed to memory, or even how much you know. It's
being able to differentiate between what you do
know and what you don't.

—Anatole France, French novelist

Too often we give children answers to remember
rather than problems to solve.

—Roger Lewin, noted science journalist
and author

This second edition of *The Backcountry Classroom* has a new look. Starting on the
cover you see the addition of two authors, Dene Berman and Mark Wagstaff.
Both bring tremendous expertise in their field to this work, and both took a leadership role in writing a number of the new chapters and rewriting many of the
existing chapters. It goes without saying that we couldn't have done it without
them.

Once you open the book you will see that the table of contents is considerably larger. There are eight new chapters: Collaboration: How We Approach
Teamwork, Crisis Management in the Backcountry, Group Orienting and Monitoring, Interpretation of the Natural and Cultural Environments, Knots: An
Introduction, Navigation: An Introduction to GPS, Rock Climbing: Leadership
Considerations for Top Roping, and Travel Technique: Canoeing and Sea Kayaking. There are also more than seventy-five new tables and illustrations. We hope
the new chapters will broaden your understanding of these topics and that the
illustrations help clarify our words.

As you explore the chapters, you'll note we've changed "Goals and Objectives"
to "Outcomes." We encourage you to examine these Outcomes carefully. These
Outcomes are our attempt to describe the knowledge, skills, and dispositions
that high-quality outdoor leaders should possess. We think these Outcomes more
accurately portray what we are trying to teach and what we should be attempting
to assess.

No doubt you will notice immediately that this edition is considerably bigger
and heavier than our previous work. We very consciously wanted to update and
expand the content of this edition, to give it a bit more heft and substance than
the first. To those of you who must carry this more "weighty" edition in your
pack or duffle, we hope you agree that it is worth the effort.

As you explore this edition in depth, you will see that our philosophy of teaching and learning has evolved considerably since 1992. The chapter on Teaching and Learning reflects this evolution. There, we engage in an extended discussion of our current thinking about the characteristics of high-quality teaching and the role that teachers play as architects of high-powered learning experiences—both in and out of doors. In this chapter we also introduce you to SPEC™ (Student-centered, Problem-based, Experiential, and Collaborative), the shorthand acronym we use to remind us of the fundamental attributes of our approach. Throughout this book, you'll see that we've appended "challenges" to various lessons that we hope will serve as useful models to those who want to try out some aspect of our SPEC methodology.

Finally, you will see my name as editor. While it was a collaborative effort and we all provided feedback on each other's work, it was my challenge, along with my assistant, Duane Gould, to pull the work of four different people together and shape it into a readable and cogent entity. For that I take full responsibility; any errors or omissions are mine.

As in the first edition, *The Backcountry Classroom* is designed to help instructors and learners master and teach about how to safely enjoy yet protect our wild places. It is designed primarily as a manual for use in the field. However, you will certainly recognize that we've taken great pains to make it useful for classroom instruction as well.

The book is presented in an outline format. It contains a body of knowledge that can be communicated any number of ways. Each lesson has specific Outcomes for each of the three domains we have labeled: knowledge, skills, and dispositions. These Outcomes are followed by the content/body of knowledge of the lesson. Finally, we include a listing of materials we have found useful in teaching the topic. We also include in each lesson our suggestions for the timing of the lesson during a typical extended expedition and some teaching strategies that we have used successfully.

We hope that both instructors and students will carry *The Backcountry Classroom* in their packs or duffles and find it as useful in the classroom as in the field. Since the first printing we have received considerable feedback on how people have used this book. As we hoped, it can be a handy reference for information, an outline for portions of a lecture or demonstration, a handout for class discussion, a reading for students preparing their own classes, and, more recently as a primary resource for more experiential "SPEC"-type lessons.

This edition is designed to be part of an expedition's mobile library. We have taken the liberty of placing the chapter on Teaching and Learning first in the table of contents because we believe it should be the starting point for determin-

Preface to the Second Edition

ing how we want both to design and deliver the learning experience. Thereafter, the table of contents is arranged alphabetically so that instructors and students can readily find topics of interest. The table of contents is intentionally not designed to suggest a specific order of subject presentation. We encourage each instructor to exercise his or her own best judgment in this regard. The reader should also note that while we include specific teaching suggestions at the end of each plan, we have sprinkled comments or useful observations within the text of the lessons as well. These comments are set in paragraph form to distinguish them from the main body of information.

We are enthusiastic advocates of the SPEC approach to learning. Having said that, we strongly believe that experience alone is not an adequate teacher. We all know that there are too many deaths and injuries in the outdoors each year along with untold damage inflicted on the natural environment because travelers do not take the time to educate themselves about the appropriate techniques for safe and environmentally safe travel in the backcountry. Much of this knowledge can be acquired nonexperientially. Yet again and again we hear the horror stories of wilderness visitors who retell their tales of close calls and wreaking environmental havoc as if these experiences were an acceptable standard for real adventure. Raw experience in and of itself may teach very little and damage quite a bit! It is experience processed in the mill of reflection and feedback that yields refined insight—the kind of insight that satisfies our hunger for understanding, develops our body of knowledge, and strengthens our capacity for sound judgment.

Although we clearly believe the lessons included herein are very useful, they are not intended to function like recipes in some wilderness-education cookbook. A novice should not sit in the comfort of his or her living room, read this volume, and then trek off into the deep woods confident in the illusion that she or he is now adequately prepared for backcountry travel. The information and suggestions in this book are no substitute for the good judgment that comes from proper instruction and first-hand experience in backcountry living. As with many of life's endeavors, reading about wilderness recreation is no educational substitute for experiencing it.

Finally, it is important to reinforce another point stated in the first edition. *The Backcountry Classroom* is not inscribed upon tablets of stone. This is of both practical and symbolic importance; we wish to stress that these plans are organic in nature. Every time we use them we still find some element, large or small, that could be changed or improved. This is completely in keeping with our philosophy of teaching and learning. We are all students of Paul Petzoldt's mantra that "immutable rules are tools for fools." Just as we do with our learners, we ask that you apply your best judgment in using this book. We urge that you approach this guide as an empiricist. If the information contained within proves accurate and our teaching suggestions work—great! If you believe that there are significant errors or omissions, by all means alter the lesson to fit your needs, and please pass your thoughts on to us. We constantly examine our ideas through the hard lens of life experience. We welcome any observation that clarifies our vision.

Jack K. Drury
Saranac Lake, NY
2005

Acknowledgments

We all know that it takes a village to raise a child, but few realize that it takes nearly as many people to create a book. We would like to thank Steve Beyer of Wilderness Drum, Chris Cashel of Oklahoma State University, Mike Kudish of Paul Smiths College, Brian McDonnell of McDonnell's Adirondack Challenges, Mary Vance, Jenny Wagstaff of Virginia Tech's Venture Out Program, and Ben Woodard of LL Bean's Discovery Schools, who made major contributions by being either primary or secondary authors to specific chapters both past and present. We would like to thank Kelly Cain of the University of Wisconsin, River Falls; Steve Campbell of Laughing Bear Expeditions; Jerry Cantwell of North Carolina Outward Bound; Kent Clement of Colorado Mountain College; Mick Daniel of North Carolina Outward Bound; Alan Ewert of Indiana University; Doug Fitzgerald of the New York State Department of Environmental Conservation; Paul Kuen of Dairyland Expeditions; Jim Lustig of San Diego State University; Leo McAvoy of the University of Minnesota; Ed Raiola of Warren Wilson College; Zoë Smith of the Wildlife Conservation Society; Cheryl Teeters of Northern Michigan University; Tom Welsh, MD, of SUNY Upstate Medical University; and Josh Whitmore of North Carolina Outward Bound for reading specific chapters and providing invaluable feedback. Peter Eppig of Education By Design and Antioch New England Graduate School was the person who introduced Bruce and Jack to what turned into the Teaching and Learning chapter. We are eternally grateful to Peter for his mentoring and leadership in our quest to be better teachers. We would like to thank Donna Wadsworth of International Paper for her assistance in securing financial support for this project. At Globe Pequot, Scott Adams deserves special thanks for exhibiting tremendous patience with us in getting him a manuscript and his assistance in getting our work into print, as well as Shelley Wolf and Justine Rathbun. David Calvin and Mary James of the Wilderness Education Association provided much needed assistance throughout our efforts. We are grateful to John A. Drury for his imaginative efforts in creating our illustrations. Kim Massari-Holmlund, who played such an instrumental role in producing the first edition of this book, was a tremendous help in creating the bibliography and providing feedback this time around. Finally, very special recognition goes to our friend and special assistant, Duane Gould, who read and reread and reread our drafts so many times and provided invaluable feedback on content, continuity, grammar, and every other aspect of our work. His analytical ability to see how each chapter fit together is uncanny. Any success this book may achieve is largely due to his efforts.

CHAPTER ONE

Teaching and Learning

What?

Since writing the first edition, we've worked with hundreds of educators from around the world. This experience has had a profound effect on our thinking about teaching—particularly our thoughts about the preparation and delivery of formal lessons, whether in the field or classroom. Predictably, this change in our "mental-model" of teaching is reflected in the way we've approached this revised chapter on teaching technique.

We are convinced that the teacher-centered, often didactic approach to formal instruction that most of us have experienced in the field and classroom needs to be reexamined. Research into the brain and learning, discussions recognizing the existence of multiple intelligences and emotional intelligence, and our increased appreciation of the constructivist theory of learning all suggest we can reach the full range of learners, each of whom have their own perspectives and style of learning, only if we expand our repertoire of teaching strategies beyond traditional chalk and talk. Didactic, direct instruction is an important tool in the tool bucket of an experienced educator. It should not, however, be the only, or, in our view, primary tool.

So What?

We all recognize the incredible potential of learning in and from the wilderness. By its very nature, wilderness travel is rich in opportunities for personal growth. Faced with the stark realities of backcountry living, students must engage fully in the struggle to meet the real challenges that confront them. In the process, they develop the knowledge, skills, and dispositions necessary to solve problems individually and as a team. When debriefed and processed appropriately, these experiences often spur leaps of individual insight and growth that are truly profound. Why is this so? And, perhaps more to our point here, why don't our many formal lessons and presentations have similar impact? What are some principles about learning that we might glean from the seemingly spontaneous learning that takes place while on the trail? How can we apply these insights in our formal lesson planning and presentations (whether inside or outside) so that we may enjoy similar results?

Now What?

In this revised chapter, we begin with a review and modest expansion of themes developed in the first edition (Part 1: Strategies and Methodologies—A and B). At that time we assumed that most formal instruction would be teacher/instructor directed. We believe our recommendations for that approach remain valid and therefore offer them once again for your consideration.

Following this review, we move on to share our most recent thinking (Part 1: Strategies and Methodologies—C). In an attempt to distill our thoughts to their essence, we will use an acronym to refer to the basic principles we've gleaned from our wilderness teaching experience. This acronym is SPEC™: Student-centered, Problem-based, Experiential, Collaborative.

Part 2: Designing SPEC Experiences attempts to describe how to design SPEC learning experiences through the exploration of seven key questions. Finally, in Part 3: The SPEC Teacher's Tool Bucket we provide a glossary of activities, tools, and techniques to help make teaching and learning more effective.

I. Outcomes

A. Outdoor leaders provide evidence of their *knowledge* and *understanding* by:

1. Describing the experiential cycle and its role in teaching and learning
2. Describing the role of a wilderness leader as teacher who creates a Student-centered, Problem-based, Experiential, Collaborative (SPEC) learning environment
3. Comparing the advantages and disadvantages of various instructional strategies, including: Student-centered vs. Teacher-centered, Problem-based vs. Content-based, Experiential vs. Theoretical, Collaborative vs. Individual
4. Describing a selection of activities, tools, and techniques that will facilitate learning in the wilderness
5. Comparing a variety of feedback strategies for assessing teaching and learning

B. Outdoor leaders provide evidence of their *skill* by:

1. Creating and coaching learning experiences that apply each of the Student-centered, Problem-based, Experiential, Collaborative (SPEC) instructional strategies
2. Providing a physically and emotionally safe environment for teaching and learning
3. Anticipating and utilizing opportunities for teachable moments
4. Using a variety of appropriate activities, tools, and techniques in "formal" lessons
5. Using appropriate strategies for assessing teaching and learning, including: observation, checklists, debriefs, sweeps, "traditional" tests, assessment tasks (i.e., stove lighting, canoe strokes, firebuilding, knot demonstration), End of the Day logs, check-ins, and rubrics
6. Facilitating a debriefing

C. Outdoor leaders provide evidence of their *dispositions* by:

1. Reflecting in journals and during debriefs about their teaching and learning experiences
2. Asking questions rather than giving answers
3. Applying the teaching activities, tools, and techniques to facilitate learning
4. Modeling Student-centered, Problem-based, Experiential, Collaborative (SPEC) lessons
5. Seeking first to understand, then to be understood

6. Struggling with and reflecting on issues of student versus instructor or leader control
7. Making value judgments about the prioritization of outcomes

II. Content

Part 1. Strategies and Methodologies

A. Reflections on the role of the teacher

1. Teaching as a sharing of power
   a) Knowledge is power. Knowledge enables learners to exercise influence and control over self, others, and the environment.
   b) When teachers use and share their knowledge, they should recognize and responsibly exercise the power that they wield. Teachers must understand the potential they have for effecting life-changing decisions in their learners.

2. Teaching as creative expression
   a) All teaching relies on effective interpersonal communication. There are as many means of communication as there are teachers.
   b) There is no "best way" to teach. All teachers must find ways that are most effective for themselves and their learners within the context of their own personalities, talents, and teaching and learning styles.
   c) Teaching is an extremely personal endeavor. It engages the individual's full repertoire of intelligence, imagination, enthusiasm, judgment, and wit in creating and effectively using educational experiences.

3. Teaching as an act of caring
   a) For learning to occur, the learner admits ignorance, at least temporarily. Learners trust and presume that this ignorance or innocence will not be unfairly exploited.
   b) The teacher should recognize the vulnerability of learners and genuinely care for their physical and emotional well-being.

B. Established strategies of outdoor educators

1. The "grasshopper" approach
   a) Teaching in the backcountry involves learning many things about a wide range of subjects in a very short time.
   b) Since the safety and comfort of expedition participants require that many subjects and skills be taught quickly, it is common for instructors to "hop" from one subject to another as circumstances permit.
      (1) In this "grasshopper" approach, the subject or skill is introduced, demonstrated, and then applied in close sequence, maximizing immediate understanding and retention.
      (2) After initially introducing a subject or skill, it can be approached at a later time and further developed.
   c) Since the "grasshopper" approach allows the sequence of subjects to remain flexible, classes can be postponed until the most effective time or environment for teaching them is encountered.

2. The "teachable moment"
   a) Teachable moments are spontaneous learning opportunities inspired by specific situations or events during the day.
   b) The use of "teachable moments" encourages learners to recognize that opportunities for learning occur constantly during a backcountry expedition. Learners should be encouraged to recognize and identify these opportunities.
   c) Teachable moments on the trail
      (1) Once a teaching opportunity is recognized, concentrate on it intensely. Make sure the entire group recognizes the opportunity for learning and is not distracted by other concerns.
      (2) Ask learners to describe the situation and its implications. This will help learners to focus attention and retain pertinent details for later discussion.
      (3) Clarify the subject right away. Repeat whatever observations and conclusions the group may reach for all to hear. Relate the observations and conclusions to the broader objectives of the course.
      (4) Though errors in skills or judgment may provide excellent "teachable moments," be sure not to subject individuals to unnecessary embarrassment or ridicule. Try to depersonalize the situation so that expedition behavior and attitude is not adversely affected. Thank the expedition member for providing an opportunity to use him or her as a constructive example.

d) Informal "teachable moments"
  (1) Many valuable insights can be shared through casual conversation or small group social discussion. When handled well, these dialogues can yield dramatic results in terms of a learner's personal growth and understanding.
  (2) Suggestions for handling informal "teachable moments":
    (a) Listen very attentively to student conversations and questions, anticipating the potential for helping to identify or clarify important points.
    (b) Evaluate the appropriateness of using specific conversations or discussions as teaching opportunities. Some feelings or questions are better left unexplored.
    (c) Assuming the moment is appropriate, ask questions that will help identify a potentially significant opportunity. Questioning should provoke simple recognition of the facts and proceed to more complex thinking, such as analysis, synthesis, and evaluation.
    (d) Be patient in reaching the desired outcome. Since learners possess different levels of intellectual ability, they will reach their own conclusions in different ways and at different times. Conversations should allow learners to explore ideas and their implications at their own pace.
    (e) The instructor must be willing to look objectively at his or her own feelings so that learners can freely express their own beliefs. The instructor may ultimately express personal views, being mindful to justify or support them, but only after students have had an opportunity to freely express themselves.
    (f) If understandings are reached during the conversation, they might be distilled and clearly articulated in a summary statement.
3. Formal presentations
  a) Organizational concerns
    (1) Selecting a site
      (a) Weather: Students should be sheltered from exposure to sun, wind, rain, or extremes of temperature.
      (b) Environmental impact: Select a natural amphitheater that is away from distracting influences and where the environmental damage from a larger group will be minimized.

      (c) Safety: Select a safe site.

      (d) Comfort: Students should be able to sit and work attentively and in relative comfort.

   (2) Timing of a class

      (a) Schedule classes early in the day when most people are fresh and alert.

      (b) When scheduling classes on travel days, do so before breaking camp.

      (c) Announce class time well in advance so that camp chores are completed.

      (d) Insist that learners be on time and start classes promptly at the announced time.

      (e) Allow for break time, stretching time, etc., during class to maintain learner attention and comfort, and try to keep classes as short as possible.

   (3) Before the class meets, make sure class teachers and learner participants are fully informed of the subject or skills to be taught.

      (a) Inform participants what materials (e.g., notebooks, equipment, etc.) will be needed for class.

      (b) Give teachers adequate time to organize their lesson plans.

b) Communication skills

   (1) Speaking skills

      (a) Speak clearly, loudly, and slowly so that all will understand. Avoid using specific words and phrases repetitively, such as "uh," "like," or "you know."

      (b) Use a vocabulary that is appropriate for the subject and the group.

      (c) Establish eye contact with learners and speak to them.

      (d) Use prepared notes as a reference as needed but avoid reading from them.

      (e) Get the complete attention of the audience before proceeding with the class.

      (f) Vary the pitch and tone of the voice frequently for emphasis.

      (g) Use nonabrasive, courteous words. Refrain from using inappropriate slang or profanity.

      (h) Refrain from using "inside" humor, as it often excludes some members of the group from a sense of participation.

(2) Listening skills

(a) Listen attentively to student questions and responses, concentrating on the main points and specifics of each. It's often helpful to repeat a question or comment to check for understanding.

(b) Listen courteously without interrupting unnecessarily and without distracting or mocking the questioner or speaker.

(c) Listen patiently and allow students sufficient time to formulate questions or respond. Silence can be the sound of a mind working.

(d) Listen empathetically and try to understand what is meant as well as what is said. Be aware of feelings and emotions, and encourage learners who are reluctant to express themselves.

(3) Nonverbal communication

(a) Allow enthusiasm, energy, and interest in the subject to show through body language. Appropriate gesticulations, facial gestures, and body movements add an element of theatrics to a presentation, focusing attention and increasing interest.

(b) Avoid physical habits that clearly distract from the presentation or limit its effectiveness (e.g., nose picking, hand over mouth, facing away from the audience, putting head down when talking).

(c) Avoid wearing clothing or equipment that unnecessarily obscures the face from the audience. Sunglasses are particularly distracting when they totally obscure eye contact.

c) Methodology skills: Select a method for presenting a lesson based on the following:

(1) Student knowledge: How much do the students already know about the subject or skill? To what extent can they contribute to the lesson?

(2) Student maturity: How long is the group's attention span?

(3) Student interest: How much interest preexists in the subject or skill?

(4) Time: How much time is available for transmitting the essential information?

(5) Nature of the subject

(a) Is the subject strictly a matter of fact, or is opinion or interpretation involved?

(b) How much emotional controversy may the subject potentially expose?

(c) Does discussion of the subject have the potential for negative impact on group morale?

(d) How abstract or concrete is the subject, and what levels of intellectual ability will be expected of students for learning to take place?

C. Exploring the SPEC approach to teaching and learning

As mentioned in the introduction to this chapter, our perspective on teaching and learning has changed. We believe we have significantly greater impact with many more learners when we adopt teaching strategies that are more student-centered (rather than teacher-centered), problem-based (rather than content-based), experiential (rather than theoretical), and collaborative (rather than strictly individual). We share our thinking regarding SPEC in the following section, recommending and illustrating some specific ways in which these principles may be applied to the design of formal lessons and presentations, both in the field and in the classroom.

1. Thoughts on selecting a teaching methodology: Selecting a teaching methodology appropriate to the context of student and teacher needs requires considerable experience and judgment. As with any complex decision, many variables must be considered to raise the probability of a successful outcome. Clearly one size fits all does not apply. While we urge readers to carefully consider our SPEC approach, we recognize the well-established value of more traditional methodologies. See table 1.2, where we share some of our thoughts regarding specific issues that may influence your choices.

A SPEC learning environment has a distinctive rhythm or feel to it. Over time, participants in this environment soon fall into its rhythm, anticipating the next stage in the pattern before it arrives. We call this rhythm the experiential cycle.

We recognize that this concept of an experiential cycle has been around for a while and that many versions of it exist. Following is our explanation of the experiential cycle as adapted from that of Education By Design, a staff development organization of Antioch New England Graduate School in Keene, New Hampshire.

Table 1.1. CHARACTERISTICS OF A SPEC VERSUS "TRADITIONAL" LEARNING ENVIRONMENT

SPEC Environment	"Traditional" Environment
Student-centered: Students learn by talking, listening, writing, reading, creating, and reflecting on content, ideas, issues, and concerns as they work in small groups or individually to engage the curriculum. Authority is shared with the teacher in many ways. Students have direct access to knowledge. They are encouraged to develop their own questions and arrive at some of their own conclusions with teacher guidance. It is presumed that students have preexisting knowledge and skill that they can contribute to the learning. Students may learn from each other as much as they learn from the teacher. (See fig. 1.1.)	**Teacher-centered:** The teacher is the center of authority. The teacher transmits most information and all knowledge to the learner. It is presumed that the teacher will ask most of the important questions and that these questions have a correct answer that must be validated by the teacher. Students are "empty vessels"—teachers are the experts that fill the vessels with appropriate knowledge. (See fig. 1.2.)
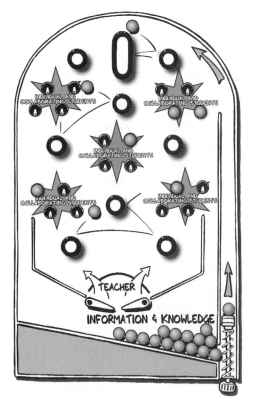	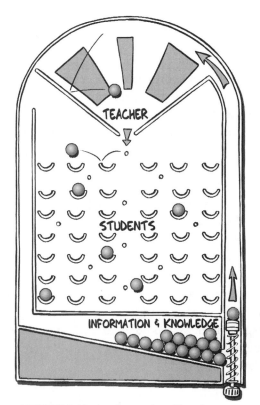
FIGURE 1.1. The student-centered learning environment	FIGURE 1.2. The teacher-centered learning environment

SPEC Environment	"Traditional" Environment
Problem-based: Teachers design complex and increasingly authentic problems for students to solve individually or in collaborative teams. Students must grapple with information (the content) as well as use skills (social, intellectual, emotional) to solve the problems successfully. Feedback and assessment is an integral and ongoing part of the process. Successful learning is assessed on multiple levels: content understanding, group process, individual skill development, etc. Students receive personalized narrative feedback regarding their performance from several sources: peers, teacher, and self-assessment. The teacher serves as a facilitator, guide, co-learner, mentor, and coach who helps students through the problem-solving/learning process.	**Content-based:** The coverage of content is the focus of the learning. Teachers create structured lessons designed to help students understand and recall important facts, concepts, and processes that they will be expected to recall on tests and examinations. Concern for skill development is often tied directly only to those skills that are required for improved mastery of the content. Assessment often comes at the end of a unit of study and is frequently evaluated in terms of percentages of correct answers or expressions of understanding as shown on pencil-and-paper tests. The teacher may have little or no opportunity to share personalized, narrative feedback with each student to provide direction for future improvement.
Experiential: Students learn by doing. All learning occurs within the context of real, firsthand experiences. Students participate, make choices, and accept some responsibility for their role in the learning process. The interactive nature of this approach creates a wealth of physical, intellectual, emotional, and social experiences. Learners construct their own meaning by reflecting on all these experiences. They are prompted to make connections to their own lives, larger contexts, and theory during this reflective stage.	**Theoretical:** Students generally learn by listening, reading, writing, or following tightly scripted activities related to the curriculum. Students have very few choices of consequence. The curriculum exists in and of itself. Passing exams is the primary context for motivation. Curricular content is often prepackaged in discrete bundles of information to be learned in a prescribed, often linear sequence. Students may or may not recognize any connection between the content and their own lives.
Collaborative: All learning takes place in a social context. Working as an individual or as part of a collaborative team, students consistently function as part of some larger "community." While competition has its place, collaboration is the fundamental value. All learners are expected to work with and show respect for others. Through multiple experiences, reflection, and a conscious attention to the emotional health of the group members, students learn to value (rather then merely tolerate) the differences in each other. Success for both individuals and the group is recognized and rewarded.	**Individual:** Individual performance is the primary measure of success. Competition is encouraged as a predominant value. Individual accountability and achievement is recognized and rewarded. Group accountability and achievement may go unrecognized or be actively discouraged. Little emphasis is placed on the development of social skills or group decision-making, management, or leadership skills. The emotional health of the group members is not as high a priority as individual grades on exams.

Table 1.2. ISSUES IN COMPARING SPEC VERSUS "TRADITIONAL" APPROACHES

SPEC	Issue	Traditional
SPEC learning usually takes more time. A powerful learning experience proceeds at the pace of the learner—not necessarily that of the teacher or some external schedule.	Time	Traditional lessons can be tailored much more predictably to time constraints as many (if not all) of the variables are under the control of the instructor.
SPEC learning definitely leads to a greater depth of understanding among a wider range of students. Living the experience at multiple levels (physical, intellectual, emotional, social, spiritual) creates the opportunity for a broad array of very powerful, long-term understandings and insights	Depth of Understanding	Traditional lessons have the potential to produce reasonable depth of understanding in the specific area of focus (physical, intellectual, emotional, social, spiritual), provided that the style of presentation matches the learning style of the specific student.
The SPEC approach may help many learners to synthesize a great deal of knowledge and experience. It is questionable whether this approach is worth the time it takes if the goal is to introduce and recall lots of information for the short term.	Breadth of Understanding	Traditional lessons can cover a wide area of information in a short amount of time. Effectively presented and reinforced, the information can be recalled successfully in short-term memory.
SPEC experiences can be life changing for some learners. Ownership implies some measure of personal investment. With the high degree of student participation and interaction, decision making, and commitment required, SPEC learning invites deep investment and therefore a tremendous amount of student ownership and pride in positive results.	Emotional Impact and Ownership	Ownership is not often a descriptor associated with very traditional approaches. Since most decision making and control is in the hands of the teacher, successful participation in a traditional learning experience may require little student investment of personal energy.
Teachers who are successful using the SPEC approach generally possess all the qualities of a solid traditional instructor. However, in addition they must: • Be comfortable with yielding some control to learners • Be comfortable not knowing all the answers • Be comfortable with the messy chaos that often attends experiential learning • Be ready to let students struggle and/or fail for the sake of the learning	Essential Teacher Qualities	Teachers consistently successful in traditional instruction usually have a complete mastery of the content, well-developed group management and organizational skills, an appreciation of learning theory, and an engaging and/or nurturing personality that develops relationships with a diverse array of students. It is important that the teacher be mature enough to put the needs and best interests of the learner first.

2. The experiential cycle: In figure 1.3 we represent the feel of a SPEC learning environment. In simplest terms, learning in the classroom or wilderness involves the interaction of three essential components: the student learner, the instructor (who also learns), and the context of challenging experiences (whether planned or spontaneous) that may yield important understanding and insights.

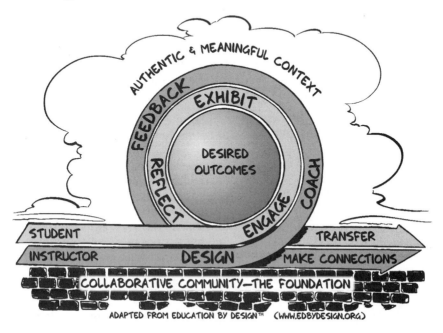

FIGURE 1.3. The experiential cycle

a) First things first

 (1) The community context: SPEC instructors recognize that all groups that stay together very long develop a kind of "culture"; i.e., a complex set of personal and group behaviors shaped by common expectation, habit, ritual, and tradition that determine how people interact with each other. In a SPEC environment, we don't want the formation of this cultural context to be haphazard. Indeed, the SPEC approach suggests that we consciously use some specific group team-building activities and processes to help shape a culture of mutual respect and trust, which we know supports high-quality small and large group collaboration. It is a given that these team-building activities and group processes are among the first experiences that the group encounters. (See Part 3: The SPEC

Teacher's Tool Bucket for an explanation of some of these techniques.)

   (a) Classroom application: SPEC classroom teachers need to go beyond simple "icebreaker" activities and do things that help learners get to know each other on a personal level and/or to form a small-group identity.

   (b) Wilderness leadership application: Wilderness leadership expeditions may start with some "icebreaker" activities. Typically, teamwork is then developed through the shared experience of living and working together in the field.

(2) Desired outcomes: A SPEC learning environment is driven by the desire to achieve a set of well-known and clearly articulated outcomes that everyone involved agrees are desirable. It is extremely important that everyone periodically revisit these outcomes: review individual and group understanding of them, review individual and group progress toward them, and reaffirm the common commitment to achieve them. Again, these desired outcomes should be discussed early on.

   (a) Classroom application: SPEC classroom teachers frequently must focus on standards or targets determined by external agencies, such as national and state governments, or by school, departmental, or organizational decision makers.

   (b) Wilderness leadership application: Wilderness leadership expeditions often focus on organizational or program outcomes. In some cases the expedition members may set their own outcomes.

b) Moving through the cycle: Teacher and student

   (1) Teacher cycle: The teacher path through the cycle tends to follow three stages. In reality, these stages are not as clearly distinct and separate from each other as figure 1.3 might suggest. Experiential learning is rarely linear and cleanly sequential. Having said that, we do recognize at least three stages an instructor will typically pass through during any one learning experience.

   (a) Design phase: SPEC instructors are architects of learning. As such, they give thoughtful consideration to designing learning experiences that require learners to develop and use the knowledge and skills they need to become better outdoor leaders. In the wilderness leadership setting, leadership, decision making, and judgment are paramount among the outcomes instructors use to guide their design process.

    i) Classroom application: SPEC classroom teachers learn to see their traditional curriculum or lessons as potential "problems to solve" (challenges). They design activities that will prepare the students to engage in these classroom challenges. (See Part 2: Designing SPEC Experiences for details.)

    ii) Wilderness leadership application: Wilderness instructors rarely need to author formal written challenges since living and working together in the wilderness itself is challenge enough. The design aspect for a wilderness leader is to anticipate upcoming challenge opportunities and thoughtfully plan how to use them for the greatest educational benefit.

(b) Coaching phase: Teachers must provide appropriate support for learners who are grappling with a challenging experience. In this case, support does not mean unnecessarily shielding the students from the power of the experience or rescuing them from the consequences of their own decisions. For many teachers schooled in traditional methodologies, knowing when to step in and actively help students versus step back to let them go on their own is one of the most difficult judgment calls to make. In either case, coaching learners through the experiences frequently requires an instructor to play many different (and sometimes seemingly conflicting) roles, including facilitator, mentor, mediator, and often that of colearner.

    i) Classroom application: Coaching in a SPEC classroom is, in fact, very similar to coaching students on a wilderness expedition. In both cases the teacher role is much more "guide on the side" than "sage on the stage." Central to the role of teacher-guide is the practice of responding to student inquiries with probing or clarifying questions rather than directive statements or answers that tell them what to do. "What do you think?" is a question fundamental to the repertoire of a SPEC classroom teacher or wilderness instructor.

ii) Wilderness application: The role of a wilderness instructor is more "guide on the side" than "sage on the stage," as described above.

(c) Feedback phase: Instructors are responsible for giving feedback to learners as they progress through a challenging experience. Feedback does not come only with a test at the end. Indeed, feedback on performance should be occurring throughout the experience. In all cases, it is important that feedback be connected to clear, quality criteria that the learners have at least discussed with the instructor. In some cases it may be appropriate for the learners to have had a hand in articulating the criteria. While teachers are the ultimate guardians of the standards of quality, it is essential that learners have some opportunity to self-assess and get appropriate feedback from peers as well. The goal of assessment should be to help learners internalize their own understanding of quality performance and thus accurately assess themselves. As Paul Petzoldt, a pioneer of wilderness education, frequently stated, "You gotta know what you know and know what you don't know."

i) Classroom application: SPEC teachers recognize that feedback in their classes should not be just about grades. Feedback, instead, is an ongoing conversation that answers the student question, "How am I doing?" with regard to known targets and clear criteria. In this sense, the feedback process in a SPEC classroom should be very similar to that of an instructor in the field.

ii) Wilderness application: Feedback in the wilderness-leadership context emphasizes instructor comment regarding skill exhibition in the field, comments on journal writing, and insights shared in group or personal debriefing sessions.

(2) The student cycle: Students respond to the design of a challenge by grappling with the essential knowledge (what Paul Petzoldt called the "must-knows") and practicing targeted specific skills that are necessary to complete the challenge and improve their capacity as outdoor leaders. Similar to an instructor, the student

passage through a challenging experience typically involves three stages.

(a) Engagement phase: Once the challenge is put before them and their understanding of its nature clarified, students set to work on solving the problem at hand. Ideally, this stage of engagement gets them involved on multiple levels (intellectually, physically, socially, emotionally, spiritually) simultaneously. A successful challenge is sufficiently well designed if it engages the whole group and each individual within the group.

    i) Classroom application: In SPEC classrooms, learners engage by working together in small teams to create products (posters, brochures, role-plays, artwork, etc.) that reveal their understanding of content while simultaneously demonstrating their use of some life-long skill.

    ii) Wilderness application: In wilderness leadership settings, engagement also reveals knowledge and skill. In this case, however, nothing need be contrived. Engagement is in evidence when learners work together to solve any kind of problem: cook a meal, set up their shelter, or use map and compass to navigate overland.

(b) Exhibition phase: Whenever learners are involved in a challenging experience, they are exhibiting some aspect of their knowledge, skills, or dispositions as individuals and as part of a group. It comes as a shock to some learners that the exhibition phase of a SPEC environment goes well beyond the limited time frame involving formal testing or presentations. In essence, the test never ends.

    i) Classroom application: In the SPEC classroom, some aspect of a student's knowledge, skills, or disposition is potentially on exhibition all the time and is therefore subject to feedback.

    ii) Wilderness application: In the wilderness "classroom," the environment is much like the SPEC classroom as described above. The idea that the test never ends is also applicable.

(c) Reflection phase: It is crucial that learners take time to think about their experience, contemplate its significance, and make connections and judgments for use in future situations. These opportunities to reflect may occur publicly in a group debrief or privately in a journal entry (see chapter 25, Group Processing and Debriefing). In either event, it must occur for the experiential cycle to be complete.

  i) Classroom application: Reflection is essential to learning in the SPEC classroom. Debriefing and journaling are excellent mechanisms for revealing student thinking.

  ii) Wilderness application: In the wilderness "classroom," reflection plays an essential role in leadership development, and debriefing and journaling play integral roles in that process.

Part 2. Designing SPEC Experiences

Once we understood the implications of the SPEC approach to teaching and learning, it became obvious that our mental model of who we are as a "teacher" had to change. Previously we saw ourselves as curriculum experts whose task was to "deliver" information to learners in the most engaging and interesting way possible. Part scholar, part stand-up entertainer, we performed on our stage whether in the classroom or in the outdoors and kept them coming back for more—in the classroom, five shows a day, five days a week, month after month, and in the outdoors, rain or shine.

Our understanding of the SPEC approach changed this mind-set and our practice. To be sure, it helps to have mastery of our discipline. It is crucial that educators who adapt SPEC methodologies be capable of differentiating between what is essential knowledge in the incredibly broad field of wilderness education and what aspects of the curriculum are of lesser importance. Because the SPEC approach typically takes more time than traditional methods, we must make judgments about which understandings and skills are worth the time and effort necessary to engage learners in a "challenge" (i.e., a SPEC lesson). Some parts of the curriculum are better approached with traditional methods. If it is easier and just as effective to "tell 'em what they need to know," then by all means do so and just deliver the information.

Although powerful learning experiences happen regularly in the wilderness—where, as an observant instructor, one only has to recognize them and help the learners reflect on them—they rarely just happen in the classroom or in formal learning situations. Over time, we've come to recognize that consistently powerful learning experiences can be and should be "designed." They can and will occur with gratifying regularity if certain principles are followed. That is why, as educators committed to the SPEC approach, we now see ourselves much more as architects of powerful learning experiences than as deliverers of information.

In the following segment, we discuss a sequence of questions we ask ourselves whenever we start to design a learning experience using SPEC principles. These questions are highlighted in the Annotated Challenge at the end of the chapter.

Designing a lesson for the classroom may be very different logistically than preparing for a learning experience in the field. In the classroom, for instance, challenges are frequently written on the chalkboard or copied on paper to hand out to each learner. In the field, however, challenges written on paper are not usually necessary or very practical. In both cases, our thought process for designing a challenge remains about the same, and thinking through the questions we discuss below helps us to clarify the intent of our teaching. Using these questions to guide us—either in the field or classroom—has given us confidence in our capacity to create engaging and enjoyable learning experiences with consistent success.

A. Considerations in designing a challenge

1. What learning outcome, standard, or course objective do you want them to "know" more fully? This needs to be expressed in terms that are observable.
    a) "Design with the end in mind" is a central principle for success when creating powerful learning experiences. It is extremely important to articulate as clearly as possible what it is you want your learners to know once the challenge is completed. At this point, it also helps a great deal to give some thought to issues of assessment:
        (1) How will you know that your learners have gained the understanding you intend?
        (2) What will you accept as evidence of their learning?
    b) If writing a challenge for the classroom, it is not always necessary that you include this "knowledge outcome" on the challenges given to the learner as too many words on the paper can easily overwhelm some learners/readers. It is necessary, however, that you, as the teacher/instructor, have this target at the forefront of your thinking when designing a challenge for use in the field or classroom.
    c) In the sample Equipment Selection challenge at the end of the chapter, the knowledge outcome is: "Participants can knowledgeably discuss the

criteria for selecting major pieces of backcountry equipment, such as backpacks, stoves, tents, sleeping bags, and sleeping pads."

2. What skill or disposition do you want them to practice? This needs to be expressed in terms that are observable.

   a) The principle of "designing with the end in mind" applies likewise to the specific skill you want the learners to develop while working on the challenge. For the same reasons cited above, be as specific as possible in describing the skill.

   b) See number 7 on page 28 for further discussion regarding targeting a skill.

   c) In the sample Equipment Selection challenge at the end of the chapter, the targeted skill is: "Decision making: analyzes and prioritizes relevant information.

3. What essential question or key issue is the focus of this challenge? What is essential about this knowledge or skill? How is it connected/relevant to both the "big picture" of the course *and* to the life of the learner?

   a) When a learner asks the question "Why are we doing this?" it would initially seem to be a fairly straightforward inquiry. Its hidden complexity is revealed, however, when the common teacher reply, "Because it is part of the course/curriculum and will be on the quiz," yields such a tepid response from learners. Successful challenges inspire the expenditure of considerable time, intellectual and physical energy, and emotion. Their reason for being must justify the expense.

   b) For the instructor, trying to articulate the core reason for doing a challenge often helps him/her to decide whether or not a challenge is worth the effort. The essential question or key issue should function as a lighthouse during the course of a challenge. When the learners, and possibly the instructor as well, are fog-bound in the confusion that attends real problem solving, both should be able to look at the essential question or key issue for enlightenment, see their task more clearly, and make decisions or plans accordingly.

   c) A detailed and/or instructive discussion about forming essential questions is well beyond the scope of this chapter. Nonetheless, following are some characteristics many educators look for in quality essential questions:

      (1) An essential question goes to the very heart of a subject or discipline. It invites exploration of a "big idea" that cannot be answered easily or sometimes even conclusively. "How can we consistently develop high-quality outdoor leaders?" is a pretty decent essential

question. Addressing this question is the focus of books with many different perspectives. Trying to answer this question adequately will invite any learner to grapple with several absolutely core issues associated with the discipline. If you address this question seriously, you'll know a great deal that is important about the topic.

(2) An essential question requires that the learner use higher order thinking skills, such as analysis, synthesis, and evaluation. Starting the question with the words *how, why,* or *which* invites a response that should cause the learner to do some research, perhaps weigh the credibility and value of different sources or bits of information, and make decisions and judgments.

(3) An essential question is usually much more complex than immediately apparent. Some experts in the field say that a good essential question will require that a learner "unpack" the issue and information. The more the learner investigates the question, the more layers of the onion need to be peeled back to get at the underlying truths or questions implicit in the study. "Can planet Earth survive humans?" might seem a simple question, but clearly it isn't.

(4) In the sample Equipment Selection challenge at the end of the chapter, the essential question is: "Running an outdoor program requires large expenditures of money on equipment. In order to ensure we get the greatest value for our dollar, what criteria should we use to guide our selection/purchase of the major pieces of equipment for backcountry travel?"

4. What challenge, task, or performance can you set before the learners that will require the knowledge and skill development you desire?
   a) The whole purpose of doing a challenge is to:
      (1) Give learners the opportunity to grapple with important information/understandings.
      (2) Practice a lifelong skill.
      (3) Provide learners an experience that engages the emotions fully because it feels "real." Part of that feeling of reality is creating a product or performance that is tangible in some way.
   b) In the field, successfully completing a difficult off-trail day hike, crossing a frigid stream, or organizing a food drop to reration the expedition are products or performances that have a firm basis in the reality of the expedition. So long as the challenge or performance is obviously related to the mission of the expedition, the "reality" of any given task with its connection to important knowledge and skill is rarely an issue.

c) In the classroom, the choice of a product that feels "real" is a bit more problematic. Here, it is often helpful for the teacher/instructor to ask himself/herself, "Where in the normal activity of daily life and commerce might a person use this information and skill?" Might someone create a brochure, make a storyboard, produce an advertisement, or author a grant proposal and employ the skill and use the information that is part of the curriculum? The possible choices of a product are endless.

d) The key, in all cases, is that the selected product does, in fact, require the use of the knowledge and skill desired. All products are not created equal, and some reveal evidence of knowledge and skill much better than others. The choice of an appropriate product for the challenge is very important.

e) In the sample Equipment Selection challenge at the end of the chapter, the task is to: " . . . create an engaging and informative print advertisement wherein you recommend a specific piece of equipment in one of the categories that is the best value for your readers."

5. What conditions (grouping, time frame, choice, positive interdependence, individual accountability, materials) must you have in place to make sure that the challenge goes well?

a) Grouping

(1) The first consideration in grouping is to make sure that the challenge actually requires more than one person to complete it successfully. Put learners in teams only when everyone will have meaningful work to do and an opportunity to contribute.

(2) Each teacher/instructor will have to learn through experimentation the advantages and disadvantages of every size group. Generally speaking, it is a good idea to start with pairs or trios and enlarge groups only as participants gain greater skill with collaborative work. Remember that adding members to the group puts one more personality into the mix. While this additional resource may help, more people in a group tends to considerably multiply the complexity of the problem solving.

(3) Groups can be formed in only five basic ways: randomly, the participants choose, the instructor designates, the group membership is matched with skill/task preferences, or the groups are formed homogeneously. Again, all of these approaches have their own positives/negatives that can be explored through experience.

(4) In the sample Equipment Selection challenge at the end of the

chapter, participants are allowed to choose when asked to form five evenly sized teams.

b) Time frame

(1) Time is and should be a limited resource, just like paper, art materials, access to the Internet, etc. Restricting time is the most common way that teachers/instructors create circumstances in a challenge that encourage all participants to work together to complete the challenge successfully. In this regard, it is better to "crunch" time (i.e., allocate a bit less than you estimate is adequate) than to be too generous. It is much easier to allow more time (assuming you have it!) when appropriate than it is to try and reclaim it once given.

(2) Teachers/instructors who are new to the SPEC approach will usually set time parameters themselves until learners get considerable experience with the collaborative process. Once learners have experience, it increases the learners' sense of ownership and control to have some input on time parameters.

(3) Teachers who are new to the SPEC approach should not be surprised if their initial estimates of time are rather dramatically off the mark. Collaborative work is a "new game" for most teachers and learners. Learning the basics, both in design and execution of a challenge, is slow at first when both the teacher and learners are just beginning to understand how to play. Most early challenges take at least one-third more time than estimated. Be patient: Everyone will become much more efficient over time.

(4) In the sample Equipment Selection challenge at the end of the chapter, the time frame is to be determined by the instructor.

c) Choice

(1) Be sure to include some authentic element of choice in the design of a challenge. Choice encourages participants to feel that they have an opportunity to exercise their creativity and "own" the results of a challenge. Lacking any element of choice, participants rightfully feel they are following someone else's agenda, and much of the emotional power of the challenge is lost. Also, a healthy dose of choice in the challenge sets up genuine individual and collective responsibility for the decision-making process and the results. If you want learners to accept responsibility for the process and product of a challenge, they must have some control over both through the authentic exercise of choice.

(2) In the sample Equipment Selection challenge at the end of the chapter, there are a number of choices:
   (a) Choosing what teams they work in
   (b) Determining what their advertisement will include and look like
   (c) Providing input on the most important criteria for each category of equipment
   (d) Determining which group will select which equipment category for the advertisement (as long as there is at least one advertisement for each category)

d) Positive interdependence
   (1) Positive interdependence is a state in which all participants in a challenge feel they genuinely need each other to get the job done successfully. Those who design challenges can use any number of strategies to foster the development of this feeling. Among the most common methods are:
      (a) Limit time
      (b) Limit access to materials
      (c) Identify very strict roles that only a designated person can play
      (d) Create a common state of responsibility for the results of the challenge (beware of group grading, however)
      (e) Raise the stakes of the challenge by having the group present or perform in front of an audience (but make sure the audience is appropriate to the experience of the performers)
   (2) In the sample Equipment Selection challenge at the end of the chapter, a factor creating positive interdependence could be time. If time is restricted, then no one person can accomplish the task within the time allowed, thus creating a need for the other group members.

e) Individual accountability
   (1) Individual accountability is the flip side of positive interdependence. A challenge that is designed well balances the needs of the group (positive interdependence) with the responsibility of the individual to do his or her best work and contribute his or her fair share. Building in conditions that promote individual accountability permits an observer to note who in fact is doing the work and who is not.

(2) Among common strategies for establishing individual accountability are setting strict task roles for each member of the group to perform, dividing research so that each participant is responsible for a different piece of the information puzzle, holding all group members responsible for responding to random questions or explanations of product or process at any time, asking group members to comment on the contribution of each member at the end of a challenge, etc.

(3) In the sample Equipment Selection challenge at the end of the chapter, individual accountability could be created by:

    (1) Having a written exam on equipment selection criteria

    (2) Having participants write in their journal their contributions to the project

    (3) Having a group debrief in which they discuss who did what on the project and perhaps write up a "group journal entry"

f) Materials

(1) Project-based learning often requires access to more resources than more straightforward chalk and talk. This can present special logistical challenges to teachers/instructors who want to use this approach, and it is especially the case when creative learners suddenly take off in a direction that is different from any anticipated by the teacher. Before embarking on a major challenge, it is always wise to check that you have access to all the "stuff" you might need to pull it off.

(2) In the sample Equipment Selection challenge at the end of the chapter, the necessary materials might include:

    (a) Easel paper

    (b) Markers

    (c) Outdoor magazines

    (d) Books

    (e) Computer with Internet access

    (f) Arts and crafts materials

6. What are the criteria for a product of "good" quality?

a) To raise the probability of learners doing good work or performing well, it is necessary that they have a reasonably clear understanding of what "good" looks like or sounds like. In the best case, learners should see or hear examples of "good," as well as examples of "not so good" and "great," so that they can begin to compare and differentiate among the various levels of quality. One good way to help learners begin to internalize a sense of "quality" work is to give them examples of a given product that represent a range of quality; then, ask the learners to arrange the samples according to quality and explain the reasons for their arrangements. The ensuing discussion is often very enlightening.

b) Lacking real-life examples, it is still helpful to use words and pictures to describe the qualities of "good" for learners. Putting this description in the form of a Product Quality Checklist (see p. 49 for details) is an excellent initial step in raising the issue of quality to a conscious level. It also gives many learners a feeling of security and accomplishment when they can check off each of the expectations for quality as they put the finishing touches on a product or performance.

c) Teachers and instructors will recognize early on the need to distinguish between at least two different kinds of criteria they set for a quality product.

   (1) Form criteria

      (a) These criteria describe expectations for how the product will look in its final form and any special parameters that must be observed in creating that final look. For instance, if the instructor requires that the product be a brochure, role-play, or poster, what are the defining characteristics that make for a quality brochure, role-play, or poster? These should be described or modeled as clearly as possible. In addition, what special parameters must be observed in the creation of the product? Is the brochure to be three folds or four, the role-play a minimum of three or five minutes in length? How large should the poster be? Time, of course, is almost always a prime concern. Let your learners know as soon as possible how much time will be allotted to work on the project. In the beginning, teachers/instructors will most commonly determine the time frame for completing the work. Later in the process, learners and the teacher may negotiate the time frame. In any event, *all these criteria should be laid out for the learners up front so there are no surprises when it comes to final evaluation.*

      (b) In the sample Equipment Selection challenge at the end of the chapter, the form criteria are:

         i) "The advertisement is on one page of poster paper."

ii) "The advertisement is engaging—it causes the viewer to look with interest, pause, and read."

iii) "The advertisement is informative—it provides the viewer with important/relevant information."

(2) Content criteria

(a) For teachers or instructors who have been disappointed by the lack of "learning" in evidence in student projects, setting content criteria addresses this concern directly. These criteria describe expectations for the message/information that is to be communicated through the product or performance.

i) Is the information accurate and relevant?

ii) Does it address the issues cited in the essential question or key issue?

iii) Is the information sufficiently detailed or comprehensive?

iv) Perhaps most important to the teacher/instructor, does the message/information communicated through the product or performance reveal understanding of the curriculum that is the target of the challenge?

(b) In the sample Equipment Selection challenge at the end of the chapter, the content criteria are:

i) "The advertisement includes a recommendation for a best value piece of equipment in one category."

ii) "The team can support its suggestions with references to specific authoritative sources."

d) One way to encourage learners to grapple with the curricular content of a challenge is to list very specific "focus questions" in the text of the challenge description. These questions may be very similar to the types of questions typically found at the end of a chapter in a textbook. Ideally, focus questions guide the learners toward the most important specific issues or points of information that must be answered as stepping stones toward dealing effectively with the overall inquiry framed by the essential question or key issue that drives the whole challenge. To ensure that learners recognize the importance of answering the focus questions and thereby grapple with the intended content, teachers/instructors often include a content criterion that states, "product addresses all the focus questions thoroughly."

7. How will you know if the learners have moved toward attaining the learning objectives you set forth for knowledge and skill? (Assessing attainment in learning is a topic of endless debate and one that is well beyond the scope of this chapter.)

   a) When we concern ourselves with the learners' development of knowledge, we want to consider the following:

      (1) What do you want the learner to know—and at what level of sophistication?

         (a) While seemingly straightforward, this question is very complex and has been the subject of philosophical debate for centuries. For our practical purposes, however, we must at least be aware that "knowing" can be expressed in many different ways, as exemplified by Howard Gardner's Multiple Intelligence theory (Gardner 1993), and at varying levels of sophistication, as exemplified by Bloom's *Taxonomy* (Bloom 1964).

         (b) One particularly useful framework we have encountered for raising our awareness on these issues comes from the work of Grant Wiggins and Randy McTighe and their program Understanding by Design. They describe the following Six Facets of Understanding, which have helped us both to design our challenges and think through what we will accept as evidence (Wiggins and McTighe 1998):

            i) Explain: Provide thorough and justifiable accounts of phenomena, facts, and data

            ii) Interpret: Tell meaningful stories, offer apt translations, provide a revealing historical or personal dimension to ideas and events; make subjects personal or accessible through images, anecdotes, analogies, and models

            iii) Apply: Effectively use and adapt what they know in diverse contexts

            iv) Have perspective: See and hear points of view through critical eyes and ears; see the big picture

            v) Empathize: Find value in what others might find odd, alien, or implausible; perceive sensitively on the basis of prior indirect experience

            vi) Have self-knowledge: Perceive the personal style, prejudices, projections, and habits of mind that both shape and impede our own understanding; they are aware of what they do not understand and why understanding is so hard

(2) What will you accept as evidence that the learner "knows" at the desired level of sophistication?

(a) Both in the classroom and the field, traditional methods of "testing" have their place. Either a written or verbal exam can provide adequate evidence of achievement for certain kinds of understanding (see *explain, interpret, have perspective,* and *empathize,* above). To the extent that words are credible evidence, written and verbal expressions (tests, interviews, journals, debriefing, Socratic dialogues, etc.) of understanding all contribute to a picture of what an individual has learned; however, when it comes to the *application* of learning, we suggest that it is important to look beyond words and focus more closely on an individual's actions in the context of real-life situations or designed challenges to find a true measure of attainment.

(b) Trying to assess a learner's capacity to apply his or her knowledge requires that the evidence of learning be manifest in behavior that is observable. In some respects, designing and observing this kind of performance assessment places a burden on the teacher/instructor that is not unlike that placed on a physician when trying to diagnose the condition of a patient. Both the physician and teacher (doctor of learning?) need to know what he or she is looking for that constitutes evidence; he or she then can either create or look for naturally occurring circumstances that may reveal the evidence (symptoms) he or she seeks. When these circumstances occur, the doctor/teacher observes and records the evidence, closely gathering significant bits of data over time and looking for a pattern. Satisfied that he or she has enough information to constitute a reasonable sample, he or she seeks to interpret it accurately. Finally, both the doctor and the teacher proceed to act on the basis of the evidence by prescribing appropriate next steps that will improve the condition of their charge.

Keeping this analogy in mind can often help us when we fashion assessment tasks or performances since it reminds us of the intent behind the design.

(c) Finally, we want to emphasize a point regarding the assessment of individual understanding. According to Constructivist Theory, learning is a highly social activity. It comes as no surprise, then, that working in teams enhances the probability that, under the right conditions, all team members will learn many different things and at many different levels of sophistication. Thus, group challenges can be a great environment for learning; however, group work is not a great environment for assessing the learning of each individual in the group. There are just too many things going on in collaborative work for an assessor to discern with reasonable certainty what each individual understands at any moment in time. Sorting out exactly who has learned what requires an assessment strategy that is much more focused on each individual than group work or a group debrief permits. We strongly advocate, therefore, that teachers/instructors separate the two experiences and plan accordingly.

(3) In the sample Equipment Selection challenge at the end of the chapter, the knowledge criteria includes participants knowledgeably discussing the criteria for selecting major pieces of backcountry equipment and adequately defending their best value choices in terms of the established criteria.

b) When we want to assess a skill, we want to consider the following:

(1) Target only one skill at a time when doing a challenge. Admittedly, any decent challenge will require that learners put a full range of skills to use; however, no instructor can possibly observe all the skills employed by all the participants during all phases of a challenge—it's not possible. The point of targeting one specific skill is to help the learner focus directly on those behaviors that will yield improved performance in the skill.

(2) For the learner to improve in a skill area, the learner must have a fairly clear mental picture of what is expected of him or her in relatively specific terms. For the instructor to fulfill the role of coach successfully, he or she must know specifically what behavior he or

she is looking for as evidence of the skill in action, have a fair chance to observe the learner's performance over time, guide the learner when necessary, and provide quality feedback to the learner throughout the process. All of these imperatives require that the instructor and the learner be focused temporarily on a relatively narrow range of expectations.

(3) Recognize that all skills are used in a specific context. For example, the decision-making skill of considering the pros and cons of different options looks very different in action when an ambulance team arrives on the scene of a multiple car accident with several victims severely injured. In this case, the consideration of options might involve a quick survey of the scene, a huddle of two key leaders to discuss their choices, and the making of a decision to implement a specific course of action. The whole process might take less than two minutes.

(4) The scene is very different when the leader and participants of an expedition sit down to consider the different routes they might take for a day hike the following day. In this context the decision might take more than an hour as all group members sit in a circle to pore over maps and guidebooks, listen patiently to the views of everyone, discuss the various possibilities, and strive to reach consensus. In both cases the targeted skill is manifest, but it looks and sounds very different according to the context. For this reason it is important to discuss the context of the challenge with learners and make sure they know what the targeted skill should "look like/sound like" for them when they are doing the challenge at hand.

(5) In the sample Equipment Selection challenge at the end of the chapter, the skill is decision making, the indicator that decision making is taking place is that the participants are analyzing and prioritizing relevant information, and the specific behavior that an observer could see or hear is, "Participants can cite information from authoritative resources that supports their choices of criteria and equipment."

Part 3. The SPEC Teacher's Tool Bucket

A. Activities, tools, and techniques. The following are what we call the AT&T, or activities, tools, and techniques, to help the SPEC teacher. We list these alphabetically, give a brief description, and provide observations about their use in both the classroom and the backcountry setting.

1. Brainstorm/distillation
   a) Description: A tool in which an individual or group first attempts to spontaneously create (brainstorm) ideas that might provide a possible solution to an issue or problem, and then narrows down (distills) the ideas to the ones that seem to be "best."
      (1) Brainstorming is used to maximize the chances of generating as many potential options as possible and improve the probability that all options will be thoroughly considered.
      (2) Brainstorming encourages creativity and provides an opportunity to "think outside of the box."
      (3) There are certain important brainstorming "rules":
         (a) Choose a facilitator who encourages the sharing of ideas and restrains the group's impulse to criticize or discount ideas.
         (b) Set a specific time frame for brainstorming. It is important to recognize that at some point you must move from brainstorming to decision making.
         (c) Have a recorder. Record ideas accurately without judging the quality of the ideas. Voicing opinions about ideas comes after brainstorming when you distill.
         (d) Only share your ideas if you are willing to let go of them. Once an idea is shared, the group owns it, and its ultimate acceptance or rejection should not be taken personally.
         (e) Work for quantity, not quality. Judging the quality of the ideas also comes after brainstorming during the distillation phase.
         (f) Do not criticize any of the ideas. All ideas must be afforded equal acceptance. To be effective, a brainstorming session must be governed by the attitude that "anything is possible." Again, evaluating the ideas comes *after* the brainstorming session.

(g) Encourage the "piggybacking" of ideas. Let ideas trigger new ideas. What some may think are crazy ideas frequently help trigger good ideas.

b) Distillation only occurs after the brainstorming process.
  (1) It is a distinct step separate from brainstorming.
  (2) It is when you narrow down the ideas to the ones you want to examine more closely or act on.
  (3) The distillation is done in relation to the established criteria of success.

c) Application: Anytime you want to explore ideas of any type, brainstorming/distillation is an excellent tool. We use brainstorm/distillation for:
  (1) Creating a Full Value Contract
  (2) Creating quality discussion and quality audience criteria.
  (3) Determining what route the group might take to their next ration point

d) Observations: The brainstorm and the distillation stages are two distinct stages. Don't try to do both at the same time. Set a time for brainstorming, and then set a separate time for distillation.

2. Carousel

a) Description: A "carousel" is where you arrange participants into groups, rotate them around, and have them respond to a series of questions or issues. Three to five people make an ideal group. You may want to decide how many groups to have based on the number of questions or issues you want to explore.
  (1) On tables around the classroom, place large sheets of chart (easel) paper, one sheet per group. (In the outdoor environment you can have a notebook at each location and have people carousel around to the various notebooks or have the notebooks move around to the groups.)
  (2) On each sheet, write one of the key questions or issues that you want to "carousel."
  (3) Try to provide a different colored marker for each group of students (so later, if anyone has questions about the comments, people will know which group made the comment).
  (4) Have each group appoint one person (perhaps one with good handwriting) to be the group's recorder.
  (5) Explain to participants that they are going to make their way around the "carousel"; i.e., they will work at each chart during the activity.

(6) Introduce each chart and explain the issue/question they will discuss when they get to that chart. As each group (or chart) moves, group members have one minute to silently review what previous groups have written on the chart. Then they will have two minutes. (You can determine whatever time limit you want, although we recommend no more than five minutes. Whatever time you set, we recommend you be consistent and keep them moving to discuss and add new thoughts to the chart.)

(7) As they work around to the different charts, they can annotate the previous groups' comments and add their own. The only thing they can't do is cross out any other groups' comments.

(8) When the groups come back to the chart they started with, they can try to distill/synthesize the comments and report out to the other groups or perhaps post the final posters for everyone to look at. This usually leads to a discussion regarding the issues. It is at this point that some lively discussions take place.

b) Application: A carousel is an effective activity when people have prior knowledge about a topic they are discussing or learning about. It relies on small-group brainstorming rather than on one large-group process that often leaves people feeling disengaged.

c) Example: See the Equipment Selection challenge at the end of this chapter. Here groups carousel around posters, writing down considerations in purchasing four major pieces of outdoor equipment. Since it is important that their comments represent "expert" thinking, they have to reference books or magazines that provide the observations they make.

3. Challenges: Challenges are SPEC learning experiences that progress with increasing authenticity, complexity, and uncertainty, requiring an increasing variety of resources and degrees of student self-direction to accomplish. We use the following types of challenges both in the classroom and in the backcountry. The following examples are brief descriptions of the types of challenges:

a) Academic challenge: Learning experiences are structured as a problem for learners to solve. They usually arise from a common area of study and are used to promote greater understanding of the subject matter. They target specified learning standards. With academic challenges, there is virtually no difference between the classroom and backcountry examples.

(1) Classroom example: Working in small teams, create a poster that graphically represents the "ideal" outdoor leader.

(2) Backcountry example: Working in small teams, create a catchy jingle that will reinforce outdoor-ethics principles.

b) Scenario: Similar to the academic challenge, the scenario's authenticity is enhanced by placing the problem within the context of a current, historic, or futuristic role play where the roles are either reality based or fictional. At this level there is virtually no difference between the classroom and backcountry examples.

(1) Classroom example: You are a group of early wilderness advocates in the 1930s. You have been asked to testify to a congressional panel on why there should be designated wilderness in the United States. You are to play the roles of the "real" wilderness advocates.

(2) Backcountry example: Create a skit that accurately represents the different interrelationships of expedition behavior. It should be creative and represent real-life situations.

c) Real life: A real-life problem is driven by a real situation that requires a real "solution." It usually comes from the larger community, is authentic, and has real-life consequences.

(1) Classroom example: You have been asked by the director of a nearby outdoor education center to create a series of evening wilderness education "fireside chats" on wilderness travel.

(2) Backcountry example: Your group is to plan and execute a day trip up a nearby mountain. In your planning be sure to include a Time Control Plan, an emergency plan, and who will serve in the task roles of leader, scout, logger, sweep, and any other appropriate task roles.

4. Check-in

a) Description: The check-in is a ritualized activity in which the group goes around to all group members and invites them to share one of two things:

(1) Anything that is going on in their lives outside of the immediate learning environment that might affect their roles as learners on that day

(2) Any observations about what they have learned or experienced that has had an impact on their learning

b) Application: We use this daily in the outdoors and on a regular basis in the classroom as a special ritual, usually at the beginning of the day, to "take the pulse" of the group in order to gauge their readiness to participate in the day's activities. The group will "circle up," and one member will start by sharing; that person then turns to the person to the right or left and says, "Good morning . . ." addressing by name the next person who will share. It works its way around the circle to the person it started with. If anyone passed, they are given another chance to share, which then ends the activity. Some mornings it is very quick, and some mornings it may take more than an hour.

- c) Special considerations
    - (1) Everyone is specifically invited to participate, but the choice to opt out or not participate is respected. People can "pass" to the next person.
    - (2) As the learning community becomes a safe environment, be prepared for emotional things to come out. If issues come up that are beyond your comfort/ability, be sure to refer them to the appropriate person who can help.

5. Chunking
    - a) Description: Chunking is a technique for getting and keeping information in short-term memory; it is also a type of elaboration that will help get information into long-term memory. For our purpose, chunking is a technique we use to break down a task or challenge into understandable "chunks"; i.e., we chunk a challenge by breaking it down into smaller, understandable units so that everyone has a clear understanding of what the task is. In one sense, it is just an oral regurgitation of the task.
    - b) Application: Whenever we give a group a challenge/task, we ask them to read (or listen) to the task, discuss it among themselves for a couple of minutes, and then report out what they think the elements or "chunks" of the task are.
    - c) Observations: We find this is a very important technique that eliminates misunderstanding and prevents a group from going in the wrong direction (sometimes literally!) with a challenge or task.

6. Collaborative learning
    - a) Definition: While collaborative learning has many features of cooperative learning (such as working in small groups, interaction with peers, active participation, and groups grappling with understanding concepts and ideas and addressing issues and producing results that would be impossible individually), collaborative learning has some unique characteristics that define it as different from cooperative learning:
        - (1) Collaboration requires more than just getting along and doing a share of the tasks. Collaboration requires an investment in the group's goals and sharing in the group vision. It means that members are willing to disagree and "bang heads" in a positive way in

order to insure that the task gets done to the highest standards possible given the resources available.

    (2) Successful collaborative learning requires learners to recognize that learners have different learning/collaboration styles and that successful teams require representation from all of these different approaches. Collaborative learners recognize that working with learners whose style is different from their own is frequently painful, but that without the diversity of styles, the team is incomplete.

  b) Application: The backcountry inherently has learners working in groups to accomplish the group's real-life tasks, so we strive to create collaborative groups whenever we work in the outdoors. We have also learned to use collaborative teams in our classrooms by implementing SPEC strategies. When efforts are structured collaboratively, we have found that students achieve and learn more, use higher-level thinking skills, and retain information more accurately. We also feel that collaborative learning promotes and builds self-esteem through more authentic experiences.

  c) Observations: We frequently describe the difference between cooperation and collaboration in this way: A person who cooperates works with all team members in a professional manner and returns to his tent at night and tells his tent partner how working with his team members drives him crazy. A person who collaborates works with all team members in a professional manner, returns to his tent at night, and tells his tent partner how working with his team members drives him crazy, but he adds one important thing: Even though his team members drive him crazy, he is extremely grateful that they are there because they all bring unique skills to the group that would be missing otherwise.

7. Cooperative learning

  a) Definition: "Instructional use of small groups so that students work together to maximize their own and each other's learning" (Hartman 2002). Cooperative learning is a team process in which members work together to support and rely on each other to achieve an agreed-upon goal. Learners work in small groups, interact with peers, actively participate, and grapple with understanding concepts and ideas and addressing issues and producing results that would be impossible individually.

  b) Application: Although we think highly of cooperative learning, we strive to work at the higher collaborative learning level.

8. Criteria for quality: The specific characteristics that we look or listen for in the tasks students take on that indicate that they have met certain

standards. They are the observable behaviors that provide evidence that learners have an understanding of the issues/information in their work or an ability to do a certain task.

   a) Content criteria: Expectations for understanding of the information they need to know to accomplish their task. (For example, if the challenge is to create a catchy jingle about outdoor-ethics principles, does the final product accurately reflect all the principles?)

   b) Form criteria: The real-world standards for this type of product. In the example above, the form criteria would be about the jingle:

      (1) Are the lyrics easy to memorize and listen to?

      (2) Does it have a tune that people remember and tend to hum or whistle?

      (3) Is it short (less than one minute)?

      (4) Does it stimulate your imagination or tickle your funny bone?

9. Debrief

   a) Definition: Reflection by group members of what has happened at the end of an experience, the day, the course, etc., in order to gain a common understanding of what happened, the significance of what happened, and what implications the experience might have for the future.

   b) Applications: Debriefing is essential in order for learners to develop higher-level thinking skills and to learn to apply what they have learned to new situations. While we don't want to create an atmosphere of "analysis paralysis," we do want to ritualize the process of reflecting on what has happened so we can learn from our experience in order to improve the outcomes of future events. Debrief strategies and techniques include:

      (1) Group debrief: A group debrief in its most fundamental form asks people to think about:

         (a) What? A clear and accurate reflection on what exactly happened so that everyone has a common understanding.

         (b) So what? What are the implications of what happened? What is important?

         (c) Now what? What do we want to remember, or what can we glean from the experience that will help us next time?

      (2) PMI debrief: A PMI debrief uses the PMI tool (see below) to debrief by asking people to consider the Positive aspects of what happened, the Minus or negative aspects of what happened, and what was not necessarily either a plus or a minus but an Interesting aspect of what happened. This tool allows you to explore specific

aspects of the experience. For example, if the group struggled to work well together to get the task done, you could frame a PMI debrief in terms of, "Let's PMI the way we worked as a team on this activity. What were the good things about how we worked as a team? What were the minuses about how we worked as a team, and what were some interesting observations about how we worked as a team?"

    (3) Pro/con or pro/delta debrief: A simplified version of the PMI where you ask a "pro" question (e.g., "What do you feel good about?") and a "con" or "delta" (Δ—the Greek symbol, in this case used to represent change or difference). The con or delta question might be, "What were you dissatisfied with?" or "What would you like to do differently next time?"

  c) Observations: We think it is important that early in a group's development you start with an emphasis on the plus or pro issues and perhaps not even address the minus, con, or delta issues. Once you have a safe learning environment where people feel comfortable giving and receiving open and honest feedback, then you can explore the minus, con, or delta issues in more depth.

10. Essential question or key issue
  a) Description: This is a statement that responds to the questions: Why should the learner do this task? What is essential about this knowledge or skill? How is it connected/relevant to both the "big picture" of the course *and* to the life of the learner?

  b) Application: We use essential questions to drive our academic and scenario challenges and also to frame most of our classroom courses. We frequently design a semester-long course based on what essential questions or key issues we want addressed.

  c) Observations: We find that many educators struggle with writing essential questions or key issues because it requires us to ask questions that we rarely ask ourselves: Why do our students really need to know this information? Why are we teaching it? What is the really essential information (what Paul Petzoldt called the "must-knows") that our learners need to master? We feel it is important to ask these questions and find ways to use our answers to create essential questions or key issues.

11. Feedback: Reflective dialogue between or among group members regarding their growth toward specific criteria. It might be between teacher and student, student and student, or student and teacher. It models that everyone is a learner. Some sample forms of feedback include:

a) Huddle feedback: Where large groups are broken down into small "huddle" groups to discuss and determine what feedback they would like to provide. We find huddle feedback much more effective than large-group feedback because it encourages more participation (it is harder to sit back and say nothing in small groups) and people are more likely to feel comfortable giving feedback in a small group than they might be in a large group.

b) Peer feedback: Where learners give each other feedback on a variety of work. It might be feedback on how they performed a task, how they contributed to a group task, or other relevant issues.

c) End-of-the-day feedback: An opportunity for learners to let the teacher know how things are going. We use "end-of-the-day sheets" both in the classroom and in the field to allow learners to give us feedback so that we can "take the pulse" of the group to help us determine if we need to modify our practice to maximize learning opportunities. The most basic, yet very effective, end-of-the-day questions are:

    (1) What are you feeling good about?

    (2) What are you concerned about?

    (3) What can I (the instructor) do to help?

12. Full Value Contract

a) Description: A social understanding that helps to create a safe place for individuals to be productive members of the community. It provides a structure for expectations of behavior that allows community members to hold each other accountable. "Full Value" refers to the idea that, "In order for us to honor our contracts, we must support one another. If we don't support one another, we are *discounting* each other" (Schoel, Prouty, and Radcliffe 1988, p. 94).

b) Application: We use the Full Value Contract in both the classroom and the backcountry. In both cases, it is created by the learners with input from instructors. We sometimes let the need for it arise and then introduce it as a way to address issues. On long backcountry trips, we spend a considerable amount of time exploring the concept and having students create their group's contract.

c) Observations

    (1) Full Value Contracts, if they are to be effective, cannot be delivered top down from the instructor. Ownership by the learners requires that they create it; however, that does not mean that the teacher doesn't have input and may even require that certain elements be included.

(2) Full Value Contracts must be living documents that are referred to on a regular basis and modified as necessary if they are to be effective. When behavioral issues arise, you may want to debrief the group in terms of how they did or did not model the Full Value Contract.

(3) The "thumb tool" (see below) is an effective way to ratify a Full Value Contract.

13. Grouping strategies

a) Do you really need to group? By far the first consideration in addressing the issue of grouping is to determine whether you really need a group to do the task or challenge. Few things undermine the authenticity of SPEC strategies more than requiring students to work in small groups when there is no legitimate reason to do so. If you can imagine one capable student meeting the parameters of the task or challenge with reasonable quality, then you need to rethink the design of the challenge. In a SPEC environment, we place students in groups because the challenge requires the diverse capacities of more than one person to engage it successfully. There must be meaningful work for everyone in the group. If there isn't, do not put students in a group.

b) How big should groups be?

(1) Fit group size to the complexity of the task and the experience level of your learners and you. When working with groups for the first time, we recommend you keep group size small—pairs or groups of three at most. This size group permits both you and your learners to begin your exploration of SPEC strategies at a lower level of risk. For you, a challenge designed for two or three should be fairly simple, directed toward reasonably straightforward outcomes, and involve a time frame that is acceptably brief. For students, a group of two or three gives them the opportunity to develop skill with SPEC group process techniques (task roles, brainstorm and distillation, sweep, etc.) while learning to handle the personality and social issues engendered by a limited number of people. When you are prepared to design challenges of greater complexity and your learners are ready to work productively with more people, then by all means increase the size of your groups.

c) How should you group them? Choose a grouping mechanism that fits your desired outcomes. There are really only five different ways to arrive at group membership. We have used all of these strategies at various times.

(1) Instructor arranges the groups: This approach gives the instructor some measure of control in balancing student strengths among the groups and perhaps to be proactive regarding the teaming of "difficult" students together. We used this approach extensively when we were first exploring the SPEC approach, and despite early resistance from some students, it worked well provided we kept the students in this configuration long enough (at least through three or four challenges) for them to adjust to each other and bond. The main disadvantage of this mechanism is that the students do not "own" the choice of group membership and therefore find it convenient to blame the instructor for any group dysfunction. Any instructor using this approach with challenging students must be prepared to "stay the course" with the group assignments and outlast student complaints.

(2) Students arrange the groups: As the instructor, this is the most challenging way of choosing groups—for a time. Less-responsible students may exploit the opportunity to team with their mates and waste all sorts of time. Frequently, some classmates may be left out of the group-formation process as well.

    (a) Anticipating these difficulties, we learned to design several simple and very brief challenges with groups formed this way. As part of each one, we insisted that *all* students be included in a group. Additionally, we were adamant that all criteria for quality be fulfilled. Finally, in the debriefing of each challenge we always asked the question: Do you feel the grouping of your team has had any impact on the quality of your work?

    (b) Predictably, some students denied there was any connection. Eventually, however, one student would break the code of silence and admit that sometimes working just with one's friends was not the best strategy for producing quality work. When other students in the class acknowledged the truth of the statement, we knew we had moved to a higher level of honesty and maturity within the class. We could then move on and honestly discuss the reasons for group work and how each challenge was an opportunity for each student to accept responsibility for his or her own behavior and learning and to demonstrate his or her increasing maturity, knowledge of content, and collaborative skill.

(c) As we became more comfortable with the SPEC approach over the years, we deliberately started each year with students choosing their own groups so that we could get at these issues early on. It wasn't always an easy strategy, but over time it has yielded great dividends.

(3) Groups are formed at random: Each year we would tell students on the first day of class, "One of my expectations for each of you this year is that before our time together is over, you will demonstrate your capacity to work productively with every other student in this class." In schools where SPEC strategies have been highly successful over a period of years, this expectation is systemwide, and random grouping is the norm in SPEC environments.

(4) Groups are formed heterogeneously by matching talents with tasks: Specific talents or capacities are identified and listed as necessary to complete the challenge successfully. Perhaps they will draw a chart (matrix) listing these abilities along a vertical axis as jobs or tasks to be led within each team. Then the students and teacher will recognize those in the class who have these special talents. The names of these students are entered along the horizontal axis of the chart. Finally, teacher and students match the entries on the horizontal and vertical axis to ensure that these talents are distributed fairly among the teams. In short, grouping is done with the requirements of the task and best interests of each team in mind, rather than the personal preferences of either the students or the teacher. Success with this approach, much like random grouping, is a clear indicator of a healthy community within the classroom. This grouping strategy also highlights the advantages of heterogeneity in a SPEC learning environment where people of various diverse talents are needed and valued.

(5) Groups are formed homogeneously: This has been done for years in the traditional classroom and is highly controversial. In theory it is supposed to allow the more capable students to excel while others get to master the basics. The research tells us that students of all ability levels benefit from homogeneous groups when compared with no grouping at all; however, students of low ability generally perform worse when placed in homogeneous groups as opposed to

students of low ability placed in heterogeneous groups. The research indicates that homogeneous grouping can have a slightly positive effect on high-ability students.

(a) Unfortunately, it often (intentionally or otherwise) promotes "labeling" among the students. Learners begin to see each other as having greater or lesser value as a person. They don't understand that group membership is often based on a very narrow range of criteria. They need to know that this is a criterion referencing a specific capacity (such as reading complex sentences, reading speed, or using fractions in math) rather than a judgment about them as a person.

(b) Keep in mind that homogeneous groups have very different effects on different students. We don't recommend it except in very special circumstances. One of us was once a student on a wilderness course where the final exam for testing navigational skills was to find our way nearly 3 miles up to the summit of a trailless peak. The instructor sorted the students homogeneously by perceived map and compass ability. The instructor had to have confidence that each group would have success and would not get lost. In this case, the students all succeeded, and the group with the "lowest" ability gained tremendous confidence in not needing help from the "higher"-ability students.

14. Huddle groups

a) Description: A small number of people who work together to accomplish a task. Usually the group gets together for a short task (thus the term "huddle") to brainstorm, debrief a specific question, or accomplish a similar task.

b) Application: We tend to use huddle groups whenever we have a simple task/question that could be addressed by the entire class. We would rather have them work on the task or discuss the question in small groups because it encourages more participation (it is harder to sit back and say nothing in smaller groups than it is in larger groups), and people are more likely to feel comfortable participating in a small group than they might be in a large group.

c) Observations: Huddle groups sometimes are effective for dealing with the occasional class "saboteur." Instead of the disruptive group member sabotaging the entire class, the person now is only sabotaging one group.

15. Initiatives games

    a) Description: Challenging activities, usually fun and cooperatively oriented, in which a group is confronted with a specific problem to solve. Initiatives games can be used for several reasons. The games can be used to demonstrate and teach leadership skills to people, which helps to promote the growth of trust and problem-solving skills in groups. Games demonstrate a process of thinking about experiences that helps people learn and practice a variety of skills and dispositions.

    b) Application

        (1) Classroom: We use initiatives games in the classroom as a metaphor for what happens in the backcountry. We have found that, between the wise use of initiatives games and well-designed challenges, we can create most, if not all, of the same learning opportunities that are created naturally in the out-of-doors.

        (2) Backcountry: We use initiatives games in the backcountry for one of two reasons (and sometimes both at the same time):

            (a) To reinforce an experience that the group has had in the backcountry so that everyone gets a deeper understanding of the topic or issue. For example, perhaps a group has struggled with group decision making during their day hikes. The instructor may have them play an initiative game such as Warp Speed (see Rohnke and Butler 1995 for more information) in order to examine how the group makes decisions and so they can improve their process.

            (b) To lighten the moment. For example, perhaps the group has been working hard trying to decide what route to take to their next ration point, and tensions are a little high as they have been unable to reach consensus. The instructor may suggest that they play an initiative game such as Elbow Tag (see Rohnke and Butler 1995 for more information) just to have some fun and release the tension.

16. Jigsaw

    a) Definition

        (1) A "jigsaw" is a cooperative learning activity that promotes the sharing and understanding of ideas or texts by creating "expert" groups, and then mixing the groups into "task" teams so they get to share and use their expertise.

(2) A jigsaw facilitates learning in two areas:
  (a) Learners acquire knowledge and understanding.
  (b) Learners develop skills and dispositions as they relate to positive interdependence and equal participation.

b) Application
  (1) Let's say you have a class of twenty-four students. You might create four groups of six each and assign each group a different chapter to read in a textbook. They would be told how important it would be to read the assignment because they will be expected to be the "experts" on their chapter and share their understanding with new groups when you reconvene.
  (2) When you reconvene, you will give them fifteen minutes in their "expert" teams to discuss their reading assignment. Encourage each person to take any necessary notes so they can share the essence of their reading assignment with their new "task" teams.
  (3) After the fifteen minutes is up, each "expert" team counts off by the number of people in the group. (In this case they would count off from one to six.) All the ones would create a new "task" team; all the twos would create another team, and so on.
  (4) Each new team would now have each person "report out" to their new "task" team for five minutes. At the end of the twenty minutes, everyone should have reported out.
  (5) In some cases the class will be over, so you may give them a written challenge to work on with the new information the next time you meet. Or, if you have more time, you give them the challenge and have them "chunk" it. (See chunking, above.)

c) Observations
  (1) A jigsaw is a great way to have learners teach each other a lot of information. Done correctly, jigsaws can be used to cover a lot of information.
  (2) It can be tricky to do your first jigsaw. You really have to be organized and plan the whole activity through. When you try this for the first time, don't be too ambitious. Choose a fairly straightforward topic. Work on the logistics; i.e., what you want the students to do and when, how long each grouping will take, how students will apply the information they teach/learn, and what happens next (an academic challenge?). Counting off or color coding sometimes helps.

      (3) Task roles are very valuable in a jigsaw. We suggest the use of a facilitator and timekeeper in particular.

      (4) Jigsaws are frequently seen by learners as fun.

17. Lecture

    a) Description: When one person delivers information verbally or visually to an audience that receives the information by listening and looking. It may also include questioning and a limited discussion.

    b) Application: Lecture is most effective when:

      (1) Factual information is presented.

      (2) Information is not available in another form.

      (3) Students have no experience.

      (4) Material must be presented in a particular way (e.g., for safety purposes).

      (5) Time is the most important consideration.

    c) Observations

      (1) Lecture is limited by the fact that:

        (a) It is a passive technique with very limited student interaction.

        (b) It only reaches one or two learning styles.

        (c) Even the shortest lecture exceeds the attention span of most learners.

        (d) It only involves the senses of sight and sound.

      (2) Lecture has been defined as "the process by which the notes of the professor become the notes of the student without ever passing through the mind of either" (www.emory.edu/EDUCATION/mfp/GreatTeacherLecture.html).

      (3) If you need to lecture, we recommend that you try to:

        (a) Keep it as short as possible

        (b) Make it as interactive as possible (e.g., ask questions)

        (c) Use visual as well as audio techniques

18. Parking lot or trash bin

    a) Description: A graphic poster, perhaps with a parking lot or trash bin drawn on it, for in the classroom, or perhaps a notebook for in the backcountry, where questions are "parked" as they arise until it is an appropriate time to respond to them.

    b) Application: We find that the use of this tool saves a lot of time. In particular, when you know many of the questions will be answered later, it allows you to acknowledge the value of the questions but "park" them for later discussion.

c) Observations
- (1) In the classroom, Post-it notes are handy to put the questions on the poster.
- (2) So you don't lose credibility, be sure to respond to the questions. If you fail to, it sends a message that they weren't important.
- (3) The use of the "parking lot" is a good way to deal with learners who want to show off their questioning ability. It allows you to acknowledge the question but not respond to it. If you have a learner who is continually asking questions, you can ask him or her to put them in the parking lot rather than ask them.

19. PMI (Plus, Minus, Interesting)
- a) Description: Using a chart with three columns, one each for P, M, and I, an individual or group can look at the plusses, minuses, and interesting characteristics of an issue or option.
- b) Application: We use it extensively for two purposes:
  - (1) In debriefing
  - (2) To weigh options in decision making
- c) Observations
  - (1) A PMI can be very helpful in providing a relatively objective analysis of an option.
  - (2) Author Edward De Bono tells the story of the use of the PMI as a decision-making tool: "Thirty youngsters aged around twelve were asked if they liked the idea of being given a small wage just for going to school. All of them liked the idea. Then they were introduced to the PMI. In small groups they scanned the Plus points of the idea and then the Minus points and then the Interesting points. At the end of this exercise twenty-nine out of thirty had changed their minds and decided it was a bad idea" (De Bono 1999).

20. Positive interdependence
- a) Description: When learners recognize that they can't accomplish a given task or challenge alone. They need each other in a way that benefits all group members, and the need contributes to the successful completion of the task or challenge.
- b) Application: We try to build conditions for positive interdependence whenever we give a classroom challenge. In the backcountry the conditions frequently exist naturally. There are a number of ways to create conditions for positive interdependence:

(1) Limit the available materials

(2) Use a jigsaw

(3) Pick one student from the group to make the group's presentation just before the presentation

(4) Require that all group members participate in the final presentation or exhibition of their work

(5) Assign and rotate roles

(6) Set criteria that necessitates intergroup decision making

(7) Require consensus decision making

(8) Give group assessments

21. Product Quality Checklist

a) Description: A Product Quality Checklist is a tool for determining whether learners met the standards on a specific task or challenge.

b) Application: We use Product Quality Checklists or something similar to them for virtually every task we give to learners. (See the Equipment Challenge at the end of the chapter for a sample and the Challenge Template, also at the end of the chapter, for a Product Quality Checklist template.)

c) Observations

(1) We think Product Quality Checklists are very handy to use, but after using them for a while you may find that they aren't detailed enough.

(2) We find rubrics are valuable in this case as they can be designed to be more detailed and allow a more refined assessment. Rubrics are descriptions of varying levels of quality for a particular complex performance task or product that guide the scoring of the task consistent with relevant performance standards.

22. Quality discussion and quality audience

a) Description: A form of Full Value Contract for how groups talk to each other and how they behave during a formal presentation.

(1) Quality discussion: A list brainstormed and distilled by the group of what a high-quality conversation among participants might look or sound like.

(2) Quality audience: A list brainstormed and distilled by the group of what a quality group of spectators of a presentation might look or sound like.

b) Application: We find both of these tools invaluable when working with groups. We have the groups create them as they need them. Creating a quality discussion list is usually the first brainstorm/distill activity we have groups do before they start working together. We then have them create a quality audience list just before the group is about to have their first presentation so that the audience understands what being a good audience looks and sounds like.

   c) Observations

      (1) No matter what the age of the group, we find these important and valuable tasks.

      (2) It is essential that the criteria be described in terms of what a person would see or hear that would be an indicator of a quality discussion/audience.

      (3) Like the Full Value Contract, if these tools are to be effective they cannot be delivered top down from the instructor. Ownership by the students requires that they create them. That does not mean, however, that the teacher doesn't have input and may even require that certain elements be included.

      (4) Like the Full Value Contract, these tools also must become living documents that are referred to on a regular basis and modified as necessary if they are to be effective. When issues arise, you may want to debrief them in terms of what they did or did not do to model the criteria.

      (5) We usually introduce the use of the "thumb tool" (see below) in order to ratify the quality discussion criteria.

23. Specific observable behaviors (look fors/sounds likes)

   a) Description: Some action that you can describe in terms of what you can hear or see.

   b) Application: We try to always create quality criteria in terms of specific observable behaviors and provide feedback in the same terms. For example, we create a quality discussion criteria list that we can observe in individuals and see or hear examples of when they exhibited specific observable behaviors. We use them when creating and providing feedback of:

      (1) The Full Value Contract

      (2) Quality discussion

      (3) Quality audience

      (4) Specific skills, such as decision making or leadership

      (5) Specific dispositions, such as collaboration or integrity

   c) Observations: Although you would think it would be easy to describe specific observable behaviors, our experience is that both learners and instructors struggle to be specific enough to describe what something actually looks or sounds like. It takes practice.

24. Sweep
   a) Description: To "sweep" is to go around and individually ask each person for input or his or her opinion on the issue or problem at hand. You sweep around the group, inviting input. Individuals respond or have the option to "pass" without saying anything. People who pass are invited to give input again once the sweep is completed.
   b) Application: We frequently sweep, particularly during large group work, to check in and see how people are feeling or what ideas they might have. It is a good tool to check in with people who don't readily volunteer information, but when asked have information to share.

25. Task roles
   a) Description: A specific job an individual takes on in order to help the group accomplish its goal or objective.
   b) Application: In the backcountry we use specific task roles, such as Leader of the Day (LOD), scout, logger, and sweep (see chapter 43, Travel Technique: An Introduction to Travel, for details) when on the trail. For our purposes here, we focus on the task roles for collaborative groups. We find them valuable in both the classroom and backcountry settings. Examples of general group task roles include:
      (1) Facilitator/leader: The person that helps the group get the task done by moderating the discussion, and expediting and organizing the accomplishment of tasks.
      (2) Recorder/note taker: The person who writes down the key information in such a way that it will help the group accomplish the task.
      (3) Timekeeper: The person who monitors time and reminds the group how much time they have left or how much time they have used.
      (4) Taskmaster: The person (sometimes the facilitator/leader) who keeps the group focused and reminds them when they are not focused.
      (5) Vibes watcher: A person who watches the decision-making process and comments on what he or she senses to be the individual and group feelings and patterns of participation. His or her job is to provide specific observations to back up his or her comments.
   c) Observations: The task roles listed above are generic examples, but there are numerous unique task roles we have used at one time or another.

For example:

    (1) Observer: Someone who watches the group (or watches an individual within the group) so he or she can share what he or she saw and heard the group (or person) do or say. It is important for the observer to do it in specific observable terms (i.e., what did it look or sound like?).

    (2) Greeter: Someone who welcomes people into the group, introduces them to group members, and makes them feel valued.

    (3) Sarcasm monitor: Someone who keeps an ear out for put-downs and caustic or cynical comments. The monitor will let people know when they are being sarcastic.

26. Thumb tool

  a) Description: The "thumb tool" is a consensus-building tool that allows each person to share his or her position on an issue. There are three ways to vote:

    (1) A thumb up means that the person enthusiastically supports the decision.

    (2) A horizontal thumb means that the person supports the decision but has reservations or doesn't have strong feelings one way or the other.

    (3) A thumb down means the person cannot accept the decision. The person giving a thumb down must provide a rationale for his or her position and provide an option that he or she would find acceptable.

    (4) For an issue to be approved, all thumbs must be either up or horizontal; there must be no thumbs down.

  b) Application: We use the thumb tool to approve a decision where we want consensus, i.e., total group ownership. For example, if you have a number of different options on how to get to your next ration point, you may want consensus on the route so no one person gets blamed for taking the "difficult" or "easy" route.

  c) Observations: The thumb tool is not a voting tool to see how many people want to do something. It is designed strictly to try to build consensus.

27. W.A.S.H. (We All Speak Here) (Mobilia 1995)

  a) Description

    (1) A technique in which four specific questions are asked to small groups. The questions are based on Dr. Bernice McCarthy's learning styles and are a what, why, how, and what if question.

(2) The four questions are designed around a common topic or concept.

(3) It can be done within a carousel or in brainstorm/distill "huddle groups" (see above).

(4) In either the carousel or huddle groups, we recommend about two minutes of brainstorming. In the huddle groups, we then recommend a one-minute distillation.

(5) If you carousel with this technique, then we recommend that you have the groups return to the question they started with and have them distill the question down to what they want to share with the large group.

(6) The distillation question can be very important and shape the direction of the discussion. For example, you could ask to distill the top three responses that are:

    (a) Most/least interesting

    (b) Most/least significant

    (c) Most/least unusual

    (d) Most/least helpful

b) Application

(1) A W.A.S.H. is a technique that allows individuals and groups to discover for themselves ideas, issues, concerns, concepts, and misinterpretations about nearly anything.

(2) W.A.S.H. can be very effective in reinforcing and examining important issues and concepts.

(3) Example: If the topic is "learning community," perhaps the questions might be:

    (a) *What* is community?

    (b) *Why* are communities important to learning?

    (c) *How* can we create a learning community?

    (d) *What if* all learning experiences took place in healthy learning communities?

III. Instructional Strategies

At the end of the chapter are two challenges. One is the sample Equipment Selection challenge referenced throughout part 2, and it is both a useful example and a good challenge to use in its own right. The second challenge, Engaging Our Learners, can be used to explore the content of this chapter.

Annotated Challenge

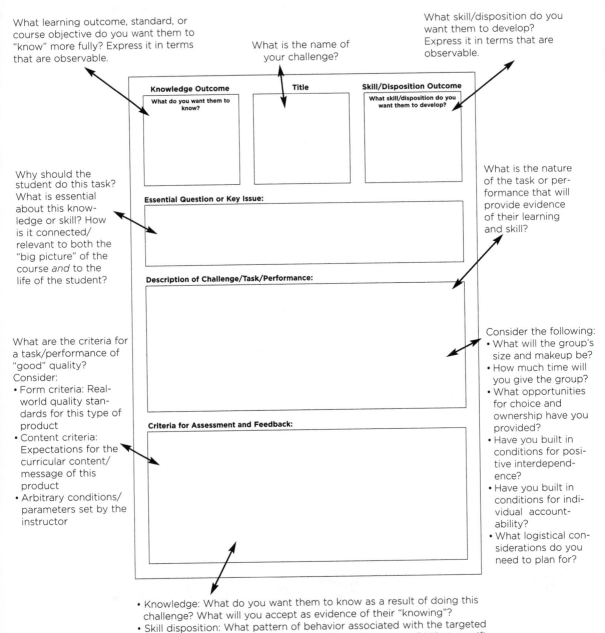

What learning outcome, standard, or course objective do you want them to "know" more fully? Express it in terms that are observable.

What is the name of your challenge?

What skill/disposition do you want them to develop? Express it in terms that are observable.

Knowledge Outcome
What do you want them to know?

Title

Skill/Disposition Outcome
What skill/disposition do you want them to develop?

Why should the student do this task? What is essential about this knowledge or skill? How is it connected/relevant to both the "big picture" of the course *and* to the life of the student?

Essential Question or Key Issue:

What is the nature of the task or performance that will provide evidence of their learning and skill?

Description of Challenge/Task/Performance:

What are the criteria for a task/performance of "good" quality? Consider:
• Form criteria: Real-world quality standards for this type of product
• Content criteria: Expectations for the curricular content/message of this product
• Arbitrary conditions/parameters set by the instructor

Criteria for Assessment and Feedback:

Consider the following:
• What will the group's size and makeup be?
• How much time will you give the group?
• What opportunities for choice and ownership have you provided?
• Have you built in conditions for positive interdependence?
• Have you built in conditions for individual accountability?
• What logistical considerations do you need to plan for?

• Knowledge: What do you want them to know as a result of doing this challenge? What will you accept as evidence of their "knowing"?
• Skill disposition: What pattern of behavior associated with the targeted skill or disposition do you want to develop in the student? What specific observable behaviors will you look for/listen for in this context as evidence that the student is practicing the targeted skill or disposition?

Developed by Leading EDGE, LLC for The Backcountry Classroom. *For more information log on to www.realworldlearning.info.*

Challenge Template

Knowledge Outcome	**Title**	**Skill/Disposition Outcome**
What do you want them to know?		What skill/disposition do you want them to develop?

Essential Question or Key Issue:

Description of Challenge/Task/Performance:

Criteria for Assessment and Feedback:

Product Quality Checklist

Date: _____   Class Period: _____

Product Author(s):	Product Title/Name:	Evaluator Name(s):

Observed	Standard/Criteria	Possible Points	Rating
	Total		

Observations:

Elements of Questionable Quality:	Elements of Exceptional Quality:

Challenge

Knowledge Outcome	Title	Skill/Disposition Outcome
What do you want them to know? The participants can discuss the rationale for choosing one or another teaching strategy in various learning settings.	Engaging Our Learners	**What skill/disposition do you want them to develop?** Teaching and transference: connects information and experience to the bigger picture

Essential Question or Key Issue:

What might we consider when choosing teaching strategies in the design of lessons and/or presentations?

Description of Challenge/Task/Performance:

You have been invited to a conference of outdoor educators. You have been asked to moderate the keynote panel discussion on the conference theme. The theme of the conference is Engaging Our Learners: Matching Methodology to Content and Context. You know there will be educational experts at the conference who are highly opinionated in their views. You also know these experts represent very different "schools of thought" regarding traditional and alternative teaching strategies.

Create a "scripted" panel discussion that is informative and entertaining. The discussion should be ten to fifteen minutes in length. The comments of the panel members should accurately represent the important issues to consider when choosing traditional and SPEC strategies for teaching various wilderness education topics. In your discussion, make sure the panelists address the following issues:

- Describe some "traditional" teaching strategies that work. What are some of the pros and cons of using these strategies for teaching various wilderness education topics? If a presenter wanted to use some of these traditional strategies, what might he/she want to keep in mind?
- Describe some SPEC teaching strategies that work. What are some of the pros and cons of using these strategies for teaching various wilderness education topics? If a presenter wanted to use some of these traditional strategies, what might he/she want to keep in mind?

Criteria for Assessment and Feedback:

Form criteria:
- Panel discussion is ten to fifteen minutes in length.
- Panel discussion is "scripted"; i.e., panel members know what they are going to say before the discussion begins.
- Panel discussion is organized around a central theme or questions.
- Panel discussion has a moderator who maintains order and keeps discussion on topic.
- All panel members contribute to the discussion.
- Panel members have the opportunity to question each other and respond to questions.

Content criteria:
- Panel members accurately describe various teaching strategies.
- Panel members indicate pros and cons of using a given strategy to teach a specific wilderness education topic.
- Panel members discuss "things to keep in mind" when using one strategy or another.
- The discussion reveals a basic understanding of a given strategy and the implications for using it.

Knowledge: Participants can discuss the rationale for choosing one or another teaching strategy in various learning settings.
- Participants make specific, credible recommendations about methodology appropriate for teaching a given topic and support each recommendation with reasons.
- Participants can adequately respond to questions that challenge their recommendations.

Skill: Teaching and transference: connects information and experience to the bigger picture.
- Participants can explain how topic and methodology move learners toward specific course/program outcomes.

Developed by Leading EDGE, LLC for The Backcountry Classroom. *For more information log on to www.realworldlearning.info.*

Product Quality Checklist

Date: _____   Class Period: _____

Product Author(s):	Product Title/Name: Engaging Our Learners	Evaluator Name(s):

Observed	Standard/Criteria	Possible Points	Rating
	Panel discussion is ten to fifteen minutes in length.		
	Panel discussion is "scripted"; i.e., panel members know what they are going to say before the discussion begins.		
	Panel discussion is organized around a central theme or questions.		
	Panel discussion has a moderator who maintains order and keeps discussion on topic.		
	All panel members contribute to the discussion.		
	Panel members have the opportunity to question each other and respond to questions.		
	Panel members accurately describe various teaching strategies.		
	Panel members indicate pros and cons of using a given strategy to teach a specific wilderness education topic.		
	Panel members discuss "things to keep in mind" when using one strategy or another.		
	The discussion reveals a basic understanding of a given strategy and the implications for using it.		
	Total		

Observations:

Elements of Questionable Quality:	Elements of Exceptional Quality:

Sample Challenge

Knowledge Outcome	Title	Skill/Disposition Outcome
What do you want them to know? The participants can knowledgeably discuss the criteria for selecting major pieces of backcountry equipment, such as backpacks, stoves, tents, sleeping bags, and sleeping pads.	Equipment Selection	**What skill/disposition do you want them to develop?** Decision making: analyzes and prioritizes relevant information

Essential Question or Key Issue:

Running an outdoor program requires large expenditures of money on equipment. In order to ensure we get the greatest value for our dollar, what criteria should we use to guide our selection/purchase of the major pieces of equipment for backcountry travel?

Description of Challenge/Task/Performance:

You are a team of editors for *Backcountry Trekker* magazine. Thousands of subscribers anticipate your annual review and recommendations regarding the quality of new gear for backcountry travel. As part of your annual process, your team reviews and reestablishes its list of criteria for making recommendations in each category of equipment: backpacks, tents, sleeping bags, sleeping pads, and stoves. This year you agree to make equipment recommendations appropriate for three-season travel in _____ (with the help of your teacher/instructor, agree on a specific region or environment and write it in here).

Follow this process to set up the remainder of this challenge:
1) Form five evenly sized teams. Each team should examine the references provided and, based on your research, begin to create a team's list of criteria for selecting each of the pieces of equipment cited above.
2) Once all the teams have completed their research, organize a "carousel" with the help of your instructor. In this carousel, acquire five pieces of blank poster paper and title each one with the label of a different piece of equipment. For instance, one poster paper is labeled "backpacks," another "stoves," etc.
3) Timed by the instructor, each team should move from one poster to another, writing down its suggestions for criteria for the equipment cited at the top of the paper. Build on or add to the suggestions of previous teams. Do *not* cross out criteria suggested by a previous team!
4) Once all teams have commented on all equipment, have the first team to comment on each poster return to that poster and distill/clarify/cull the language so the list of criteria is clear to all. Post these clarified lists for viewing, discussion, and common agreement, if possible. Each team must be able to support any of its suggestions with references to specific authoritative sources if challenged to defend what the team has written.

Your task: Using the criteria established, your group is to create an engaging and informative print advertisement wherein you recommend a specific piece of equipment in one of the categories that is the best value for your readers. There must be at least one advertisement created for each category of equipment. Your selections must be currently available for purchase. Be prepared to share both your advertisement and the rationale behind your choices with others in the group on _____ (insert day and time the project is to be ready).

Criteria for Assessment and Feedback:

Form criteria:
- The advertisement is on one page of poster paper.
- The advertisement is engaging—it causes the viewer to look with interest, pause, and read.
- The advertisement is informative—it provides the viewer with important/relevant information.

Content criteria:
- The advertisement includes a recommendation for a best value piece of equipment in one category.
- The team can support its suggestions with references to specific authoritative sources.

Knowledge:
- Participants can knowledgeably discuss the criteria for selecting major pieces of backcountry equipment.
- Participants can adequately defend their best value choices in terms of the established criteria.

Skill: Decision making: analyzes and prioritizes relevant information
- Participants can cite information from authoritative resources that supports their choices of criteria and equipment.

Product Quality Checklist

Date: _____   Class Period: _____

Product Author(s):	Product Title/Name:	Evaluator Name(s):
	Equipment Selection	

Observed	Standard/Criteria	Possible Points	Rating
	The advertisement is on one page of poster paper.		
	The advertisement is engaging—it causes the viewer to look with interest, pause, and read.		
	The advertisement is informative—it provides the viewer with important/relevant information.		
	The advertisement includes a recommendation for a best value piece of equipment in each category.		
	Total		

Observations:

Elements of Questionable Quality:

Elements of Exceptional Quality:

CHAPTER TWO

Backpacks: Pack Fitting

I. Outcomes

A. Outdoor leaders provide evidence of their *knowledge* and *understanding* by:

1. Comparing and critiquing internal and external frame packs
2. Describing the process of properly fitting a backpack
3. Describing the process of adjusting a loaded pack while on the trail
4. Identifying and describing the function of each of the major component parts of a pack's suspension system
5. Comparing and critiquing the capacity of pack suspension systems to provide comfort and stability under heavy loads

B. Outdoor leaders provide evidence of their *skill* by:

1. Fitting a pack to themselves and assisting in properly fitting packs to others
2. Adjusting their packs for stability and comfort while on the trail

C. Outdoor leaders provide evidence of their *dispositions* by:

1. Modeling proper fit and adjustment of the pack to maximize comfort
2. Modeling the choice of function and comfort over popular trends or styles when selecting a backpack

A. Types of backpacks. Backpacks vary significantly to meet the needs of a wide range of outdoor users. Among the wide varieties of packs on the market, the outdoor leader must be familiar with the two basic designs.

1. The external frame pack
   a) Purpose:
       (1) It is designed to hold a heavy load with sufficient stability and rigidity, allowing the packer to walk in safety and relative comfort.
       (2) The rigidity of the frame allows the weight of the load to be distributed evenly to the body of the packer through the suspension system.
       (3) This pack is a good choice for comfortably carrying heavy loads over moderate terrain or designated trails because the pack bag and frame may rise far above one's head.
       (4) Some external frame designs tend to keep you cooler due to more air space between your back and the frame.
       (5) This type of pack tends to be less expensive and lighter in weight.
   b) Components
       (1) Frame: Usually constructed of welded tubular aluminum, tubular aluminum with fitted joints, or "high-tech" plastics.
       (2) Waist belt: Fits snugly around the waist of the packer so that the padded portion of the belt rests squarely on the hips. This transfers the weight of the load to the pelvic girdle and onto the skeletal frame of the packer. The pelvis and legs are among the strongest parts of the body and best designed to carry weight; the more the pack frame can ride on the skeletal system and the less it relies on the muscular system, the less fatigued the hiker will be.
           (a) The belt should be heavily padded and is usually contoured.
           (b) The belt is usually attached to the pack frame with nylon webbing straps, clevis pins, or cinch belts.
           (c) The waist belt usually comes in various sizes (e.g., small, medium, or large) and is usually equipped with an adjustable length of nylon webbing that can accommodate a variety of waist sizes.
           (d) The waist belt has a quick-release buckle of metal or hardened plastic.

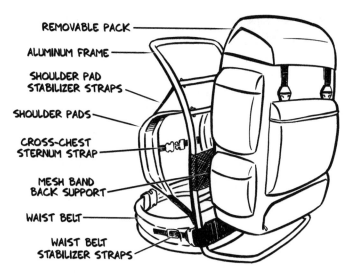

REMOVABLE PACK

ALUMINUM FRAME

SHOULDER PAD
STABILIZER STRAPS

SHOULDER PADS

CROSS-CHEST
STERNUM STRAP

MESH BAND
BACK SUPPORT

WAIST BELT

WAIST BELT
STABILIZER STRAPS

FIGURE 2.1. The external frame pack

(3) Waist belt stabilizers: If included on the pack, these are located near where the belt will ride on the user's hips.

    (a) These short lengths of nylon webbing and buckles connect the waist belt directly to the pack frame.

    (b) When tightened, these two stabilizers pull the pack frame toward the packer's hips, creating a snug, stable fit while walking.

(4) Shoulder pads: These heavily cushioned nylon pads are attached to a crossbar on the upper third of the pack frame and to the base of the pack frame by adjustable webbing straps and clevis rings and pins.

    (a) When properly fitted over the packer's shoulders, the shoulder pads assist in carrying some of the pack's weight.

    (b) More importantly, they help stabilize the pack by drawing the frame and load close to the back so that most of the weight will ride directly on the pelvis.

(5) Shoulder pad stabilizers: These nylon webbing and buckle assemblies connect each of the shoulder pads to a crossbar on the upper third of the pack. When these straps are pulled tight, the pack frame is brought snug against the upper back and shoulder area of the packer. When tightened, these straps help minimize some of the rocking and swaying of the pack frame when walking.

(6) Mesh back band: This wide nylon mesh band is drawn tightly across the two vertical legs of the external frame. The mesh band can either be one wide band or several narrower bands.

    (a) When properly taut, this back band presses against the shoulder blades and prevents the packer's back from coming in contact with any of the metal tubing of the pack frame.

    (b) On some packs, this band creates enough space to allow for some air circulation between the pack and the person wearing the pack.

(7) Cross-chest sternum strap: This nylon webbing with a quick-release buckle is attached to the front and middle of each of the shoulder pads.

    (a) When this strap is drawn across the chest and pulled tight, the two shoulder pads are pulled toward the packer's sternum.

    (b) This keeps the shoulder pads securely in place, increases comfort, and helps reduce some of the side-to-side rocking motion common to many external frame packs.

2. The internal frame pack

  a) Purpose:

    (1) It's ideal for activities such as mountaineering, skiing, snowshoeing, off-trail hiking, and scrambling over rugged terrain.

    (2) An internal frame pack is more flexible, rides closer to the body, and is more responsive to the packer's subtle turns and shifts than an external frame pack but as a result provides less ventilation.

    (3) The absence of a frame and its corresponding lower profile make this pack preferable in heavy brush, where it is less likely to catch or snag on branches.

    (4) As the pack tends to be positioned lower on the back compared to an external frame pack, it provides a lower center of gravity for better balance.

    (5) This design is usually more expensive due to its greater complexity and more labor-intensive construction.

  b) Components: (Most internal frame packs have suspension systems made up of basically the same components as those of better external frame packs; i.e., waist belt, waist belt stabilizers, shoulder pads, etc.)

    (1) Frame: As the name suggests, the frame of the internal frame pack is not visible because it is contained inside the pack itself. Depend-

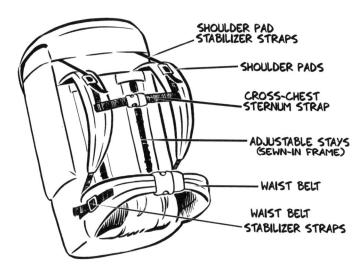

SHOULDER PAD
STABILIZER STRAPS

SHOULDER PADS

CROSS-CHEST
STERNUM STRAP

ADJUSTABLE STAYS
(SEWN-IN FRAME)

WAIST BELT

WAIST BELT
STABILIZER STRAPS

FIGURE 2.2. The internal frame pack

ing on the specific design of the pack, the staves (made of metal, plastic, or sometimes fiberglass) that give the pack its rigidity are usually located in concealed pouches within the wall of the pack bag that is closest to the packer's back.

(2) Torso adjustment: Internal frame packs usually have fairly sophisticated adjustments for properly fitting the torso length of the packer. Each model's apparatus must be understood and adjusted to ensure a proper fit.

(3) Stave fitting: For a proper fit, if the pack has metal staves, they should be removed from their pouches, bent to conform to the curves of the packer's back, and then returned to their pouches. Simply hold the stave against the pack where it normally rides and bend it to conform to the curve of the shoulder blades and back. Helpful hint: Trace a line from the top of the pelvis around to the spine. The bottom of the stave should be approximately 4 inches below this line when measured against the packer's spine.

B. Fitting the pack. Ideally, packs should contain at least thirty to thirty-five pounds (fourteen to sixteen kilograms) of equally distributed weight close to the body and between the shoulder blades when being fitted to the packer. It helps to go through the fitting process in front of a mirror or with a knowledgeable partner.

1. Fitting the waist:
   a) Loosen shoulder straps and slide arms through shoulder straps first to get the pack on your back.
   b) Loosen the waist belt stabilizers so that the waist belt is free to wrap around the waist and conform to the packer's body. The padded sections of the hip belt should not touch in front when wrapped around the waist; if they touch, the belt is too big. Try adjusting the buckles, or try a different hip belt or pack.
   c) Adjust the waist buckle so that, when fastened, it is located just below the belly button.
   d) Suck in the stomach and pull the waist belt tight. The top of the waist belt should be above the pelvic crest.
   e) Pull the waist belt stabilizers tight. The bottom section of the pack should feel comfortably secure against the hips.
2. Fitting the shoulder straps:
   a) Once the hip belt is positioned, cinch the shoulder straps tightly and then back them off slightly.
   b) Look in a mirror, if possible, and check to see if the shoulder strap height is correct.
      (1) Shoulder straps of external frame packs without load-lift straps should attach to the pack frame at a point roughly even with the top of your shoulders.
      (2) Shoulder straps of external and internal frame packs with load-lift straps should wrap around the top of the shoulders and attach to the frame about 1 inch below them.
      (3) Ideally, the shoulder straps are covering as much surface area of the back and shoulders as possible.
   c) Check shoulder strap length and width by making sure the buckle is far below the armpit to prevent chafing. They should be far enough apart so the neck is not squeezed, and close enough together so they do not slip off.
   d) Load-lift straps should begin just below the tops of your shoulders (near the collarbone) and angle back toward the pack body at roughly a forty-five-degree angle.
   e) Position the sternum strap where it is comfortable, usually about 2 inches below the collarbone, making sure breathing is not affected when the strap is buckled. Most people find a sternum strap helpful in increasing comfort and preventing the shoulder straps from sliding off

the shoulders, though some find them confining and uncomfortable. Its use is optional.

3. Fitting the torso:
   a) The pack suspension system must fit properly between the shoulder (where it meets the base of the neck) and the top of the hipbone. This distance is known as torso length.
   b) After fitting the waist belt to the hips:
      (1) Check to make sure that one of the existing back bands passes squarely across the points of both shoulder blades. This should keep the packer's back off the frame of an external frame pack or maximize comfort of an internal frame pack.
      (2) Check for good torso fit by slightly loosening and tightening the shoulder straps. You should be able to redistribute the weight between the shoulders and hips by doing this.

C. Pack adjustments on the trail

1. Someone not accustomed to carrying a pack for extended distances over varied terrain can expect to experience some discomfort until the body adjusts to carrying the weight. It is a myth that a heavy pack will be perfectly comfortable for an inexperienced hiker.
2. While walking, packers should frequently be adjusting the waist belt, the shoulder pads, and the stabilizers to improve the level of comfort. For example:
   a) Should the hips get tired or sore, loosen the waist belt to allow the shoulders to carry more of the weight.
   b) Should the shoulders become sore, tighten the waist belt and loosen the shoulder pads so that weight is transferred to the pelvis. By alternating the loosening of each shoulder strap, one shoulder can rest and then the other.
3. Packers should avoid cinching the shoulder straps so tight that the arms tingle and lose sensation.
4. If a pack leans significantly in one direction, it may be due to improper packing as opposed to pack adjustment.
5. Consider loosening one or both shoulder straps when taking a heavy pack off so it will be easier to remove, and also so it is easier to put back on once the rest break is over.
6. Plastic buckles break, especially waist belt buckles on heavy packs! Be sure to carry extra buckles within the group when you lead a trip.

III. Instructional Strategies

A. Timing

1. This lesson can be taught very early so that individuals enter the field with properly fitted packs.
2. Pack adjustments are usually taught using teachable moments on the trail as problems naturally arise.
3. Rest stops are a particularly good time to introduce pack-adjustment terminology and make suggestions for fine-tuning a pack for proper fit.

B. Considerations

1. Begin with a brief lecture/demonstration of pack components and proper fitting techniques. Have participants partner up, try on their packs, and adjust their packs properly. Once packs are adjusted properly, take turns and have the group critique each pair's work.
2. If possible, have a variety of pack designs available for participants to try out. Put participants in pairs or groups of three and provide a variety of pack designs for people to practice the fitting process. Have a discussion afterward of what they like and dislike about each of the designs.
3. On the first or second day of the trip, have participants pack their packs to the best of their ability and put on their packs. Hike them around for five to ten minutes. Most of the time, several participants will complain of all sorts of aches and pains. Have participants partner up, adjust the packs properly, and repack them for proper weight distribution if necessary. This exercise usually demonstrates dramatic differences in the way a pack is fitted, loaded, and balanced.
4. Challenge participants of equal size and weight to switch off and carry each other's fully loaded packs. This will encourage proper strap-adjustment techniques and provide an opportunity for students to provide each other with feedback on comfort, balance, etc. This also allows participants to teach one another and to share individual expertise. *Be aware that this exercise can create potential conflict when participants discover some packs are heavier or lighter than others.*

C. Materials

1. Full-length mirror, if available
2. Packs of various designs
3. A packed external frame pack
4. A packed internal frame pack

CHAPTER THREE

Backpacks: Pack Packing

Although packing the backpack may seem like an obvious and simple task, it is important for travelers to learn this skill early and practice it throughout their time outdoors. Campers with poorly packed packs lose things much more frequently than those who pack their packs well. In addition, a poorly packed backpack has a greater chance of injuring the carrier and will generally cause greater discomfort. C.B.S., which stands for Conveniently Balanced System, is a mnemonic device that can be used to remind participants of the basic considerations in efficient pack packing.

I. Outcomes

A. Outdoor leaders provide evidence of their *knowledge* and *understanding* by:

1. Describing considerations in packing for convenience and accessibility
2. Describing considerations for packing a well-balanced pack
3. Describing considerations for establishing a consistent, efficient system of packing
4. Describing considerations for weight distribution in a pack to meet the demands of various terrains
5. Critiquing a packed pack using the C.B.S. (Conveniently Balanced System) criteria

B. Outdoor leaders provide evidence of their *skill* by:

1. Packing items for accessibility on the trail
2. Packing a well-balanced pack that is safe for travel over a variety of different terrains
3. Developing a system of pack organization that allows for efficient packing and inventory of gear

1. Modeling use of the C.B.S. criteria when packing
2. Modeling a neat, organized pack
3. Modeling a minimal amount of gear secured to the outside of the pack

II. Content: C.B.S. (Conveniently Balanced System)

A. Convenience. A pack that is organized so that it permits access to its most needed contents greatly enhances the packer's efficient use of time and energy.

1. The itinerary for the day should be considered when organizing the pack.
   a) Arrangement of equipment in the pack should reflect the probability of that equipment's use during the day.
   b) External pockets should hold items that will be used most frequently during the day. Such items might include water bottle, shovel, toilet paper, trail snacks, foot care items, sunglasses, bug repellent, camera, etc.
   c) Other equipment that will be used for traveling or weather changes should also be secured in an easily accessible place. Such items might include rain and wind gear, hat, pack raincover, ice axe, climbing rope, crampons, etc. In cold or wet weather, rain gear and extra insulating clothing should be packed near the top of the pack or in a sheltered external pocket so that they can be reached during rest breaks.
2. Equipment that may be needed in an emergency should be easily accessible.
   a) Such items might include first-aid kit, important medications, repair kit, water purification system, rain fly, flashlight, etc.
   b) All members of the group should know the location of these items.
   c) Keys to the emergency evacuation vehicle should be packed in a safe location that is known to all, or hidden at the vehicle.
3. Items not usually needed until arrival at the campsite can be packed deeper inside the pack bag. Such items might include extra clothes, stove, pots and pans, food bags, personal toilet kit, tent, etc.
4. Items or gear requiring special protection should be packed inside waterproof or water-repellent stuff sacks.
   a) Extra clothing can be stuffed into waterproof, coated nylon or plastic sacks and packed near the bottom of the pack.
   b) Cameras and eyeglasses, for example, should be packed in cases and stored in the pack when not in use.
   c) Sleeping bags and sleeping pads can be stuffed inside a waterproof sack and packed in the bottom of the pack.

B. Balance. A well-balanced pack with properly distributed weight adds to the safety and comfort of the packer.

    1. Weight distribution and comfort

        a) Heavy loads are most comfortably carried when the weight is placed directly in line with the largest and strongest bones and muscles of the body (i.e., the pelvic girdle and upper thigh bones and the muscles of the thighs and buttocks).

            (1) The heaviest part of the pack should be centered as close to the body and as near to the top of the spinal column/base of the neck area as possible. The load should be centered between the shoulder blades.

            (2) When packing the pack, the single heaviest item of equipment (e.g., tent or food) should be packed in the top half of the pack and as close to the packer's back as possible.

        b) Heavy loads are most comfortably carried when they are balanced left to right, top to bottom, and front to back.

            (1) Balance left to right: Items of similar weight should be packed on opposite sides of the pack so that neither side of the body is uncomfortably overburdened. For example, if a fuel bottle is packed in the upper left external pocket, a water bottle can be packed in the upper right external pocket.

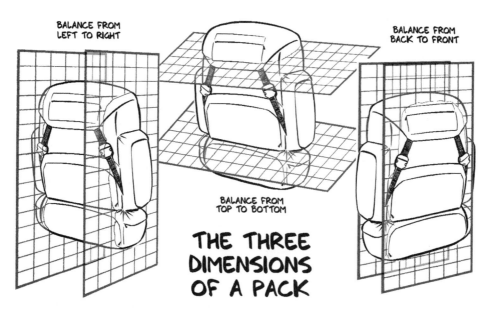

BALANCE FROM LEFT TO RIGHT

BALANCE FROM BACK TO FRONT

BALANCE FROM TOP TO BOTTOM

THE THREE DIMENSIONS OF A PACK

FIGURE 3.1. Pack weight distribution and balance

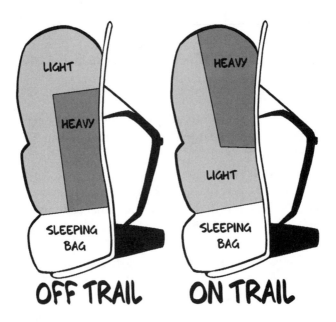

FIGURE 3.2. Pack weight distribution on trail versus off trail

(2) Balance front to back: Heavier items should be placed as close as possible to the packer's back to minimize pulling the packer backward.

(3) Balance top to bottom: Relatively even distribution of weight from top to bottom is desirable. If in doubt, pack heavier items toward the top of the pack.

(a) Heavy items should not be placed so high in the pack that they tip the packer forward.

(b) Sleeping bag stuff sacks on the bottom of a frame pack should not be so overloaded that they pull the packer backward.

c) With internal frame packs that lack protective cushioning, an ensolite pad or clothing item can be placed along the interior pack wall closest to the packer's back to protect it from the edges of rigid equipment (e.g., pots, stoves, plastic food containers, etc.).

2. Weight distribution and safety

a) Terrain should influence the way that weight is distributed in the pack.

(1) Flat, easily traveled terrain: For maximum comfort, pack the heaviest weight high and close to the shoulders. The center of gravity is higher, and the legs bear most of the weight.

(2) Rough terrain, steep inclines, dead falls: The pack weight should be

distributed slightly lower toward the middle of the back, allowing for greater balance and mobility while twisting or turning.

    (3) Boulder hopping, river crossing, traversing: The weight of the pack should be low on the back to lower the body's center of gravity and maximize balance. Some comfort may be sacrificed with the weight in this position. The shoulders will tend to bear more of the weight. Be careful not to pack the weight so low that the traveler is pulled backward.

b) Items that should be isolated from food and clothing, such as fuel bottles and stoves, should be packed in the outside pockets of the pack or in leakproof containers below the food to minimize the possibility of contaminating food with leaked fuel.

c) It is important to minimize the amount of gear secured to the outside of the pack. Ropes, cords, clothing items, pots, cups, etc., cause a variety of problems. These items can become snagged on branches, throwing the hiker off balance. This may cause the hiker to be injured. In addition, items tied onto the outside of the pack are more liable to fall off and be lost en route. Excessive noise can be created from the "banging" and "clanking" of dangling gear, adversely impacting other users and observation of wildlife. This practice also presents a less than professional image.

    (1) Examples of items you should avoid tying on the outside:
        (a) Pots and pans (noise)
        (b) Water bottle (too important to risk losing if it falls off)
        (c) Sleeping pad (can be shredded or punctured easily)
    (2) Examples of items that are more appropriate to be securely tied on, if necessary, might include:
        (a) Tent
        (b) Tent poles
        (c) Shovel
        (d) Climbing rope
        (e) Crampons

C. System. A pack that is organized with an efficient and consistent system speeds the process of daily packing and aids in maintaining an accurate inventory of equipment.

1. A personal "system" of pack organization allows the packer to load the pack easily, locate individual or group equipment quickly, and keep track of gear. A well-established system even allows you to find something quickly in complete darkness without the aid of a light.

2. Some individual items can be grouped together and packed in separate stuff sacks.
   a) Toilet kit: toothbrush, toothpaste, comb, hand cream, etc.
   b) Clothes bag: socks, underwear, bandannas, etc.
   c) Food bag: rations, food hanging rope, spice kit, etc.
   d) Personal repair kit: pack parts, nylon cord, wire, small tools, etc.
   e) Ditty bag: flashlight, extra batteries, shoelaces, playing cards, etc.
3. Packers should strive to keep their packs streamlined and neat.
   a) All equipment should be placed either inside the pack bag, in pockets, or securely lashed to the pack frame of an external frame pack. No odds and ends should protrude from the pack to catch on branches, poke other hikers, or wriggle free. All extra lengths of pack cord and webbing, or stuff sack drawstrings, should be doubled up, tied off, and tucked in so they do not hang loosely from the pack and catch on branches, etc.
   b) Soft items such as clothing should be stuffed between rigid equipment in the pack. This maximizes the efficient use of space and minimizes rattling, squeaking, or shifting of contents while walking.
   c) Anything to be carried on the outside of the pack should be tightly and very securely lashed. Nylon webbing straps with appropriate buckles work well for this. A clove hitch is particularly useful for securing sleeping bag straps to a pack frame.
   d) Compression stuff sacks, though more expensive than conventional stuff sacks, can be helpful in reducing the bulk of sleeping bags and clothing.
   e) Tent poles, ice axes, etc., should be lashed or strapped securely so the packer can fit through a gap between trees or rocks and the pack can easily follow.
4. Packing an internal frame pack
   a) More technique is typically required to pack an internal frame pack to ensure a neat, streamlined pack.
   b) Filling all space within the main compartment using the stuff sack system of packing can be a challenge. Packers tend to leave spaces and unfilled crevices within the pack and often find that all the gear will not fit.
   c) Packing suggestions for an internal frame pack:
      (1) Take the sleeping bag out of the stuff sack and stuff it directly into the pack, which can sometimes save space.
      (2) Take the tent out of the stuff sack and stuff it directly into the

pack, which can also help, for the reason cited above. Tent parts can be split up and distributed among group members.

(3) Use clothing and soft items to fill spaces.

5. Once a system has been developed that suits a packer's needs, it should be used consistently. Items can be packed the same way, allowing for occasional minor adjustments due to itinerary or terrain.

III. Instructional Strategies

A. Timing

1. Pack packing is usually taught very early in the course, preferably before the first full day on the trail.

2. If the first campsite is close to the trailhead, this lesson can be taught experientially by creating the need to know. Let the group pack their packs with minimal or no instruction, struggling to fit everything in and make their way to the campsite. With this experience fresh on their minds, they will have plenty of questions when the lesson is taught before the next travel day.

B. Considerations

1. This lesson may be taught as a lecture/demonstration in which the instructors display all of their own gear, describe their own system, and pack their packs while explaining the reasons for what they are doing. Immediately after the class, participants should pack their own gear.

2. A second method of teaching this lesson may be used with more experienced packers. After being on the trail for one or two days, have one or two group members lay out their gear and explain their ideas about packing. Participants may discuss the pros and cons of various approaches and arrive at many of the same understandings that would come through a more direct approach.

3. For younger participants a discussion may be initiated by using a very poorly packed pack as the focus for a contest (e.g., "find ten things wrong with this pack"). Use the ensuing discussion to highlight the main points of packing theory.

4. Participants can also be taught by having them pack by "rooms" of the "house." For example, they can pack the "kitchen," which would include pots, pans, food, stove, utensils, etc. This method tends to inject humor into the lesson.

5. Use teachable moments to point out positive and negative qualities of various packing strategies used by members of the group. With younger participants, a "Pack-of-the-Day" prize may be awarded to encourage the proper technique.

C. Materials. A backpack and all of its contents. If the group is using internal and external frame packs, it is best to demonstrate with both.

CHAPTER FOUR

Bathing and Washing

I. Outcomes

A. Outdoor leaders provide evidence of their *knowledge* and *understanding* by:

1. Describing why washing with soap in lakes and streams is physically and aesthetically harmful to the environment
2. Describing the importance of bathing and washing regularly while living outdoors

B. Outdoor leaders provide evidence of their *skill* by:

1. Bathing with minimum impact on the water sources and surrounding environment
2. Washing clothes with minimal impact on the water sources and surrounding environment

C. Outdoor leaders provide evidence of their *dispositions* by:

1. Modeling proper bathing and washing practices
2. Minimizing the physical and aesthetic impact of bathing and washing on water sources and surrounding environments

II. Content

A. Bathing and washing clothes: Why a special approach? Few will argue that water sources need protecting, but many do not realize or stop to think of the physical and aesthetic impact of washing in a water source.

1. Physical impacts: Most people are familiar with biodegradable soaps versus nonbiodegradable soaps, but what are their impacts? Whether a soap is biodegradable or not, it can have a negative impact on the environment. The chemicals that make up soaps can be broken into two general categories: those that are nutrients and those that are toxic to plants and animals. One consequence of introducing soaps into the water ecosystem is called *cultural eutrophication.*

   a) Cultural eutrophication: Occurs in an aquatic environment in which the amounts of nutrients are abnormally high. It causes rapid growth of plant life, eventually reaching a point where the plant life blocks the sunlight and diminishes the oxygen content of the water. Without sunlight the plants cannot carry out photosynthesis and they die. The plants stop producing oxygen when they die, and this loss can result in the death of many species, essentially by suffocation (Vivian 1973). It is unknown what role wilderness users contribute to this phenomenon, but every effort should be made to minimize it.

   b) Intestinal illness: Drinking water that is contaminated with soaps can cause diarrhea and other intestinal irritations or ailments.

2. Aesthetic impacts: Who wants to drink water downstream of someone who has just washed in it with soap or shampoo? Using soap leaves a physical as well as an aesthetic or psychological impact. The wilderness is an area where human impact is intended to be minimal; seeing soap suds floating down a stream does not fit this ideal.

3. Legal considerations: In most areas, it is illegal to put any foreign substance into the water ecosystem, whether directly or indirectly through runoff.

B. Bathing: how?

1. Preparation

   a) Fill two or more containers (cook pots, billy cans, or collapsible water jugs) with water.

   b) Select a washing site with good drainage at least 200 feet (65 meters) from the water source.

   c) If possible, have a partner available to help pour water over your head and back.

d) Bandannas can be used as washcloths.

e) Protect your feet from cuts by wearing your camp shoes.

f) A water bag or jug hung from a tree limb can serve as a shower.

g) Water can be warmed up by laying a water bag or placing a billy can in the sun for a few hours.

2. Bathing

a) Enter the lake or stream to get wet in preparation for bathing.

b) Walk up to the washing location, then soap and wash thoroughly.

3. Rinsing

a) Once thoroughly washed and ready to rinse, have a partner slowly pour water over head and body, rinsing the soap off.

b) If necessary, have a partner get more water to finish rinsing off.

c) Once thoroughly rinsed with no trace of visible soap remaining, enter the stream or lake for a final rinse.

4. Other considerations

a) If you are bathing alone, consider staying in shallow water (e.g., less than knee deep) for safety reasons.

b) In arid climates where water is scarce, or in cold climates where you might want to minimize your exposure to the cold, limited "sponge baths" are recommended. Wash critical areas with a moist bandanna, using little or no soap.

C. Washing clothes: how?

1. Preparation

a) Prepare as for a bath, except a partner is not necessary.

2. Washing

a) Rinse clothes thoroughly in a lake or stream, but use no soap.

b) Take the clothes up to the washing site and wash them in a container (cook pot, billy can, etc.), using small amounts of soap as necessary.

3. Rinsing

a) In a container of clean water, rinse the clothing. Keep replacing the soapy water with clean water until the clothing is completely rinsed. (It is not necessary to rinse clothing in a stream or lake.)

b) It is important to realize that most soaps do not rinse well in cold water, and soap residue in clothing may cause skin irritation.

c) Hang clothing out to dry.

d) Use care in disposing of the soapy water—choose an area with good drainage at least 200 feet (65 meters) from your water source.

D. Bathing and washing clothes: when?

1. Bathing
   a) If possible, it is wise to bathe every day to help maintain spirits, sanitation, and good health.
   b) If bathing is not possible, daily regular hand washing is essential (see chapter 37, Personal Hygiene).
2. Washing clothes
   a) Often, just rinsing clothes will help remove perspiration and body salts.
   b) Washing with soap can be done occasionally, but be sure to rinse clothing items thoroughly to prevent skin irritation due to soap residue.

III. Instructional Strategies

A. Timing. This class is best demonstrated early in the trip to set a tone of bathing regularly and demonstrating care for the environment. Especially early in the trip and for less experienced students, the instructor may want to set aside time specifically devoted to hygiene.

B. Considerations
1. This is a good class to be taught by students via demonstration.
2. When teaching this class, an emphasis should be placed on making sure participants understand why certain procedures are followed.
3. Baths can be taken with swimsuits on, or males and females can go to different areas for privacy. This may be a good time to discuss public nudity, as well as the course policy regarding coed bathing and the importance of being discreet with other groups and individuals.

C. Activities. See the "Harry Hygiene" challenge in chapter 37.

D. Materials
1. Water containers (two or more)
2. Biodegradable soap
3. Bandanna or towel

CHAPTER FIVE

Campsite Selection

I. Outcomes

A. Outdoor leaders provide evidence of their *knowledge* and *understanding* by:

1. Describing considerations in selecting a low-impact campsite
2. Describing considerations in selecting a safe, comfortable campsite
3. Explaining factors related to making decisions about when to camp
4. Explaining the importance of following rules and regulations related to campsite selection
5. Describing considerations in breaking camp

B. Outdoor leaders provide evidence of their *skill* by:

1. Selecting safe, comfortable, low-impact campsites
2. Choosing when to camp based on factors that will minimize environmental damage and maximize safety
3. Selecting campsites that conform to land management agency rules and regulations
4. When breaking camp, leaving campsites in a natural state

C. Outdoor leaders provide evidence of their *dispositions* by:

1. Modeling selection of safe, comfortable, low-impact campsite
2. Modeling conformity to rules and regulations in campsite selection
3. When breaking camp, leaving campsites in a natural state

II. Content

A. The low-impact campsite. Selecting a low-impact campsite may appear at first to be determined by rules, but instead should be based on an ethic, using guidelines as a framework in making decisions. Low-impact campsite considerations include:

1. Established campsites versus pristine campsites: One of the first decisions to be made is whether impact will be minimized by camping at an established campsite or by camping at a pristine campsite where no one has ever camped before. When choosing to camp in either an established or pristine campsite, consider the following:
   a) Selecting a campsite that has never been used before provides a more genuine wilderness experience.
   b) Having participants select a pristine campsite takes a higher level of decision making, thereby providing another opportunity to develop leadership skills.
   c) Using an established campsite is perhaps a better choice for campers who may not have the knowledge or skills to select a pristine site.
   d) Using an established campsite is required when safety or environmental considerations dictate its use.
   e) Selecting a pristine site requires that it be at least 200 feet (65 meters) from water, trails, and other campsites.
2. Aesthetics: The group should camp out of sight and sound of trails, shorelines, and other groups because:
   a) It provides a higher-quality experience for others if they don't see evidence of another group camped there and increases the social/psychological carrying capacity of an area.
   b) It is illegal to camp within these areas in most regions, unless the local agency has designated campsites within these limits.
3. Water: Can the group camp at the selected location and protect the quality of the water source?
4. Ground cover
   a) Can the ground cover on the selected site withstand the impact it will likely receive during the intended length of stay?
   b) Can tents be pitched and a campsite established without disturbing the existing cover (i.e., moving rocks or logs, pulling up vegetation, etc.)? This is especially critical when canoe camping since it is very easy to destroy vegetation along the shore when hauling canoes and packs out of the water.

c) Will participants conscientiously "walk lightly," watching where they walk to avoid trampling ferns, flowers, and other delicate flora?

5. Wildlife: Will use of the site have an adverse effect on wildlife and their habits?

6. Slope: Will the group subject the site to erosion?

7. Wood: Can wood for fires be used without having an adverse impact on the area's fuel supply?

B. Safety and comfort. It is critical from a liability standpoint and for the group's emotional well being that the site is safe and reasonably comfortable. Safety and comfort considerations include:

1. Weather: Is the site reasonably protected from elements of wind, precipitation, lightning, and flash floods?

2. Water: Is a suitable water source within a reasonable distance?

3. Widowmakers (a dead tree or tree limb[s] that could potentially fall and cause injury): Are tent sites free of dangerous widowmakers?

4. Slope: Can reasonably comfortable tent sites and meeting areas be found?

5. Aspect (the direction the campsite faces): What is the camp's location in relation to the sun, weather, views, etc.?

6. Geology: Is the campsite safe from things like falling rocks, landslides, mudslides, etc.?

7. Privacy: Is there sufficient space available to afford privacy for individuals in the group and the group as a whole (also considering the social/psychological impact on other groups).

8. In bear country, considerations to be aware of include:
   a) Avoid setting up tents in bear habitat or bedding areas. Bears are attracted to secure, cool areas that provide thick, low ground cover (e.g., thick woods or brush, under deadfall, near water, etc.). Extreme care should be taken in choosing a site in bear country, since virtually all areas may be habitat (Peacock 1990).
   b) Set up tent sites away from areas where food has been eaten, stored, or prepared. Also avoid putting tents between these areas and bear habitat.
   c) Where possible, group the tents together in a line so bears can easily avoid the area and not become inadvertently surrounded by tents.

C. When to camp

1. Before the group is overtired
   a) If the leader has to ask if the group is ready to camp, it is probably time to do so.

b) Group members may be afraid to admit they are tired, or others may not realize how tired they are.

c) The potential for accidents, injury, and environmental damage increases when the group is tired; therefore, if in doubt, set up camp.

2. Before darkness

   a) Few enjoy setting up camp in the dark, especially after a hard day.

   b) The potential for physical injury and environmental damage increases after sunset.

   c) Setting up camp in the early afternoon allows the group to:

     (1) Enjoy the area

     (2) Explore

     (3) Get personal and group chores done and replenish energy and enthusiasm

     (4) Get a good campsite in more crowded areas

D. Rules and regulations. Local rules and regulations are usually implemented to protect the wilderness user or the wilderness resource; therefore, every attempt should be made to follow them.

1. If the group does not follow rules, a double standard results and sets a tone of "do as I say, not as I do."

2. If for some reason rules cannot be followed, be sure to discuss the reason with the group so they understand the justification.

Discuss local rules and regulations pertaining to campsites at this time.

E. Breaking camp

1. Make sure that every attempt is made to minimize signs of the group's presence. When breaking camp, it is the group leader's responsibility to do a sweep of:

   a) Every tent site

   b) Kitchen areas

   c) Meeting areas

   d) The latrine site (if one was used)

2. Have campers restore trails and other areas to hide signs of the group's presence. Restoring the site should leave the area with as natural a look as possible.

III. Instructional Strategies

A. Timing

1. While safety and low-impact considerations in campsite selection need to be taught immediately, campsite selection as a class should be taught after students have had an opportunity to select campsites and have had a little experience with a variety of campsites. This reinforces the information in this lesson and gives it more meaning.

2. Early safety and low-impact considerations can be taught informally on a small-group basis, but it is essential to have a formal class on campsite-selection considerations to reinforce this knowledge.

B. Activities

1. Let the group leader or his or her delegate select the campsite and have the group critique it at the next debriefing.

2. Take the whole group through the campsite just before leaving and ask them to assess how well they camouflaged their sites and how they could improve on their efforts.

3. See the Campsite Selection challenge at the end of this chapter.

Challenge

Knowledge Outcome	Title	Skill/Disposition Outcome
What do you want them to know? The participants can describe considerations when selecting a safe, environmentally friendly, and comfortable campsite.	Campsite Selection	**What skill/disposition do you want them to develop?** Decision making: uses resources in the gathering and analysis of information

Essential Question or Key Issue:

What are the essential things to consider when choosing, setting up, and breaking a backcountry campsite?

Description of Challenge/Task/Performance:

You are the owners of a guide service that is committed to educating your clients in the philosophy and skills of safe, environmentally friendly, and enjoyable wilderness travel. The regional office of your state Department of Environmental Conservation has hired you to design a brochure that will inform novices of the proper techniques for selecting, setting up, and breaking a campsite. This brochure will be distributed at trailheads.

Working in your small group, create a two-sided, tri-fold, 8-by-11-inch brochure that will inform travelers new to the backcountry of the basic principles of responsible campsite selection and use. The brochure should be accurately informative, easy for the general public to understand, and presented in a way that attracts reader interest and encourages application of its contents.

As you design the brochure, please include information about the following:
- What are the essential considerations in selecting an environmentally responsible, safe, and comfortable campsite?
- What are the essential things to remember when establishing the campsite?
- What are the essential practices to follow when breaking the campsite?

Criteria for Assessment and Feedback:

Form criteria:
- The brochure is double sided, tri-fold, and 8 by 11 inches in size.
- The brochure is accurately informative. The information contained is essential to the purpose of the brochure and can be substantiated by an authoritative resource if necessary.
- The brochure is easy to understand. The message is communicated with language and graphics that are accessible to an audience possessing basic literacy.
- The brochure is interesting to read and encourages application of its contents. The images and language attract positive attention and use.

Content criteria:
- The brochure contains information essential to selecting an environmentally responsible, safe, and comfortable campsite.
- The brochure contains information essential to establishing an environmentally responsible, safe, and comfortable campsite.
- The brochure contains information essential to breaking an environmentally responsible, safe, and comfortable campsite.

Knowledge:
- Participants can describe considerations when selecting a safe, environmentally friendly, and comfortable campsite.
- Participants can respond adequately to questions regarding the content of their brochure.

Skill: Decision making: uses resources in the gathering and analysis of information
- Participants can cite authoritative resources when asked to clarify or expand on the "essential" nature of the information included in the brochure.

Product Quality Checklist

Date: _____   Class Period: _____

Product Author(s):	Product Title/Name:	Evaluator Name(s):
	Campsite Selection	

Observed	Standard/Criteria	Possible Points	Rating
	The brochure is double sided, tri-fold, and 8 by 11 inches in size.		
	The brochure is accurately informative. The information contained is essential to the purpose of the brochure and can be substantiated by an authoritative resource if necessary.		
	The brochure is easy to understand. The message is communicated with language and graphics that are accessible to an audience possessing basic literacy.		
	The brochure is interesting to read and encourages application of its contents. The images and language attract positive attention and use.		
	The brochure contains information essential to selecting an environmentally responsible, safe, and comfortable campsite.		
	The brochure contains information essential to establishing an environmentally responsible, safe, and comfortable campsite.		
	The brochure contains information essential to breaking an environmentally responsible, safe, and comfortable campsite.		
	Total		

Observations:

Elements of Questionable Quality: | **Elements of Exceptional Quality:**

CHAPTER SIX

Catholes and Latrines: Proper Disposal of Human Waste

In traveling through the wilderness, we want to have as little impact as possible. In doing so, special attention must be paid to the human waste we create. While we create many types of waste, this chapter deals with the proper disposal of human waste, toilet paper, and feminine hygiene products. Many campers can tell stories of experiences finding human waste in strange and inappropriate places with no consideration for aesthetic or environmental consequences. Human waste has been seen in the middle of the trail, on rocks in the middle of streams, and even in the crotch of a tree 4 feet off the ground! Humans are generally animals of convenience, and unless the impact of these actions is understood, change is unlikely. This lesson has the potential of having an incredibly positive impact on the quality of the wilderness experience.

Like many wilderness activities, the disposal of human waste requires good judgment. The air temperature, soil type, relative humidity, annual amount of precipitation, and amount of recreational use all contribute to deciding what method might be "best" for disposing of human waste. While this chapter is consistent with the Leave No Trace (LNT) program, it also takes into account that, ultimately, how you dispose of your waste should be determined by your own specific circumstances.

I. Outcomes

A. Outdoor leaders provide evidence of their *knowledge* and *understanding* by:

1. Describing the physical, environmental, and aesthetic consequences of not properly disposing of human waste
2. Describing how to dispose of human waste with minimal impact in a variety of conditions and environments
3. Describing the consequences of not properly disposing of waste
4. Comparing and critiquing disposal methods in a variety of conditions and environments
5. Describing the issues of pollution, privacy, proximity, and depth and how they influence choice of location for a latrine

B. Outdoor leaders provide evidence of their *skill* by:

1. Making and using a cathole
2. Properly constructing and using a latrine
3. Urinating and defecating a safe distance from water, trails, and campsites
4. Taking into account the issues of pollution, privacy, proximity, and depth when locating latrines
5. Appropriate disposal of toilet paper and feminine hygiene products

C. Outdoor leaders provide evidence of their *dispositions* by:

1. Modeling proper human waste disposal techniques
2. Leading discussions regarding the issues of human waste disposal

II. Content

A. Consequences of not properly disposing of human waste

1. Aesthetic impact: Aesthetics is the study of beauty and its appreciation. Someone who leaves human waste in visible sight of others is insensitive to beauty and inconsiderate of other users. Wilderness users must make an effort to preserve the beauty of the outdoors.
2. Physical impact
    a) Human waste has the potential to adversely affect water sources profoundly by contributing to the spread of waterborne diseases such as giardia, cholera, typhoid fever, and other similar diseases.

b) A variety of illnesses caused by human contamination have been documented in wilderness waters. The most prevalent, giardiasis, is caused by a protozoan. Its symptoms are severe diarrhea, stomach cramps, and nausea. Properly disposing of human waste, along with practicing good hygiene, helps to minimize the spread of this illness. (See chapter 47, Water Treatment.)

c) The presence of fecal bacteria in water systems is an indicator of contamination. Deer, coyote, sheep, beaver, and cattle are examples of other mammals that may also be affected by waterborne organisms.

3. Safety: Failure to properly dispose of waste can attract animals to campsites, creating unnecessary risks for participants and adversely affecting wildlife habits.

B. Disposal of urine. Urine is a mostly harmless bodily product (Hampton and Cole 1995). Because of its salt content, however, urine can attract animals that may then dig up or ingest vegetation to get the salts. Another possible problem is that, in some regions of the world, urine is a carrier of parasites.

1. Taking care to urinate in nonvegetated areas and away from water minimizes potential harm to the wilderness environment.

2. There are some environments in which this general rule does not apply. When traveling in canyons with fast-moving rivers or in certain coastal areas, urinating directly in the water has less impact.

C. Disposal of feces. Disposal techniques vary from one environment to another. The method for disposal of feces that has the least environmental impact is to carry them out. In some areas, this method is mandated. For example, portable toilet systems are required for river trips on the Colorado River through the Grand Canyon. This method is hardly practical for most backpackers.

1. Outhouses: Use wherever they are provided.

2. Catholes: A cathole is a small hole in the ground meant for a single use by one person. Use of a cathole is the preferred way of properly disposing of feces in most environments.

a) A cathole can be dug with a trowel (use the trowel only to move dirt, not the feces). Dig a hole 6 to 8 inches (15 to 20 centimeters) deep and 4 inches (10 centimeters) in diameter.

b) Catholes should be located well away from trails and water sources (200 feet or 60 meters; approximately seventy adult steps).

c) Squat over the hole and, when done, use a small stick to stir in soil. Cover with 2 inches (5 centimeters) of soil and disguise the hole as well as possible with natural materials.

d) After using a cathole, properly dispose of the toilet paper by putting it in a plastic bag, and then cover the waste and restore the site as naturally as possible.

e) Catholes should not be used in heavily camped areas because of the increased likelihood of the cathole being uncovered by others.

f) Consider the environment when determining whether or not to dig a cathole and how deep to dig it. Consult local guidebooks when considering trips to special environments.

3. Latrines: A latrine is a large hole in the ground designed for multiple uses.

   a) Determining whether latrine use is appropriate: Check with local land managers regarding latrine use in your area of travel. The use of latrines is not a desirable option, except in certain circumstances where:

      (1) The number of potential cathole sites is limited.

      (2) A group plans an extended stay in one area.

      (3) Campers are not capable of choosing appropriate cathole locations.

   b) Considerations in latrine construction: Constructing a latrine requires a balance of various needs. No two latrines will ever be the same. Individuals should strive to be creative while taking into account the considerations that follow. It may help to remember these considerations, using the first letter of each, as the three Ps and a D of latrine construction.

      (1) Pollution: Make sure all latrines are located at least 200 feet (60 meters) from water sources and in well-drained soil. They should not be located in an area prone to flooding during wet weather.

      (2) Depth: Latrines should be dug to a depth where good biological action will help break down waste. In most environments, the duff layer provides the best depth (8 to 16 inches [20 to 40 centimeters] maximum) for latrines.

      (3) Privacy: Our society has conditioned us to desire privacy in disposing of our waste. If privacy is not provided, group members might not use the latrine and instead leave their waste randomly in the woods with little or no concern for the environment.

      (4) Proximity: While privacy must be maintained, it is just as important to make sure latrines are close enough to the campsite for group members to use. If they are too far away and not convenient, group members are once again more likely to leave their waste randomly in the woods.

   c) Latrine construction

      (1) Considering the three Ps and a D described above, find a location

that is comfortable, and be sure that the next camper who uses the campsite would not consider it a good spot for a tent site or cooking area.

(2) Decide on a shape. Square is the conventional shape, but many prefer a rectangular trench, which some find easier to straddle. Rounding the corners of the latrine makes it easier to restore the site to a natural appearance when closing it up.

(3) Cut out the sod and set it aside. Water the sod if necessary to maintain any vegetation growing in it. Leave the soil next to the latrine along with a shovel or spade.

(4) After each use of the latrine, sprinkle just enough soil on the waste to keep flies and odor to a minimum—more than that will fill up the latrine too quickly.

(5) To assure privacy while using the latrine, a marker such as a bandanna can be tied around a nearby branch to indicate that it is occupied.

(6) Close the latrine when waste gets to within 3 or 4 inches (8 to 10 centimeters) of the top. Replace the soil and then carefully replace the sod, aiming to restore the site to its natural condition.

(7) One way to minimize the use of latrines is to encourage the use of catholes while traveling during the day before getting into camp.

4. Marine environments

   a) Feces and urine degrade more quickly in salt water than in topsoil. Select a secluded site in the intertidal zone on a sand beach, dig a shallow cathole, and cover it after use.

   b) Try washing with salt water as an alternative to toilet paper; otherwise, all toilet paper should be burned or packed out.

D. Toilet paper and its alternatives

1. Toilet paper

   a) Only white, nonperfumed brands of toilet paper should be used. It should be used sparingly and must be disposed of properly.

   b) We recommend bagging toilet paper and packing it out, but in some circumstances it is okay to bury it thoroughly in the cathole or latrine. Judgment should dictate your decision.

   c) The practice of burning toilet paper in a cathole or latrine is not recommended due to the fire danger.

2. Alternatives to toilet paper: The following are some alternatives to toilet paper. While at first they may seem unappealing to the novice, these

alternatives are found to be quite practical once one is accustomed to their use. Natural alternatives to toilet paper are convenient, and you needn't pack them out.

> a) Some prefer the use of leaves—but make sure you are not picking poison ivy, poison oak, or nettles!
>
> b) Pinecones or sticks with a rounded end and no bark will both work.
>
> c) Flat, rounded stones work well, as do large seashells with smooth edges.
>
> d) In the winter, snow (depending on the conditions) works extremely well as it is hygienic and readily available.

E. Feminine hygiene products

1. Tampons, napkins, and pads need to be packed out as they don't decompose readily and also attract animals. Store them in single or doubled plastic bags, with crushed aspirin, inside a small stuff sack until you can properly dispose of them.
2. Consider the use of applicatorless tampons. They require much less space to store. Avoid using sanitary pads as they take up even more space.
3. When menstruating, consider carrying daily needs around in a small container that is close at hand (e.g., a locking plastic bag). You don't want to have to search through your pack for tampons every time you need one.
4. Some women prefer to use cervical caps or natural sponges in the backcountry.

III. Instructional Strategies

A. Timing. This class is an excellent one to be taught via the grasshopper method (see chapter 1, Teaching and Learning). Teach enough to ensure proper waste disposal early and revisit the topic until the material has been covered completely.

B. Considerations

1. As the group enters a campsite, ask participants where they could go to the bathroom and how they would store food at night. Depending on the age level and motivation, instructors may have to monitor the group closely to insure compliance with proper waste-disposal techniques.
2. This is a good class for students to instruct. Although relatively simple, it requires good communication skills and the ability to give a demonstration. Depending on the course location, special environmental considerations for disposing of human waste should be mentioned.

C. Materials

1. Trowel for digging a cathole
2. Toilet paper
3. Tampons or pads
4. Plastic bag and stuff sack to pack out waste

CHAPTER SEVEN

Clothing Selection

I. Outcomes

A. Outdoor leaders provide evidence of their *knowledge* and *understanding* by:

1. Describing the broad concept of thermal regulation and the major considerations for selecting a backcountry clothing system
2. Describing thermal homeostasis and how body heat is maintained or lost
3. Comparing and critiquing strategies for thermal regulation to maintain thermal homeostasis
4. Describing, comparing, and critiquing the characteristics of common fabrics and materials that are designed to maximize the effectiveness and versatility of a clothing system
5. Comparing and critiquing various clothing items for inclusion in a backcountry clothing system

B. Outdoor leaders provide evidence of their *skill* by:

1. Selecting and properly using appropriate clothing for safe backcountry travel in temperate climate zones during the spring, summer, and fall seasons
2. Developing a clothing list for a multiday backcountry trip in a temperate environment
3. Applying thermal regulation concepts by demonstrating the ability to use the "Dress W.I.S.E." layering system

II. Content

A. Physiological considerations. Backcountry travelers must select clothing that will allow them to maintain a stable body core temperature, retain or dissipate excess body heat and moisture, and protect themselves from the elements. This concept is known as *thermal regulation*.

1. Temperature control: Clothing must permit the body's core temperature to be maintained within a relatively narrow range above or below 98.6°F (37°C) for proper physical and mental functioning.
2. Humidity control: Clothing must allow the water vapor (perspiration) produced by the body to dissipate readily from the body's surface.
3. Protection from the elements: Clothing should protect the wearer from exposure to sun, wind, rain, and snow.
4. Protection from injury: Clothing should protect the wearer from common injuries associated with travel in the backcountry, such as sunburn, blisters, insect bites, skin irritation from poisonous plants or briars, etc.

B. Understanding the need for thermal regulation. The body is constantly trying to maintain internal equilibrium, which includes a constant body temperature of 98.6°F (37°C), known as thermal homeostasis. Depending on the environment, conditions, and level of activity, the body's natural heat loss through radiation and evaporation helps or hinders the process of maintaining thermal homeostasis. Important strategies of thermal regulation, such as proper clothing selection and layering, play key roles in safety and comfort in the backcountry by helping the body retain or dissipate heat while controlling humidity, thus maintaining thermal homeostasis. The backcountry traveler must understand the following basic principles:

1. Conduction
   a) Definition: Conduction occurs when fast-moving (warm) molecules hit slower-moving (cool) molecules and transfer energy in the form of heat

to the slower molecules. Heat loss occurs by means of this energy transfer when the skin comes into contact with cooler objects; heat gain occurs when the skin comes into contact with warmer objects.

b) Examples:

    (1) If we sit on a cold rock, we cool rapidly because the heat moves from our body to warm up the cold rock.

    (2) If an object is hot, like a metal cup or backpacking stove, the transfer of heat from the hot cup or stove to the cooler hand can burn the skin.

c) Countering conductive heat loss/gain:

    (1) Sitting on an insulation pad will prevent heat loss to a cold surface.

    (2) Wearing gloves will protect the hands and fingers, preventing heat gain (and possibly a serious burn) from contact with an extremely hot object, such as a stove.

2. Radiation

a) Definition: Radiation is the transfer of thermal energy (in the form of heat) from one object's surface to the surface of another object without physical contact and without any warming of the space between the two.

b) Examples:

    (1) Exposed skin radiates heat, especially from the head and neck areas, where blood vessels close to the skin carry large amounts of warm blood.

    (2) Radiant heat transfer can also work against us when the skin absorbs radiant heat from the sun, potentially causing sunburn.

c) Countering heat loss/gain through radiation:

    (1) In cold environments and conditions, clothing items such as insulated footwear, hats, and gloves serve to prevent heat loss from radiation. It is especially important to cover areas of the body—such as the head, neck, wrists, and hands—that have a high number of blood vessels near the surface of the skin, making these areas particularly susceptible to radiant heat loss.

    (2) In hot environments, hats and long-sleeved shirts help prevent radiant heat transfer to your skin (i.e., sunburn) and heat-related illnesses from exposure to direct sunlight.

3. Convection

a) Definition: Convection is the exchange of heat between hot and cold objects by physical movement in a liquid or gas.

b) Examples: Wind travels through our clothing and blows away heat trapped between skin and clothing. The same dynamic applies when we are immersed in moving water.

   c) Countering convective heat loss/gain:

     (1) In cold environments, windproof clothing, flaps over zippers, and drawstring closures with cord locks are useful in maintaining thermal homeostasis.

     (2) In hot climates, loose clothing designed with optimal ventilation will help prevent overheating.

4. Evaporation and respiration

   a) Definitions:

     (1) Evaporation occurs when perspiration or sweat on the skin's surface passes from a liquid state to a vapor, causing a cooling of the skin. Some perspiration is caused by physical activity, and some is part of the body's natural process of emitting vapor through the skin while the body is at rest or during sleep.

     (2) Respiration is the process by which the body exchanges oxygen and carbon dioxide through inhaling and exhaling (breathing). During this process, heat loss occurs both through evaporation (taking dry air into the moist lungs) and convection (warming cold air taken into the lungs).

   b) Examples:

     (1) "For short periods, you can sweat up to four liters per hour; for longer periods (up to 6 hours), 1 liter per hour is common" (www.rwc.uc.edu/koehler/biophys/8d.html).

       (a) Under cold conditions, too much moisture from perspiration is dangerous once exertion slows down or stops because the excessive moisture cools quickly, contributing to loss of body heat that can lead to hypothermia.

       (b) Under hot conditions, too much sweat buildup will cause the skin to become saturated. Saturation leads to general failure of the cooling process and can contribute to onset of heat-related illnesses and/or injuries, such as heat exhaustion and heat stroke.

     (2) "The volume of air which you inhale with each breath must be humidified by your body to saturation in order to be used efficiently. This vapor is then exhaled, resulting in an evaporative loss which at high altitudes can rival sweat as a cooling factor" (www.rwc.uc.edu/koehler/biophys/8d.html).

c) Countering heat loss/gain through:
  (1) Evaporation
    (a) Breathable, nonwaterproof fabrics allow body moisture to escape and block the wind very effectively; waterproof, breathable fabrics such as Gore-tex are able to provide for some evaporative heat loss during periods of precipitation when they function as designed.
    (b) Decreasing the level of physical activity will decrease the level of perspiration, thus decreasing the level of evaporative heat loss as well.
  (2) Respiration
    (a) Decreasing the level of physical activity will decrease the amount of heat being lost through respiration.
    (b) Breathing through an item of clothing (e.g., face mask, neck warmer, or scarf) can prevent some heat loss caused by cold air being taken into the warmer lungs during respiration.

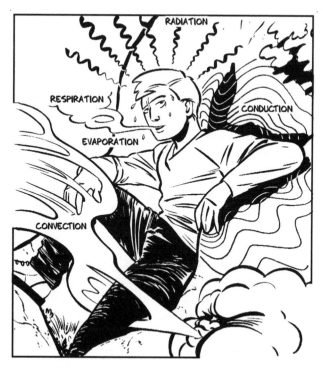

FIGURE 7.1. A person losing all forms of heat

C. Psychological considerations. Clothing must be selected based on function while taking into consideration the environment, multiple users, and other group members. Style and looks should always be of secondary importance to the clothing's function.

1. Wearing brightly colored clothing is considered obtrusive and may negatively affect the wilderness experience of other users. Wearing natural, earth-tone colors brings less attention or no attention to the wearer. There are exceptions to this rule for obvious safety reasons, such as the use of blaze orange when traveling during hunting season, orange personal floatation devices, etc.
2. Contemporary outdoor clothing can be quite expensive and serve as a status symbol for the wearer, sometimes causing feelings of inequity among other group members. In an institutional setting, this issue should be an administrative consideration based on program goals and objectives. For example, the same type of rain gear could be issued to all participants in order to promote a sense of group equality.

D. General principles of clothing selection

1. Clothing should be roomy and comfortable, allowing for reasonable freedom of movement.
2. Clothing must allow for unhindered circulation. Tightly bound, elasticized cuffs around ankles or wrists should be avoided since they tend to restrict circulation.
3. Clothing must meet thermal regulation needs; i.e., keep the user warm or cool depending on the environment or conditions.
   a) Some articles must be capable of providing the wearer with "insulation" (i.e., dead air space that creates a thermal barrier between the body of the wearer and the colder environment). The thermal conductance of the material should be low. Thermal conductance refers to the ability of the fabric to allow the transfer of heat and is measured in kilocalories per square meter ($Kcal/m^2$). The smaller the number, the better the material can insulate from the cold because it is a poorer conductor.
   b) Layering involves wearing a variety of clothing articles over one another. Clothing should be selected so that it can be "layered." This allows the wearer to respond to changing environmental conditions and levels of exertion by putting on or taking off layers.
   c) In cool or cold conditions, clothing must maintain its ability to insulate even when wet from perspiration or external sources of moisture, such as rain or accidental immersion in a body of water.

d) In warmer environments and during periods of vigorous activity, clothing should allow "ventilation" of excess body heat. Clothing should have a variety of adjustments that allow for ventilation (e.g., zippers, Velcro, snaps, armpit zippers, drawstring closures with cord locks, etc).

4. Clothing should keep the wearer dry when required.
5. Clothing should provide protection from plants (e.g., poison ivy, briars, nettles, etc.) and insects (e.g., mosquitoes, ticks, black flies, chiggers, etc.).
6. Clothing must be dependable and durable.
   a) Zippers, buttons, stitching, etc., should be of heavy-duty quality that can withstand the rigors of wilderness travel.
   b) External layers of clothing should be of rip/tear-resistant fabric and reinforced or doubled in areas such as elbows, knees, and seat to withstand heavy wear.
7. Clothing should be relatively easy to maintain and launder.
8. Clothing should be versatile and have multiple uses whenever possible to minimize the weight of clothing carried (e.g., shorts doubling as swimsuit, long underwear doubling as nightshirt).
9. Clothing should be lightweight and compressible. One should be able to "stuff" clothes into sacks or in crevices within a pack, duffel, or dry bag.
10. Clothing should be properly designed for its function (e.g., external garments should have large pockets that are conveniently located and can be securely fastened).

E. Clothing fabrics

1. Technological advances in outdoor clothing design have revolutionized outdoor adventure pursuits. Because of the rapid advances and changes in fabrics, fibers, and yarns within the clothing industry, we have not attempted to provide an exhaustive list of synthetic materials. For the most up-to-date information on synthetic materials, we suggest you explore the excellent Web site www.thetechnicalcenter.com/.
2. Choosing apparel can be an overwhelming task for the average backcountry traveler. Understanding the advantages and disadvantages of basic fabrics (cottons, wools, synthetics, and blends) is a good place to start. (See table 7.1.)

F. Fabric construction. After gaining an understanding of the four primary fabrics (cotton, wool, synthetics, and blends), the backcountry traveler should decide which is most appropriate for the intended use. Complex technology is employed in fabric design and construction, especially among the synthetics. Innovative technology has been used to produce various woven, knit, or nonwoven fabrics.

Table 7.1. FABRIC PROS AND CONS

Advantages	Fabric	Disadvantages
• Comfortable against the skin • Breathable and conducts heat away from body in warm conditions • Readily available to purchase • Easily laundered in all temperatures • Tightly woven cotton fabric blocks some wind	Cotton	• Absorbs water readily (7 percent of its weight in moisture); becomes heavy and dries slowly • Great conductor (6 Kcal/m^2), making it a poor insulator, especially when wet • Tends to mildew under constant wet, humid conditions • Dangerous—major contributor to hypothermia in chilly, wet, or windy weather
• Conducts (2 Kcal/m^2) little heat (one-third as much as cotton) and has wicking properties • Insulates even when wet (fibers are resilient and spring back, allowing air to be trapped • Is somewhat hydrophobic (sheds water) because of residual animal oils left in the unprocessed fibers • Can be bought for a cheap price at used clothing stores (be sure to tear out cotton liners)	Wool	• Too scratchy for some folks • Wet-dog smell when wet • Can be heavy and bulky • Don't wash in hot water and dry in your dryer—it shrinks!
• Very lightweight (fraction of the weight of wool) • Absorb very little water yet will function as a wicking layer • Poor thermal conductor, therefore an effective insulator • Dry rapidly (especially when worn) • Comfortable against skin • Nonallergenic • Less prone to mildew and rot • Come in a variety of colors, weights, and blends	Synthetics	• Tend to be expensive (have to shop for the bargains) • Will melt or burn readily when exposed to extreme heat • Some tend to hold body odor ("poly pro" becomes "smelly pro" or "poly pew") • Will wear out quickly if proper care instructions are not followed • Many insulators provide little protection from wind and must be worn with a wind shell
• Combine the best qualities of each fabric, frequently adding to the strength and abrasion resistance • Can be a combination of a number of fabrics (nylon, cotton, wool, synthetics, and others)	Blends	• Blending can combine weaknesses of each fabric • Blends containing cotton absorb water readily and freeze in cold weather

1. Woven fabrics
    a) Woven fabrics have interlacing yarns that intersect at ninety-degree angles.
    b) If the fibers are interlaced too tightly, the dead air space is reduced and thermal insulation is minimal (Gonzalez 1987). An advantage of a very tight weave, however, is its wind-blocking ability.
    c) Examples: rip-stop nylon and nylon taffeta.
2. Knits
    a) Knits are composed of interlocking loops of yarn and tend to be bulkier than woven fabrics.
    b) The interlocking construction traps air and makes it a better insulator (Gonzalez 1987).
    c) Examples: thermal underwear, sweaters, and pile jackets with a knit backing.
3. Nonwoven fabrics
    a) Consist of fiber material that is bonded or matted together chemically or by pressure. Polyesters, acrylics, and polypropylene fibers are used to produce nonwoven fabrics.
    b) For example, Thinsulate is a polypropylene product spun into a microfiber construction, and, like all nonwoven fabrics, it is a good insulator because it traps air (Gonzalez 1987).
    c) Example: felt.

G. Outer layer (shell) fabrics that protect from wind and precipitation. There are four different categories to consider when choosing your outer layer.
1. Breathable, uncoated nylon fabrics
    a) Highly breathable, tightly woven nylon fabrics are wind resistant yet still allow moisture from perspiration to escape. Garments made of these fabrics may repel, but will not stop, penetration by rain or melting snow.
    b) Compared to the coated and bonded nylon fabrics, uncoated nylon is typically more comfortable to wear during strenuous activity because of its superior breathability and lighter weight.
2. Waterproof, coated nylon fabrics
    a) Made essentially waterproof with a sealant such as urethane or neoprene. Moisture can neither pass in or out of a garment made of coated nylon.
    b) Garments made of coated nylon repel rain but trap body moisture. During periods of physical activity, the wearer will become soaked with perspiration unless the garment is extremely well ventilated.

3. Breathable nylon fabrics with water-resistant membranes
   a) Garments made with this fabric technology, such as Activent, are highly breathable and water resistant. Patagonia has used this technology for many years and continues to use this technology under the name Pneumatic.
   b) DWR (durable water-repellent finish) is applied to virtually all waterproof/breathable clothing. DWR causes water to bead up on the clothing; it will wear off in time and need to be replenished with spray-on or wash-on solutions. DWR will greatly increase the functionality of all waterproof, breathable clothing.
   c) These garments are ideal when ventilation is more important than shedding precipitation, such as high aerobic activity and light rain or snow.
4. Waterproof nylon fabrics with breathable laminates
   a) These fabrics consist of waterproof/breathable laminates or coatings and repel precipitation while allowing body moisture to pass through. Maximum rain protection is achieved, but some breathability is lost. Gore-tex is the best-known technology in this category.
   b) There are other common coatings used to achieve waterproofing and breathability. For example, jackets and pants can be Schoeller-WB coated (WB refers to waterproof, breathable coating) and will tend to be less expensive compared to Gore-tex products. The Lowe Alpine Company, for example, has developed their own WB-coated clothing line that has tested well.
   c) These garments are ideal when shedding precipitation is more important than ventilation, such as during light to moderate physical activity and heavy precipitation.

H. Footwear
1. Socks (four to six pairs):
   a) They should be medium to heavy, wool/synthetic blend socks.
   b) Two pairs of socks should normally be worn with boots to minimize blisters. While two pairs of socks of equal weight is more versatile (i.e., inner and outer socks can be readily exchanged), a light synthetic inner sock is popular due to its ability to minimize blisters and wick moisture away from the foot.
2. Camp shoes
   a) Nylon tennis shoes, canvas wading shoes, or other lightweight footwear is highly recommended for wearing around camp. They should fit over heavy socks.

3. Boots (general guidelines)
   a) Weight of the boot should be appropriate for the ruggedness of the terrain, for the amount of weight a person will be carrying, and for the size and weight of the person.
      (1) Lightweight boots are suitable for day hikes, carrying very little weight on easy to moderate trails.
      (2) Medium-weight boots with heavier soles and more rugged construction are good for supporting moderate loads (twenty to forty-five pounds) over moderate terrain.
      (3) Heavyweight boots (for heavy loads and rough terrain) generally have full-grained leather uppers (not split leather with a suede nap) for strength, support, durability, and weatherproofing (Drury and Holmlund 1997). Soles are thick and rugged and attached to uppers with cement or a stitched welt. The sole often has a shank made of metal, fiberglass, or plastic to stiffen the boot; shanks protect the bottom of the foot from sharp rocks and rugged terrain.
   b) Boots must fit comfortably over two pairs of hiking socks and allow for foot expansion late in the day under heavy loads. Two pairs of socks will minimize blisters and maximize the wicking action of moisture away from the foot.
   c) Boots should be well constructed. Check to see that stitching, grommets, seams, soles, and insoles are of good quality material capable of withstanding extended heavy use.
   d) Boots should "breathe." Waterproof rubber boots are generally a poor choice for three-season hiking, although they may be practical in extremely wet environments.
   e) Fitting boots:
      (1) Put the boot on a bare foot or with a thin liner sock only.
      (2) Slide the foot forward in the boot.
      (3) It should be possible to insert two fingers between the back of the boot and the Achilles tendon.
      (4) Put on two pairs of socks of the type that will actually be worn.
      (5) The sides of the foot should just touch the inner sides of the boot.
      (6) Toes should be able to wiggle comfortably.
      (7) One finger should fit between the heel of the foot and the back of the boot.
      (8) Lace the boot comfortably and walk.
      (9) The heel should lift just slightly off the bottom of the boot.
      (10) The arch of the inner sole should conform to the arch of the foot.

(11) The ball of the foot must conform to the slight depression in the inner sole.

(12) Kick the boot toe against a solid object several times. The big toe should not come in contact with the front of the boot.

(13) If the feet are of uneven size, always fit the longer foot. Use an extra-thick insole or an extra sock for the smaller foot.

4. Footwear for water-based activities

   a) Paddling footwear, another rapidly evolving branch of the outdoor clothing industry, can be very practical for water-based activities. Items of specialized paddling footwear (e.g., wetshoes, hybrid sandals, and neoprene boots, booties, and socks) are likely to be made of nylon, neoprene, and other quick-drying synthetics.

   b) Sport sandals with padded, sticky bottoms and ankle straps have become extremely popular footwear for water-based outdoor activities. But, a word of caution: Although comfortable and appropriate for some water travel, sandals provide minimal or no protection to the feet from cuts, burns, insect bites, punctures, toe injuries, ankle injuries, and sunburn. Judgment is required to determine the appropriateness of this footwear.

I. Putting it all together. What is the ideal clothing system? By taking into account the concept of layering and the other considerations discussed in this chapter, each backcountry traveler can adapt a functional clothing system using the following simple guidelines. Remember: "If you can't always dress smart, always dress W.I.S.E."

1. W = wicking layer: The first layer worn against the skin, its function is to wick moisture away from the skin and insulate. Inner layers of clothing should be of materials that absorb minimal amounts of moisture and allow moisture to readily evaporate from the body's surface (e.g., polypropylene, Thermax, CoolMax, Capilene, wool). These fabrics typically come in various weights/thicknesses.

2. I = insulation layer: The primary job of this layer is to insulate by trapping body heat. Fleece, pile, bunting, wool, or goose down can serve as an effective middle layer. Names of common synthetic insulating fabrics are: Polarlite, Polarplus, Synchilla, etc. Synthetic insulating fills such as Hollofill, Quallofill, Polarguard, Thinsulate, etc., are also used in coats, pants, footwear, hats, gloves, and outerwear designed for extreme cold and for sedentary activities. The synthetics insulate when wet, dry out relatively quickly, and are competitively priced. Goose down is lightweight and very compressible; however, these attributes are outweighed, so to speak, by

goose down's poor insulating capability when wet and its long drying time.

3. S = shell layer: The outer layer protects from wind and precipitation. Garments can be made of coated or uncoated nylons or a specialty fabric such as Gore-tex.

4. E = extra layers: Be prepared by carrying extra layers to deal with the diverse conditions experienced by all backcountry travelers.

J. Clothing lists. See the end of this chapter for a typical clothing list for a backpacking trip in the Sierra Nevada, California, and for sea kayaking trips in Alaska and Baja, Mexico.

III. Instructional Strategies

A. Timing

1. Clothing requirements for a trip should be communicated well beforehand and, when possible, reviewed in a pretrip orientation. It is essential for staff to ensure that participants are properly outfitted through a pretrip clothing and equipment check. Staff should conduct a "clothing shakedown," actually looking at clothing (and other gear) and not relying on students' memories or perceptions of what they have packed.

2. Information concerning clothing selection is reinforced informally throughout the course. A more formal presentation on the subject should be part of a classroom course or held near the end of an expedition when participants have had the opportunity to formulate their own views on the clothing requirements.

B. Considerations: assessment strategies

1. Later in the course, a participant-oriented clothing debrief may be very beneficial. The students can critique personal clothing brought on the trip, compiling a list of advantages and disadvantages in their journals and then discussing together the pros and cons of particular items of clothing.

2. Have students create (from memory) a personal clothing list designed to be sent out in registration material to a group of novice teenagers about to embark on a ten-day wilderness expedition. The environment, time of year, climate, and adventure activities should vary slightly from the current experience so that students apply their knowledge in a different context.

3. The knowledge section of this lesson can readily be taught in the classroom and assessed through traditional tests. The skills and dispositions need to be observed throughout the trip.

C. Activities

1. This lesson may be taught early in a course as an instructor-directed lecture/demonstration in which each article of clothing is presented and the rationale for its selection explained. One method of involving the students in an instructor-directed session is to have students attend the class dressed "W.I.S.E." The students can conduct comparisons of fabrics, designs, and brands.

2. Experiential activities to supplement a lecture are very important to engage all types of learners.

    a) Example 1: Have students bring clothing and create a jumbled pile of clothes in the middle of a student circle. After the instructor has given a brief lecture on fabric comparisons and the W.I.S.E. system of dressing, take turns having blindfolded students randomly pick a piece of clothing, determine the fabric, and tell for which layer they think the article of clothing would be best suited.

    b) Example 2: Another activity is the best-dressed contest. Divide students into smaller groups, and then have each group choose one individual to model the most appropriate outdoor clothing found among the membership of the small group. Have a contest to see which group member is the best dressed. Have the group systematically explain the merits of the clothing system to a judge or panel.

3. See the Selecting Clothing for Backcountry Travel challenge at the end of this chapter.

Clothing List for an August Backpacking Trip in the Sierra Nevada, California

(courtesy of Aztec Adventures of San Diego State University)

Footwear

- **Hiking boots:** Select footwear appropriate for the type of terrain, amount of weight to be carried, and for the size and weight of the hiker.
- **Camp shoes:** Lightweight tennis shoes or sport sandals for minimizing one's impact in camp. (Tennis shoes are preferable for greater safety and comfort.)
- **Socks:** Two to three pairs of heavy ragg wool hiking socks and two to three pairs of polypropylene liner socks.
- **Gaiters:** Worn over the top of hiking boots to keep scree, dirt, and snow out. Gaiters should be long enough to cover the lower leg (just below the knees) and should be as "maintenance-free" as possible. Gaiters with zippers should have a back-up closure system (Velcro, snaps, etc.)

Lower-Body Garments

Two insulation layers, plus a wind/rain layer, which must fit comfortably over each other so they can be worn at the same time. If you tend to get cold easily, add the secondary layer of expedition-weight bottoms in addition to the primary midweight layer and pile pants.

- **Midweight long-underwear bottoms:** One pair, made of polypropylene, Capilene, etc.
- **Lightweight or expedition-weight long-underwear bottoms:** One pair, which must fit over/under midweights.
- **Rain/wind pants:** Must be roomy enough to fit over all lower-body garments.
- **Hiking shorts:** Loose-fitting nylon athletic or river shorts—abrasion-resistant with pockets.
- **Cotton underwear:** An excellent choice due to breathability.
- **Bathing suit:** For bathing when there is little privacy. It may or may not be possible to swim in alpine lakes or streams due to very cold water temperatures.

Upper-Body Garments

Three insulating layers, plus a wind and rain layer, which must fit comfortably over each other so they can all be worn at the same time. If you tend to get cold easily, add the pile vest in addition to the other three layers.

- **Parka:** Coated material is mandatory. Parka must provide a waterproof barrier as well as a shell for insulation from the cold and wind.

- **Cotton shirts:** Cotton is excellent for hiking on warm days. Lightweight, button-down cotton shirts with breast pockets and collar offer flexibility in ventilation and dry out quicker than cotton T-shirts.
- **Midweight top:** A turtleneck with a zippered or button-down collar is excellent for ventilation. Fabric can be polypropylene, Capilene, or any other synthetic—absolutely no cotton blends!
- **Lightweight or heavyweight top:** Again, depending on your comfort level.
- **Pile jacket:** A 200- or 300-weight jacket would be adequate.

Head Garments

Two insulating layers for your head.
- **Balaclava or stocking cap:** This garment covers both the head and neck portions of the face. Made from wool or pile, it is very comfortable and effective to wear while sleeping at night.
- **Shade hat:** Indiana Jones/Bermuda tourist styles are better than baseball caps because they keep the sun off the back of your head and neck.
- **Bandannas:** Have multiple uses besides covering your head. Bring at least two!
- **Mosquito bug net:** The mosquitoes can be fierce in some areas of the Sierra Nevada.
- **Sunglasses:** With 100 percent UV protection, or glacier glasses, with straps to prevent loss. Traveling across snowfields in the bright sun without protective sunglasses is dangerous, causing snow blindness in a matter of minutes.
- **Sunglasses case:** To keep those valuable glasses from getting scratched or crushed.

Hand Garments

Your hands are as important as your feet. Expect your hands to become dry and chapped, sunburned, and scratched and scraped. Some students have worn a lightweight pair of cotton gloves while hiking to keep the intense rays of the sun from burning their hands.
- **Gloves or mittens:** Lightweight wool or synthetic.

Clothing List for Sea Kayaking in Baja, California

(courtesy of Aztec Adventures of San Diego State University)

Head

- **Shade hat:** Side-brimmed is best, but a baseball cap with bandanna covering the back of your head and neck will work in a pinch.
- **Warm hat:** A wool or fleece stocking cap or balaclava can be worn while sleeping or in the evening when it is cool and windy.

Upper Body

- **Cotton T-shirt/shirt:** Cotton is wonderful to put on after a long day of paddling. Keep a shirt designated only for "camp" to avoid the saltwater chafe.
- **Synthetic long-underwear top:** Midweight (Capilene, polypropylene, etc.) will keep you warm even when wet. Nice to wear under your spray jacket as added insulation.
- **Wool sweater or fleece jacket/pullover:** Great for in camp or if conditions get cold.
- **Windbreaker or rain jacket:** This will keep you warm in the evenings.
- **Paddling jacket:** Protection from wind and water spray.
- **Wetsuit**

Lower Body

- **Nylon shorts:** Better than cotton because nylon dries more quickly.
- **Synthetic long-underwear bottoms:** Midweight.
- **Cotton sweat pants:** Nice to have in camp for the cool evenings.
- **Bathing suit**
- **Underwear**

Hands

- **Paddling gloves** (weightlifting/cycling gloves can be substituted): Some people like them to prevent calluses/blisters.

Feet

- **Sport sandals and/or neoprene booties:** The terrain around camp is very rugged. In warmer weather, sport sandals are nice to wear all the time. In cooler weather, neoprene booties keep your feet warm when you are getting in and out of the kayak.
- **Hiking shoes:** Essential for day hikes.
- **Hiking socks:** Wool or wool/nylon blend.

Clothing List for Sea Kayaking in Alaska

(courtesy of Aztec Adventures of San Diego State University)

Do *not* bring cotton (once it's wet, it's useless). Bring wool or synthetics (polypropylene, fleece, etc.) instead. It's likely that you'll end up with one set of wet clothes (your paddling clothes) and one set of dry, warm clothes for camp, so keep this in mind as you make your clothing selections.

- **Camp shoes:** When it is dry, a lightweight pair of hiking shoes or sturdy tennis shoes will be nice.
- **Wool and/or fleece socks:** Bring a minimum of four pairs.
- **Midweight long-underwear bottoms:** Two pairs.
- **Fleece pants or expedition-weight long-underwear bottoms**
- **Nylon shorts**
- **Midweight long-underwear top:** Two pairs.
- **Expedition-weight long-underwear top**
- **Fleece jackets or wool sweaters:** Bring two.
- **Nylon-blend camp shirt**
- **Wool or fleece stocking caps:** Bring two.
- **Baseball cap**
- **Rain hat:** Waterproof hat with brim.
- **Mosquito head net**
- **Bandannas**
- **Waterproof gloves:** "Pogies," or neoprene or rubber kitchen gloves.
- **Lightweight fleece or wool gloves**
- **Rubber boots**
- **Waterproof rain pants**
- **Waterproof rain jacket or parka with hood**
- **Paddling jacket**

Challenge

Knowledge Outcome	Title	Skill/Disposition Outcome
What do you want them to know? The participants can describe the broad concept of thermal regulation and the major considerations for selecting a backcountry clothing system	Selecting Clothing for Backcountry Travel	**What skill/disposition do you want them to develop?** Decision making: brainstorms ideas or options to consider

Essential Question or Key Issue:

What should we take into consideration when choosing clothing to wear on a backcountry expedition?

Description of Challenge/Task/Performance:

You and your college-age friends are members of the outing club at a prestigious university. The young daughter of your faculty sponsor has asked her dad if he would come to her sixth-grade class at school and teach her classmates about selecting appropriate clothing for an upcoming three-day camping trip. Because of a schedule conflict, he is unable to attend. Instead, he has asked that you and your outing-club peers conduct the class in his place.

Create and conduct a highly informative, interesting, and engaging classroom experience for a class of sixth-grade boys and girls (eleven and twelve years old) that addresses the essential question cited above. The classroom experience should last about thirty to forty minutes.

As you design the class, please consider the following:
- Twelve-year-olds have an attention span that is notoriously brief. Consider a lesson that is interactive, hands-on, learning by doing.
- Your lesson should help the students understand both "what" to wear and "why" to wear it. In your lesson, be sure to integrate the most important concepts of thermal regulation with the practicalities of clothing selection.
- Twelve-year-olds need very concrete examples to support their learning. Be sure to provide your learners with very specific real-world examples whenever possible.

Criteria for Assessment and Feedback:

Form criteria:
- The lesson is appropriate for sixth-grade boys and girls (eleven and twelve years old).
- The lesson lasts about thirty to forty minutes.
- The lesson is highly informative: It communicates information essential to the purpose of the task.
- The lesson is interesting and engaging: It involves learners directly through hands-on activity.
- The lesson provides learners with specific real-world examples to support learning.

Content criteria:
- The lesson addresses the issue of clothing selection for backcountry travel using accurate information.
- The lesson integrates concepts of theory (thermal regulation) with examples of practice (specific choices of clothing) so that learners understand both "what" to wear and "why" it is important to wear it.

Knowledge:
- Participants can describe the broad concept of thermal regulation and the major considerations for selecting a backcountry clothing system.
- Participants can adequately respond to questions that challenge or further explore their recommendations.

Skill: Teaching and transference: brainstorms/distills ideas or options to consider
- Participants use a formal brainstorm/distillation process to consider different ways of making the lesson engaging to sixth-graders.

*Developed by Leading EDGE, LLC for **The Backcountry Classroom**. For more information log on to www.realworldlearning.info.*

Product Quality Checklist

Date: _____   Class Period: _____

Product Author(s):	Product Title/Name:	Evaluator Name(s):
	Selecting Clothing for Backcountry Travel	

Observed	Standard/Criteria	Possible Points	Rating
	The lesson is appropriate for sixth-grade boys and girls (eleven and twelve years old).		
	The lesson lasts about thirty to forty minutes.		
	The lesson is highly informative: It communicates information essential to the purpose of the task.		
	The lesson is interesting and engaging: It involves learners directly through hands-on activity.		
	The lesson provides learners with specific real-world examples to support learning.		
	The lesson addresses the issue of clothing selection for back-country travel using accurate information.		
	The lesson integrates concepts of theory (thermal regulation) with examples of practice (specific choices of clothing) so that learners understand both "what" to wear and "why" it is important to wear it.		
	Total		

Observations:

Elements of Questionable Quality:	**Elements of Exceptional Quality:**

CHAPTER EIGHT

Collaboration: How We Approach Teamwork

Most people have a distinct and dominant approach to working in groups, and that in turn impacts their decision making, leadership, and interaction with others. Just as some of us are left-handed and some are right-handed, we have a dominant or preferred collaborative tendency, which is our natural predilection when working with others. The understanding and recognition of our own dominant approach and that of those we interact with will help us collaborate effectively, understand group dynamics, maximize learning experiences, and become better leaders and decision makers.

I. Outcomes

A. Outdoor leaders provide evidence of their *knowledge* and *understanding* by:

1. Describing the four distinct approaches to collaborative work
2. Describing the contributions of each approach to collaborative work
3. Describing the downsides of each approach to collaborative work
4. Describing how to communicate in the language of each approach to collaborative work
5. Describing the implications of each approach to collaborative work for debriefing, assessing, planning lessons, and expedition behavior
6. Describing the link between each approach to collaborative work and leadership
7. Describing how conflict and pain are inherent to collaborative work

B. Outdoor leaders provide evidence of their *skill* by:

1. Recognizing the characteristics of each approach to collaborative work
2. Communicating effectively in the language of each approach to collaborative work
3. Debriefing and assessing from the perspective of each approach to collaborative work
4. Planning and delivering lessons that reflect an understanding of each approach to collaborative work
5. Using the IP3 to create a Full Value Contract
6. Analyzing and addressing group conflict through the lens of each approach to collaborative work

C. Outdoor leaders provide evidence of their *dispositions* by:

1. Modeling empathy and appreciation for the contributions of each approach to collaborative work
2. Modeling patience, tolerance, acceptance, and, ultimately, support of individuals with different approaches to collaborative work
3. Modeling awareness of the dynamics of group conflict as it relates to approaches to collaborative work
4. Recognizing that diversity includes differences of opinion, philosophy, style, and personality, and not just culture, ethnicity, and religion

II. Content

A. The four collaborative tendencies (see fig. 8.1)

1. Ideas: "Ideas" group members see the big picture and are frequently visionary and creative. "Ideas" group members want to know what the possibilities are, and their favorite question is, "What if?" They need flexibility and dislike rigidity.

   a) How "ideas" group members contribute to collaborative work:
   - (1) They are visionary.
   - (2) They are risk takers.
   - (3) They are flexible and comfortable with chaos.
   - (4) They operate intuitively.
   - (5) In the extreme, their greatest strength is their ability to come up with visionary and creative ideas.

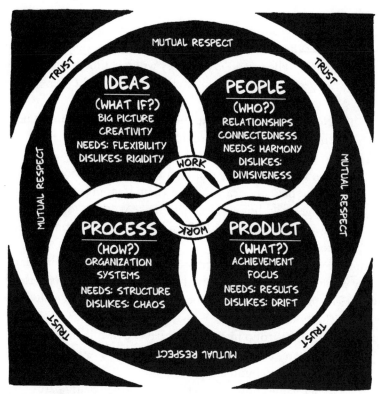

FIGURE 8.1. The four collaborative tendencies

b) How "ideas" group members sometimes hinder collaborative work:
   (1) They sometimes don't follow the rules.
   (2) They frequently struggle to focus on just one idea and follow
       through on it. As a result, they may look unorganized or inconsis-
       tent.
   (3) They are not too concerned with details and frequently struggle to
       work with people who are.
   (4) They need their ideas validated by others.
   (5) They can be perceived as impulsive and unrealistic.
   (6) They tend to be impulsive and dramatic.
   (7) In the extreme, their greatest weakness is their tendency to be an
       "arsonist"; i.e., they go around planting ideas (starting fires)
       but not following through and frequently not allowing others to
       follow through, thus preventing problem solving or task accom-
       plishment.

c) How "ideas" group members communicate:
   (1) Yes: When "ideas" group members say yes, they actually mean maybe. The reason is that they will most likely come up with a new idea, one they think is better, shortly after they have okayed the existing idea or project.
   (2) No: When "ideas" group members say no, they mean no because they already have a better idea in mind.
d) How to communicate with "ideas" group members:
   (1) Ask them what they think and ask for their ideas.
   (2) If you have an idea you want them to approve, try to get them to come up with it and let them make it "their" decision.
   (3) Avoid disagreeing with them if possible. They tend to need people to support their ideas.
2. People: "People" group members value people and focus on relationships. They want to know *who* is involved in the decision and *whom* the decision will affect. "People" group members crave harmony and dislike divisiveness and conflict.
   a) How "people" group members contribute to collaborative work:
      (1) They are sensitive to people's feelings.
      (2) They like to build community.
      (3) They value cooperative efforts and enjoy being part of a team.
      (4) They bring a sense of inclusiveness to a group.
      (5) In the extreme, their greatest strength is caring about people.
   b) How "people" group members sometimes hinder collaborative work:
      (1) They sometimes appear wishy-washy because others don't know where they stand.
      (2) They don't want to offend people, and as a result they don't always share their true feelings.
      (3) They don't like hard and fast rules that can divide people.
      (4) They tend to be slow to react until they have checked everyone else's opinion.
      (5) They avoid risk taking and tend to avoid pressure situations.
      (6) In the extreme, their greatest weakness is their tendency to be a "soaped fish"; i.e., no one can get a handle on them and see where they stand.
   c) How "people" group members communicate:
      (1) Yes: When "people" group members say yes, they usually mean maybe. They don't want to commit to something until they have checked with others.

(2) No: When "people" group members say no, they also mean maybe for the same reason. They don't want to commit to a decision until they have checked with others.

d) How to communicate with "people" group members:
(1) Let the person know who already supports your idea or plan.
(2) Speak in terms of consensus building regarding your task.

3. Product: "Product" group members value achievement, focus, and quality. "Product" group members want to know *what* needs to be done. They need results and dislike drift or indecisiveness.

a) How "product" group members contribute to collaborative work:
(1) They value performance and producing a quality product.
(2) They are committed to getting the job done.
(3) They take pride in being task-oriented and getting many things accomplished.
(4) They value expert knowledge.
(5) In the extreme, their greatest strength is getting high-quality results.

b) How "product" group members sometimes hinder collaborative work:
(1) They are often stubborn and tend to work alone and do things their way.
(2) They tend to hate meetings and would rather just get on with the job.
(3) They can be authoritative.
(4) They tend to see one "right" answer and don't like to "waste" time exploring creative alternatives.
(5) They are considered insensitive because they worry more about getting the job done correctly than people's feelings.
(6) They can be too rigid and defeated by their own perfectionism.
(7) In the extreme, their greatest weakness is their tendency to be a "Lone Ranger" workaholic. Since they believe they have the best solution and can do the best job, they tend to want to do it all.

c) How "product" group members communicate:
(1) Yes: When "product" group members say yes, they mean yes. They are very literal and have difficulty understanding why others aren't.
(2) No: When "product" group members say no, they mean no for the same reason as explained above.

d) How to communicate with "product" group members:
(1) Speak in clear terms of the task or "problem to solve."
(2) Propose clear solutions that can be approved and implemented.
(3) Be clear, be succinct, and don't waste time.

4. Process: "Process" group members value procedure. They want to know *how* something is going to be done. They need structure and dislike chaos.

    a) How "process" group members contribute to collaborative work:

        (1) They usually are well organized and self-disciplined.

        (2) They attend to details and get things running smoothly.

        (3) They are practical and direct.

        (4) In the extreme, their greatest strength is bringing order out of chaos.

    b) How "process" group members sometimes hinder collaborative work:

        (1) They don't like surprises or changes to plans.

        (2) They generally are not tolerant of "rule breakers."

        (3) They tend to be insensitive to people and allow rules to be more important than people.

        (4) They sometimes appear inflexible.

        (5) They are reality-oriented and can be impatient with those who are considered to have their "heads in the clouds."

        (6) In the extreme, their greatest weakness is the tendency to become a "bean counter," where details become more important than the overall goal.

    c) How "process" group members communicate:

        (1) Yes: When "process" group members say yes, they mean yes. They are satisfied that rules have been followed, criteria met, and individuals have worked within the system.

        (2) No: When "process" group members say no, they mean maybe. If the rules are followed and if the criteria are met and if you work within the system, you can change a no to a yes.

    d) How to communicate with "process" group members:

        (1) Make an appointment and be on time.

        (2) Talk of solving problems and accomplishing tasks within the existing system.

        (3) Allow time for the person to reflect and process your proposal.

        (4) Have a clear plan.

B. Conflict, discomfort, and pain inherent to collaborative work

1. The four collaborative tendencies naturally create conflict and pain. When the needs of one person are being met, then others are in pain. It is virtually impossible to meet everyone's needs at the same time.

2. Conflict: As the four types of collaborative tendencies work together, their differences are amplified and conflict results. Conflict is not bad; in fact, it

actually appears to be essential if groups are to work to their highest potential.

3. Trust and mutual respect: Appreciation of and respect for the collaborative tendencies of others creates an atmosphere of mutual respect. Over time, mutual respect builds trust and a willingness to put up with the pain inherent in collaborative work, knowing that, at some point in the process, everyone's needs are going to be met.

4. Collaboration versus cooperation: Collaboration is a higher level of cooperation. Cooperation is the ability to work together for a common goal. In cooperation there is an understanding and willingness to tolerate the pain of group work. In collaboration there is not only an understanding and willingness to tolerate the pain, but there is a recognition and celebration of the diversity necessary for the highest levels of collaborative work. In other words, in cooperation there is a tolerance of people's differences, but in collaboration there is a celebration of differences.

C. The link between collaborative tendencies and leadership, group dynamics, lesson planning, and debriefing

1. Leadership

   a) Understanding your own collaborative tendency allows you to realize Paul Petzoldt's axiom, "Know what you know and know what you don't know." As usual, Paul was ahead of his time. This concept is now called "metacognition" or "thinking about thinking." This allows you to clarify your own areas of strength and weakness.

   b) Understanding group members' collaborative tendencies allows you to gauge your group's strengths and weaknesses. It will ultimately assist you in decision making because you will have better knowledge of your group.

2. Group dynamics/expedition behavior

   a) Group development and conflict: Understanding these tendencies allows group members to better understand conflict and its role in group development (see chapter 23, Group Development). Participants will be better prepared to anticipate where conflict will come from. It will not eliminate the "storming" stage of group development, but it will permit leaders to understand it and strive to create an atmosphere that celebrates diversity and breeds mutual respect and trust.

   b) Creating a Full Value Contract: Understanding collaborative tendencies can help create a Full Value Contract. Using the IP3 planning tool (see table 8.1, as well as a sample Full Value Contract in table 8.2), you can

Table 8.1. THE IP3 PLANNING TOOL

Group members: Project Name/Date:

IP3 PLANNING
COLLABORATION

DIRECTIONS: Please consider past challenges as opportunities to learn about effective collaboration. Based on these experiences, please respond to each of the following questions as you plan for this upcoming collaborative effort.

IDEAS	PEOPLE
What will you do to ensure that all ideas are heard and considered?	What will you do to invite all group members to participate actively and feel valued?

PROCESS	PRODUCT
What will you do to ensure that your group is well organized and that you use available resources efficiently?	What will you do to ensure that your final product is of the highest quality given the resources available?

Table 8.2. SAMPLE FULL VALUE CONTRACT USING THE IP3 PLANNING TOOL

Group members: Project Name/Date:

IP3 PLANNING
COLLABORATION

DIRECTIONS: Please consider past challenges as opportunities to learn about effective collaboration. Based on these experiences, please respond to each of the following questions as you plan for this upcoming collaborative effort.

IDEAS	PEOPLE
What will you do to ensure that all ideas are heard and considered?	**What will you do to invite all group members to participate actively and feel valued?**
• Whenever we have to gather ideas, we will use the brainstorm rules, and we will sweep around at least twice to make sure everyone has an opportunity for input. • We will strive to make sure only one person speaks at a time, and the rest will be active listeners; i.e., we will have eye contact and appropriate body language toward the speaker. • We will keep an open mind to others' ideas.	• We will respect the need for and give one another personal space and privacy as needed. • We will use "I" messages and provide feedback on ideas and actions, but not pass judgment on people. • We will use "check-ins" to see how people are doing. • We will speak only for ourselves and not for others. • We will treat everyone with respect even when we don't agree with their ideas or behaviors. • We will not use "put-downs."

PROCESS	PRODUCT
What will you do to ensure that your group is well organized and that you use available resources efficiently?	**What will you do to ensure that your final product is of the highest quality given the resources available?**
• We will be prepared for and on time for all group gatherings. • We will strive to keep our personal gear organized and in good working order. • We will use organization tools like timelines to help us be efficient. • We will use task roles like scout, logger, and sweep to help us be more efficient (see chapter 43). • We will pledge to participate in all activities or explain why we don't want to. • We will set clear and achievable goals. • Whatever rules we create by consensus, we agree to follow.	• We will be willing to receive and give open and honest feedback in an appropriate manner. • We will do what we promise/commit to do. • We will establish clear criteria to measure our success. • We will support what is "right" over what is popular. • We will put aside differences in order to get the job done well.

Table 8.3. THE IP3 DEBRIEFING TOOL

Group members: Project Name/Date:

IP3 DEBRIEFING
COLLABORATION

DIRECTIONS: Please consider the quality of your collaboration in the challenge just completed. Please respond to each of the following questions.

IDEAS	PEOPLE
Were all ideas heard and considered?	Were all group members invited to partici-pate and valued when they did so?
What might you/we do differently next time?	What might you/we do differently next time?

PROCESS	PRODUCT
Was your group well organized, and did it use available resources efficiently?	Was your final product of the highest quality possible given the resources available?
What might you/we do differently next time?	What might you/we do differently next time?

have the course participants brainstorm each of the four IP3 planning questions (see chapter 10, Decision Making, for more on brainstorming) and distill them down to a Full Value Contract. It is important that the criteria are clear, unambiguous, and observable.

    c) Planning collaborative work: The IP3 planning tool can also be used for planning any activity that requires the group to carefully consider their process.

3. Lesson planning: Knowledge and understanding of collaborative approaches is invaluable in planning learning experiences. The challenge is for the instructor to be able to explicitly describe how the lesson will meet the needs of those with each type of collaborative tendency.

4. Debriefing: The IP3 debriefing tool (table 8.3) is an excellent tool to explore how the group feels and gives team members ideas on how to improve. It can be used in a large group setting but is often more effective when it is used as follows:

    a) Ask group members to respond individually to the two questions in each quadrant. Encourage them to find a quiet spot to reflect on how they want to respond and then write out their responses.

        (1) Ask them not to put their names on the tool.

        (2) Let them know that the tools will be shared anonymously with other group members.

    b) After all the participants have completed the eight questions, have the participants form groups of three or four people each.

    c) Give each person in the small groups one of the completed tools, making sure they don't have any of the tools filled out by their own small groups' members.

    d) Ask them to reflect on the responses on the tool and compare the responses with how *they* felt about the questions.

    e) Have the small groups report out, totaling the numbers of "yes" responses and "no" responses and what they thought they needed to do next time to improve.

    f) Next time you have a group activity, start it by reminding the group what it wanted to do differently to be better than they were previously.

D. Cautions and reminders about collaborative tendencies

1. Don't pigeonhole people. We all use some of each approach to collaboration.

2. Don't use this information as a crutch. We all have to learn to stretch.

3. Stretch during practice and play to your strengths at crunch time.

4. High-functioning teams need representatives who use each of the collaborative approaches. Understand the difference between cooperation and collaboration.

5. Conflict is an essential ingredient when producing the highest quality product possible, but it is only valuable in an atmosphere of mutual respect and trust.

6. Learn to celebrate people who are strong in quadrants other than yours rather than complain about them.

7. To *empower*, make decisions by consensus. For *quality*, implement decisions autocratically.

8. Use sarcasm with great caution. It is very destructive and can frequently bring harm to the sense of community within a group.

III. Instructional Strategies

A. Timing. This activity is ideally taught before the participants go out into the field. On the other hand, if it is taught after students have experienced the challenges of working together it helps explain why their collaboration is so challenging. In either event it will help them understand expedition behavior and group dynamics better and will assist participants when they prepare learning experiences.

B. Considerations

1. It is very important to remind and reinforce the cautions and reminders about collaborative tendencies (see II. D.) in order to avoid stereotyping and utilizing this information inappropriately.

2. This information needs to be reinforced on a regular basis. Using the Collaboration challenge (see the end of the chapter) is one way to do this.

C. Activities. See the Collaboration challenge at the end of the chapter.

D. Materials. Understanding Collaboration—Collaboration Profile Questionnaire (optional; available from Leading EDGE, www.realworldlearning.info).

Challenge

Knowledge Outcome	Title	Skill/Disposition Outcome
What do you want them to know?		**What skill/disposition do you want them to develop?**
The participants can describe/depict the characteristics of various approaches to collaboration and discuss the implications of each.	Collaboration	Decision making: draws conclusions from available information

Essential Question or Key Issue:

How does each of the four approaches to collaboration contribute to the successful solution of a complex problem?

Description of Challenge/Task/Performance:

With the assistance of your teacher/instructor, brainstorm a list of common problem-solving situations encountered on a typical backcountry trip. Each of these problems should require the collaboration of three or four people to solve (e.g., hanging a food bag, crossing a stream, setting up a rain fly, route finding on an off-trail hike, etc.). Create small teams. Each of the teams should select (or draw randomly) a different backcountry problem to solve through a role play.

Review the positive attributes of each of the four approaches to collaboration. Create a role play that illustrates how the four different approaches to collaboration, working together, contribute positively to the solution of the selected problem chosen by your team.

At the conclusion of your role play, please lead a short discussion of how the role play actually illustrated the contributions of each approach to collaborative process.

Criteria for Assessment and Feedback:

Form criteria:
- The role play has a story to tell. The plot line is obvious as it relates to the problem being solved.
- Actors portray their characters convincingly.
- The actors stay in character throughout the skit.

Content criteria:
- The role play depicts a common problem typically faced on a backcountry expedition.
- The positive attributes/contributions of each approach to collaboration are apparent in the solution of the problem.

Knowledge:
- Participants can describe/depict the characteristics of various approaches to collaboration and discuss the implications of each.
- Participants can accurately discuss the characteristics and implications of each approach to collaboration depicted in the role play.

Skill: Decision making: draws conclusions from available information
- During preparation for the role play, each participant accurately describes some specific way each of the approaches to collaboration contributes to problem solving.

Developed by Leading EDGE, LLC for **The Backcountry Classroom.** *For more information log on to www.realworldlearning.info.*

Product Quality Checklist

Date: _____   Class Period: _____

| Product Author(s): | Product Title/Name:

Collaboration | Evaluator Name(s): |
|---|---|---|

Observed	Standard/Criteria	Possible Points	Rating
	The role play has a story to tell. The plot line is obvious as it relates to the problem being solved.		
	Actors portray their characters convincingly.		
	The actors stay in character throughout the skit.		
	The role play depicts a common problem typically faced on a backcountry expedition.		
	The positive attributes/contributions of each approach to collaboration are apparent in the solution of the problem.		
	Total		

Observations:

Elements of Questionable Quality:

Elements of Exceptional Quality:

CHAPTER NINE

Crisis Management in the Backcountry

Emotional crises occur in wilderness settings when a participant's usual strategies to cope with stress are ineffective. An understanding of crisis management and acquisition of the basic skills to deal with a variety of behavioral and emotional crises is essential for today's wilderness leaders. When leaders have these skills, potentially disruptive situations can be minimized. This chapter is designed to provide an overview of some of the tools necessary to empower leaders to deal with these crises, but in no way is the information provided here an adequate substitute for the specialized training required, and often provided, by wilderness therapy programs.

I. Outcomes

A. Outdoor leaders provide evidence of their *knowledge* and *understanding* by:

1. Defining an emotional crisis and identifying behaviors that are likely to be evident during a typical crisis found in wilderness settings
2. Describing the Wilderness Risk Managers Committee (WRMC) criteria for charting a crisis
3. Describing the five-step model of crisis intervention
4. Describing nonviolent crisis intervention and appropriate intervention strategies
5. Describing the difference between, and when to utilize, defusings and debriefings

B. Outdoor leaders provide evidence of their *skill* by:

1. Assessing when a crisis has occurred
2. Eliciting feelings from people in crisis
3. Brainstorming solutions with people in crisis

4. Intervening, without escalating, when people are verbally or physically threatening
5. Conducting a defusing

C. Outdoor leaders provide evidence of their *dispositions* by:

1. Establishing a positive relationship built on trust with participants who are upset
2. Providing the support needed for people in crisis to restabilize
3. Responding with firm, enforceable limits to aggressive participants
4. Dealing with emotional as well as physical aspects of unanticipated events
5. Using good judgment when calling for backup or deciding to evacuate a participant who is in crisis

II. Content

A. Overview. Crisis management is designed to prevent a crisis or minimize its impact. Crisis intervention is used during a crisis. Nonviolent interventions are used to de-escalate crises from becoming violent. If many individuals are affected and the situation has been a traumatic one, defusings and debriefings are frequently needed to help groups cope with the aftermath of traumatic events.

B. Important terms and definitions

1. Crisis management is designed to prevent or minimize the effects of a critical incident. It aims to help individuals work through their problems, or, at the very least, to keep their disruptive and destructive tendencies from affecting others. Crisis intervention is used when individuals are experiencing inner turmoil, such as debilitating anxiety or depression.
2. Nonviolent interventions are used to de-escalate crises before verbal or physical violence can occur.
3. Defusings and debriefings are techniques to manage traumatic stress on a preventative basis.

C. Defining crises

1. Crises are narrow moments in time when a person is not able to cope effectively. Crises are sudden and short in duration and may trigger unacceptable behavior (in that it compromises individual or group values or goals) that may endanger self or others. The person in crisis experiences anxiety,

fear, panic, or a host of other potentially debilitating emotions (disequilibrium). Crises that may lead to a state of emotional turmoil occur in all types of wilderness programs where people experience high levels of stress. Crises are both normal and expected and can be experienced by anyone whose usual ways of coping with stress are unsuccessful.

Example: A student on a thirty-day course receives feedback during a debriefing that her peers are not happy with her behavior. They feel she hasn't done her share of work, and what work she has done has been done poorly. They accuse her of not living by the Full Value Contract they had all agreed to at the beginning of the trip (see chapter 8). Instead of accepting the feedback, she blows up and starts screaming, "I hate the Full Value Contract! I hate all of you, and I wish I had never come on this course!"

2. At the extreme, some people experience Acute Stress Disorders (ASD) (American Psychiatric Association 1994), the symptoms of which include:
   a) Exposure to a situation in which there has been death or serious injury in which the person experienced intense fear, helplessness, or horror
   b) Experiencing at least three of the following symptoms:
      (1) The feeling that the situation is not real (derealization)
      (2) The feeling that you are distant and removed from your feelings (depersonalization)
      (3) Amnesia
      (4) Flat or constricted range of emotions
      (5) A dazed feeling
   c) Anxiety or increased excitement
   d) Avoidance of stimuli that triggered the event
   e) Reexperiencing the event over a few days or longer
   f) Experiencing disruption in areas of life functioning

      Example: On an expedition up Mount McKinley, one of the group members unropes in camp, takes two steps, and falls 120 feet through a small snow bridge to his death. His tent partner reacts by experiencing restless sleep and nightmares, and he has a hard time taking care of routine responsibilities. With a blank expression on his face, he says that he still can't believe what happened, and he expresses a desire to leave the expedition immediately.

3. When Acute Stress Disorder lasts more than six months, it becomes Post-Traumatic Stress Disorder (PTSD) (American Psychiatric Association 1994). Participants may experience the symptoms listed above, which were caused by a previous traumatization but are triggered by circumstances in the field. ASD and PTSD require *professional mental-health care*.

4. A final framework for defining a crisis incident is suggested by the WRMC. While some of the criteria for reporting incidents are limited to physical problems, most are applicable to emotional or behavioral events. The criteria for reporting incidents appear to be sufficiently broad to cover a variety of mental-health incidents. A reportable crisis incident involves one or more of the following, and:

  a) Requires more than cursory staff attention
  b) Requires follow-up care by staff in the field
  c) Interferes with participation
  d) Requires evacuation
  e) Is a lost-day case; i.e., when one participant cannot partake in planned activities for one day

D. Crisis intervention steps

  1. This model is useful for helping individuals who are experiencing an inner state of turmoil. Examples may include debilitating anxiety or withdrawal and/or depression. The following is a five-step model designed to resolve the state of disequilibrium (Dixon 1979).

  a) First, the leader must quickly try to establish a positive, trusting relationship with the person in crisis. This kind of initiative requires confidence, assertion, and experience on the part of the leader.

  b) The leader should try to get the person to express and ventilate his or her emotions by using such techniques as listening with empathy, accepting without judgment, asking open-ended questions, and clarifying feelings.

    (1) Although this process may be frightening for some leaders, it is essential to the resolution of the crisis.

    (2) The leader should separate the person in crisis from the group and listen to and support the person in crisis—for as long as it takes.

  c) If the person begins to return to a normal emotional state after being given the opportunity to share and vent his or her feelings, the leader should then try to facilitate a discussion identifying the cause of the crisis.

    (1) The leader must be active and in control, yet let the participant explore and describe his/her immediate perception of the cause of the crisis.

    (2) The leader must remember that people's perception of events is unique and that passing judgment should be avoided.

    (3) One of the worst things that a leader can do is to imply that the event was really not that serious, or that it was not truly the cause

of the crisis. Doing so can trigger a variety of responses, including causing the person to close down and withdraw.

   d) The leader should next attempt to help the participant move from venting feelings to making sense of the event and his or her crisis reaction.

   e) Finally, the leader must, after the person is out of immediate crisis, decide on how to bring the person back into the group or elect to evacuate the person.

      (1) The leader must determine if the person is a threat to self or others, is emotionally unstable, or is otherwise unable to continue with the trip.

      (2) There are benefits to having the person continue, as long as the person and/or the group is not at further risk. If there is a risk of physical or emotional harm, evacuation is necessary.

E. Nonviolent intervention

1. Individuals in crisis may need a leader's immediate attention and response. However, crises do not manifest themselves independently; rather, they are often the defining moment in a series of occurrences that lead to harmful behavior.

   a) A model developed by the Crisis Prevention Institute (CPI) (Caraulia and Steiger 1997) provides an understanding about intervening in crises before they reach the level of verbal or physical violence. This model considers anxiety, disruptive behavior, and harmful behavior.

   b) Anxiety

      (1) Anxiety and apprehension are likely to occur anytime one enters a new situation. In order to cope, familiar responses and behavior patterns are often used. However, when multiple stressors occur, a potentially explosive situation is at hand.

      (2) Anxiety is often manifested by a change in nonverbal behavior. In order to respond to this, a leader must recognize and respond in a supportive manner. A leader should:

         (a) Recognize that an anxious person requires personal space. In times of crisis, the need for such space may dramatically increase.

         (b) Reinforce supportive statements with body language.

         (c) Pay attention to tone, volume, and rate of speech to both alleviate anxiety and communicate meaning effectively.

      (3) As anxiety increases, humans are less responsive to words and respond more to the tone, volume, and rate of speech.

(4) Intervention in a crisis is safest at the anxiety stage; unfortunately, it is also the most difficult stage at which to intervene.

(5) Example: It is the first day of the course, and activity is very hectic as participants are being issued equipment, having their clothing checked, and meeting new people. Chris is very anxious about the day and struggling to maintain composure with all that is going on. Group members are given an hour to get lunch and told to return promptly at 1:00 P.M. to finish packing the expedition rations. Chris returns ten minutes late and receives a stern rebuke from one of the course instructors. Chris's anxiety peaks, and he decides to withdraw from the course and go home.

c) Disruptive behavior

(1) When a participant's anxiety is not dealt with appropriately, there is a tendency for negative behavior to escalate.

(2) This phase is characterized by increasing noncompliance, hostility, and belligerence, with volatility increasing and rational thought diminishing.

(3) A continuum of verbal escalation occurs at this point, elements of which include:

(a) Questioning the leader's authority to set boundaries

(b) Noncompliance with behavioral directives

(c) Irrational verbal release

(d) Verbal threats toward others

(e) Release of tension following outbursts

(4) Leader's response:

(a) The leader should attempt to help the participants regain composure and also empower them to help themselves.

(b) This is often most effectively accomplished by:

i) Setting clear limits (it is most helpful to try to set limits at the start of the trip before events occur)

ii) Explaining and discussing inappropriate behaviors

iii) Allowing simple choices

iv) Enforcing consequences for inappropriate behaviors

(5) Example: For a few days, tensions have been building among a group of four participants who have not been convinced that the course leadership goals are valid, and they question the entire model of outdoor leadership that the course is based on. It finally comes to a head when they confront the instructor, belligerently

stating, "Who are you to say what leadership is? You can't tell us what to do!"

d) Harmful behavior

    (1) If the crisis situation escalates through the anxiety and disruptive behavior phases, a leader must prepare to deal with a person exhibiting physically harmful behaviors. This requires the use of extremely careful judgment.

    (2) Physical restraint

        (a) Intervening with physical restraint is only used to keep the person and others safe.

        (b) The decision to use restraint can sometimes be anticipated, but it must always be made with great care.

        (c) It is only a temporary measure until the person can regain control.

        (d) Using physical restraint requires specialized training to insure that it is safely used. Wilderness therapy programs usually offer this training, although more often than not only for their own staff. It is important to know the policies and procedures of your employer or potential employer.

    (3) Example: A group of "youth-at-risk" boys on a two-week wilderness trip is having a rest day in a remote wilderness area. The boys are doing laundry and other personal maintenance tasks. Sammy has hung his laundry out to dry by the nearby pond. Juan starts splashing water on the nearly dry clothing. Sammy loses it and starts chasing Juan while both verbally and physically threatening him with a large stick. It appears that he is serious. The staff restrains Sammy for about five minutes until he appears to calm down. When they let him up, he goes after Juan again. They restrain him again, this time for about fifteen minutes, until he finally calms down and becomes more rational.

F. Defusings and debriefings

1. Victims of, or even witnesses to, serious injury or threat to physical integrity are at risk for Acute Stress Disorder (ASD) and Post-Traumatic Stress Disorder (PTSD).

2. Two techniques, Traumatic Stress Defusing ("defusing") and Critical Incident Stress Debriefing (CISD, or "debriefing"), were developed as techniques to manage traumatic stress on a preventative basis (Mitchell and

Everly 1995). Debriefings and defusings may be required when there are incidents that harm or threaten the welfare of participants and which cause an emotional impact that outstrips participants' ability to cope. The efficacy of these techniques has recently been questioned, but they remain the standard for post-traumatic care.

a) Defusings

    (1) What are defusings?

        (a) Defusings are sessions that occur sooner than debriefings (less than eight hours after an incident), do not delve into the emotional issues with as much depth, are less structured, and are aimed at smaller groups.

        (b) Defusings often are conducted in twenty to forty-five minutes. Defusings follow three steps: introduction, exploration, and information.

        (c) Defusings can be conducted by peer support personnel, mental-health professionals, or a combination of the two.

        (d) Individual counseling or other follow-up services may be indicated for some participants.

    (2) When to use defusings:

        (a) Defusings can often replace debriefings.

        (b) Defusings are the technique of choice in most situations due to the fact that most adventure-education activities involve small numbers of participants.

        (c) Defusings can occur within a few hours of the incident and when staff training requirements are less than for debriefings. Defusings can occur in the field.

b) Debriefings

    (1) What are debriefings?

        (a) A debriefing, used in the current context, is a meeting or discussion, employing a group format, that uses education and crisis intervention to relieve or resolve psychological distress that is the result of a critical and traumatic event (Mitchell and Everly 1995).

        (b) Debriefings are a formal, technical group process that should not be confused with the more common use of the term "debriefing" to connote a more informal discussion of events as they relate to experiential education participation.

        (c) Debriefings involve a mental-health professional and a

few peers of those affected. (All CISD personnel should be specifically trained to utilize this model. "Mental-health professionals" are defined as those with at least a master's degree.) It takes place days after an event, and its intent is to minimize PTSD.

(2) When to use debriefings:

   (a) Debriefings are the method of choice when defusings are ineffective, when the group size is too large, or when there is a delay in the ability to provide services to the group.

   (b) In order to provide such debriefings, it is necessary to have a mobilization team to convene with victims when traumas occur.

   (c) Debriefings employ a seven-step model that includes the following steps, included here to give outdoor leaders an overview of the process:

      i) Introduction: This phase introduces team members, explains the purpose and process of the meeting, and tries to put participants in a good frame of mind to go through the process.

      ii) Fact: During this step, the facts of the situation are established from multiple points of view.

      iii) Thoughts: This is a transition phase to help participants move toward their emotional responses.

      iv) Reaction: Often the most powerful phase; when participants talk about the worst parts of the situation.

      v) Symptoms: The participants are asked about their symptoms, and the focus turns more toward cognition.

      vi) Teaching: During this phase, symptoms are discussed, as are ways of coping with them.

      vii) Reentry: Here, participants are prepared to reenter the outside world. Some participants may need individual counseling.

III. Instructional Strategies

A. Timing. This is an advanced topic for mature and capable learners. Special thought needs to be given as to whether the group is ready for this information and where and when it might be taught.

B. Activities. Role plays are good ways to simulate crises in the field. The following short vignettes provide enough background information and are conducive to using crisis management, nonviolent intervention, and defusings.

1. Scenario 1: After three days of rain on a backpacking trip, Tom can be heard talking with other participants about his desire to leave the trip if it doesn't stop raining soon. As the leader, how might you intervene? Pick someone to play Tom, someone to be the leader, and others to be the other group members.

2. Scenario 2: Suzy continues to fall behind the other participants, and as the day goes on, she has become increasingly more sullen and withdrawn. What, if anything, do you say or do? Pick someone to be Suzy and someone to be the leader.

3. Scenario 3: Two teenagers in an adventure program have been arguing about cooking the evening meal. As you approach them, you hear verbal threats and gestures. How do you intervene? Why did you choose this strategy?

CHAPTER TEN

Decision Making

In order to give the subject of decision making the attention it deserves, we have divided this chapter into two parts: An Introduction to Decision Making and A Process for Making Decisions. We have provided one set of overarching outcomes for the two parts and two scenarios, Decision at High Mountain and Adventure of Hair Worm Pass. The Hair Worm Pass scenario is designed to be used with part 1 of the chapter and is intended to provide an opportunity to practice recognizing decisions, "defining the problem" in decision making, and understanding the range of complexity in decisions. We suggest that you read the Decision at High Mountain scenario before you use part 2 of this chapter as the scenario is referenced throughout it. We explain how to use the scenarios in the Instructional Strategies section.

I. Outcomes

A. Outdoor leaders provide evidence of their *knowledge* and *understanding* by:

1. Describing the steps in a decision-making process
2. Describing the role decision making plays in leadership training
3. Describing the transferability of decision making to nonwilderness settings
4. Explaining the roles emotion, preference, prejudice, intuition, and personal style play in decision making
5. Comparing the different kinds of decisions and their characteristics, ranging from "simple" to "complex"
6. Critiquing the decisions made by themselves and others

B. Outdoor leaders provide evidence of their *skill* by:

1. Implementing the steps in a decision-making process
2. Making, implementing, and evaluating decisions
3. Articulating a rationale for their decisions

4. Consistently making quality decisions

5. Using various decision-making tools and strategies appropriately

C. Outdoor leaders provide evidence of their *dispositions* by:

1. Ritualizing and modeling the decision-making process

2. Putting the group's needs above their own interests when making decisions

3. Making the ethically right decision versus making the easy or popular decision

4. Supporting a group decision that conflicts with their own personal opinion in appropriate instances

II. Content

Part 1. An Introduction to Decision Making

A. Variability in decision making

1. All decision-making situations are not created equal.

   a) Every decision-making situation comes with its own set of circumstances and variables that make it unique. No matter how often a typical decision-making situation arises, some variable has changed since the last time it was encountered. If nothing else, the variable of time has changed. It is important that decision makers recognize this variability and take it into account when making or evaluating decisions.

   b) Decision-making situations range in complexity. Some decisions are very simple and easily made. Other decisions are exceedingly complex and difficult. Every decision lies somewhere along an imaginary continuum that ranges from simple to complex. Knowing the characteristics that distinguish a simple from a complex decision can be helpful in developing strategies for responding effectively to different decision-making situations.

2. Characteristics that help determine whether a decision is simple or complex (see table 10.1).

   a) Let's take a look at two typical wilderness decision-making scenarios, one being simple and the other complex. We will use these scenarios to demonstrate various points in decision making. The scenes take place in

Adventure of Hair Worm Pass

It was a beautiful fall day in the Northeast. The leaf colors were near their peak, and the temperature looked like it would reach a high in the mid-sixties yet might produce a frost some morning very soon. The days were getting noticeably shorter, but that was only a minor consideration for outdoor leaders Glenn and Naheed as they reached the halfway point in the twenty-eight-day wilderness training they were instructing. The students had learned a lot during the two weeks they had been living and traveling outdoors, and at this point they were fairly competent campers. They could camp and canoe with relative ease, although they had a lot to learn to master their navigation skills. They had just begun to backpack, so they were learning a lot as they worked their way across the 210,000-acre Cold River Wilderness Area. After dropping off their canoes, they had a short hike up the Calkins Brook horse trail to an undeveloped campsite on the northern side of the small brook near the 2,200-foot benchmark. They planned a two-day layover there in order to practice their map and compass skills, taking a short off-trail hike tomorrow, and, if all went well, doing an ambitious hike up Tahawus Peak on the next day. After debriefing the events of the day that evening, small groups of students got together to plan tomorrow's day hike.

The students were to hike up the trail to the intersection with the Trout Brook Trail (horses were allowed on the Trout Brook Trail, but not on the trail going up Tahawus Peak), then hike down the Trout Brook Trail an appropriate distance until they could follow the outlet of String Bean Pond. From there they were to hike back to the Calkins Brook horse trail and then back up to their camp. Two teams of five students each planned their route and wrote up their Time Control Plans. Both teams had a first-aid kit and packed extra clothing, rain gear, flashlights, and food. They felt prepared and well equipped. In addition, they made emergency plans and left them with the instructors. The instructors were going to stay in camp, catch up on course assessment paperwork, and provide an emergency reference point in case either of the groups had any problems.

One group, made up of student leader Dana, along with Helena, Pat, Jo, and Kris, appeared less confident in their map and compass skills, so the instructors worked very closely with them to make sure they had an accurate Time Control Plan and went over it very carefully with them. The biggest concern was how would they know when to leave the Trout Brook Trail to head up to String Bean Pond. They decided to leave the trail a little early and take a diagonal compass bearing to the outlet of String Bean Pond. They figured once they hit the outlet, they would just have to follow it upstream to the pond. They also felt that the terrain would help them. If they hit a hill by leaving the trail too early, it would have to be the hill to the east of the pond. When they were ready to leave the pond for their campsite at 2,200 feet, they figured that if they headed slightly to the west of camp that they would then have to head east when they eventually hit the trail, and the trail would then lead them to camp. It was well thought out, and the staff was impressed with their forethought. The instructors checked their mileage computations and their compass bearings. The students took into account declination and appeared to be accurate. The staff felt that the other group, made up of student leader Jan, along with Billie, Dale, Kim, and Lee, had enough experience to figure out the route without their help and that, even if they did make some mistakes, they could find their way in any event. They intentionally did not check their Time Control Plan and told the students that they weren't going to. They told this group that they should go ahead if they had complete confidence in their ability to successfully complete the trip without instructor support. The group was confident.

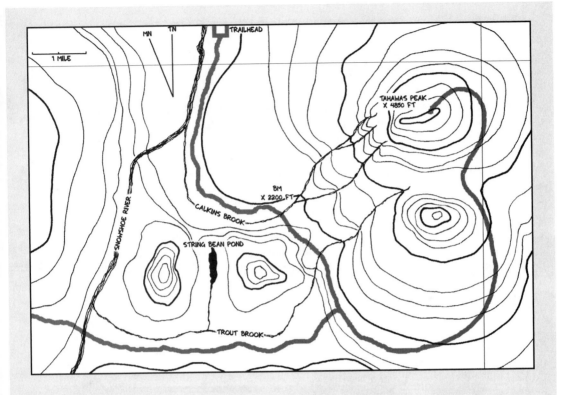

Dana and Jan got up at 7:00 A.M. and started heating up water for morning drinks before they woke up their group members. Dana's group got on the trail earliest but was passed by Jan's group before too long. Jan's group was hiking at a rapid pace and seemed eager to "beat" the other group back to camp. Dana's group was methodical and carefully followed their planned hiking pace of hiking forty minutes and resting ten. At each rest break they checked where they thought they were on the map. They didn't see the other group, but they found the south end of the pond by lunchtime. It wasn't much of a pond—it was more like a former beaver pond where the dam had been partially breached, leaving a smaller pond with open meadow surrounding it. It was beautiful in its stark contrast to the heavily forested woods where they were camped. They reveled in the sunshine as they ate their trail lunch.

Jan's group made great time traveling through the woods but struggled to find their landmarks. They figured they would be able to easily find String Bean Pond Outlet from the trail and then follow it up to the pond. When they got down to the general area where the outlet should be, they headed off trail. It took them nearly five minutes to find Trout Brook, and, once they did, they didn't see the outlet and had no idea whether it was to the left or right. They decided to send two people (Jan and Lee) upstream on Trout Brook to look for the outlet and three people (Billie, Dale, and Kim) downstream. Each group was to hike five minutes out and then turn around and come back. About three minutes out, Jan and Lee found the outlet. They immediately headed back, waited for the rest of their group to return, and then gave them the good news. They quickly headed up the stream and were just north of the pond by noon when they decided to eat lunch.

Meanwhile, as Dana's group finished up their lunch, they double-checked their compass bearing and headed northeast toward the Calkins Brook trail and their campsite. They found the trail within a reasonable time and headed east to their campsite. They arrived back at the campsite in the midafternoon and were surprised that Jan's group had not arrived yet. The instructors were glad to see Dana and the other group members, but they, too, were surprised that Jan's group had not returned before them.

Jan's group checked their compass bearing as they left the north end of String Bean Pond, but their confidence in their ability was a bit deflated as a result of their difficulty in finding the pond. Jan was from northern Michigan and Billie was from North Carolina, areas where there is no difference between true north and magnetic north (i.e., the declination is 0 degrees). As a result of their previous navigation experience, they didn't pay much attention when Naheed taught the group on the first week of the course how to compensate for declination. As a result, even though the group had checked their compass bearing, they did not compensate for declination. When they headed due north from String Bean Pond, they thought they were heading directly toward the Calkins Brook horse trail. Instead they were hiking 15 degrees west of true north. After hiking nearly an hour and not finding either Calkins Brook or the trail, they stopped and tried to figure out where they were. They were certain they were hiking in the correct direction, so the only thing that made sense to them was that they must have been hiking slower than they thought. They decided to hike another thirty minutes to see if they would hit the brook or trail. After hiking nearly thirty minutes they came to a brook that, according to the compass, was flowing north! They couldn't figure it out. If they were at Calkins Brook, why was it flowing north, and why did it take them so long to get there? After talking it over for nearly fifteen minutes, Kim blurted out, "I've got it! We forgot declination. We are between the trail and the Snowshoe River. If we head due east, we have to hit the trail!" The group talked it over at length and studied their map to look for other alternatives. Eventually they all agreed and decided to travel due east (105 degrees). They crossed the brook, and within five minutes they had found the trail running in a generally north/south direction.

After hiking about fifteen minutes down the rutted and mucky horse trail, they decided to take a break. By this time it was late afternoon, and they had been hiking for more than three hours since they had filled up their water bottles at String Bean Pond. Their water bottles had been emptied long ago, and the stress of "getting lost" had made them even thirstier than normal. They took a break to estimate how long it would take them to get back to camp. They figured it was at least an hour, and they wanted water before that. While discussing what to do about the water, Billie looked down and saw a 3-foot by 1-foot puddle in the horse trail that was at least 6 inches deep. Billie exclaimed, "We could use our water filter and drink the water from this puddle!" The group's thirst overcame any reservations they had, and they put the filter in the puddle and pumped away. They filled two water bottles and, as they nearly filled a third, ran the puddle dry. A horsehair worm was found wriggling in the bottom of the puddle. Again, their thirst outweighed any concern about horsehair worms. They drank their water and headed down the trail. Within an hour they were back at camp, much to Glenn and Naheed's relief.

What a debrief they had that night!

the area covered by the Adventure of Hair Worm Pass map located on page 144.

    (1) Simple decision scenario: Your group of moderately experienced hikers is hiking east on the Trout Brook Trail and comes to an intersection. You have defined the problem as the group being at the intersection and now wanting to travel to a campsite you know exists just off the trail near the 2,200-foot benchmark by Calkins Brook on your map.

    (2) Complex decision scenario: Your group is camped at the 2,200-foot benchmark by Calkins Brook. This is your first visit to the area, and your group wants to hike to the top of Tahawus Peak and back.

Found in table 10.1 are characteristics that help determine how simple or complex a decision is, along with a short synopsis of each characteristic. Descriptions of how each characteristic applies to both the simple and complex scenarios are in the columns to the right. See table 10.2 for a continuum of decision complexity.

  b) Observations on making simple decisions:

    (1) The more one strives to make simple decisions consciously, the more likely using the steps in the decision-making process will become second nature.

    (2) Like any skill, the more we practice good decision making, the better we get at it.

  c) Observations on complex decisions:

    (1) As decisions become more complex and the implications of their outcomes more uncertain, group members are more likely to want to have some control over the process. While accommodating this impulse may not always be possible (as in a life-threatening emergency), decision makers are well advised to be aware of this tendency and proceed accordingly.

    (2) Brainstorming is a technique that raises the probability that all viable options are recognized. It also increases a sense of ownership if all participants have had opportunity to put their ideas before the group.

  d) The role of judgment in complex decision making:

    (1) When information is incomplete and knowledge uncertain, analysis must give way to judgment as the driving force of decision making. Judgment fills the gap of missing information. Rarely do "correct" answers or solutions emerge from complex decisions.

Table 10.1. RECOGNIZING THE COMPLEXITY OF DECISIONS

CHARACTERISTIC	SIMPLE SCENARIO	COMPLEX SCENARIO
Predictability of the outcome: In simple decisions, the outcome is virtually certain. As the decisions become more complex, the outcome is less certain.	The decision has few variables, and the outcome is extremely predictable. One option will definitely take the group toward the campsite, and one definitely will not. Predictability is pretty high that if they make the right decision, they will be heading toward their campsite.	Due to the many variables in this scenario, it is almost impossible to predict the outcome. There are multiple routes of varying degrees of difficulty.
Information available: In simple decisions, information is readily available. As decisions become more complex, information is less available, less complete, and/or less reliable.	Assuming the group has a map and the ability to read it, they have all the information they need to make their decision.	Because there are so many variables, and because the group hasn't visited the area before, it is almost certain that they won't have all the information they would like or need.
Time: Simple decisions rarely take much time and often take little effort. As decisions become more complex, time is desired to realize a thorough and satisfactory process.	Time to make the decision should not be an issue in this scenario. The group should have plenty of time to make this simple decision.	Because there are so many variables and so little information is available, the group would probably like to take as much time as possible to make this decision. Unfortunately, they can only take so much time to decide, or they will never have time to make it up the mountain and back.
Options or choices: In simple decisions, the options are clear and distinct. As decisions become more complex, the options are less apparent.	There are only two real options: either turn left or turn right.	There are at least four viable options for going up and the same for coming down. Many of the options have suboptions or contingency options.

CHARACTERISTIC	SIMPLE SCENARIO	COMPLEX SCENARIO
Analysis: In simple decisions, the analysis is seemingly objective—i.e., it is "black and white"—and you can easily separate facts from assumptions. As decisions become more complex, the role of emotions may have a greater impact on the interpretation of variables that impact the selection of options.	The analysis is fairly basic: The campsite is north of where the group is, and, according to both our map and our compass, the trail to the left (north) should lead there. Outside factors (i.e., weather, how tired the group is, etc.) have virtually no impact on whether the group should go left or right.	Selecting an option in this scenario will require extensive analysis. Does the group have the skills necessary to navigate an off-trail route? How thick will the forest cover be? Will the weather hold up for the duration of the trip? Is the group physically fit enough? The questions are nearly endless.
Values: In simple decisions, values are not an issue. As decisions become more complex, values play a much more visible role in the identification and selection of options.	As long as the group agrees with the goal of getting to the campsite, then values have little impact on this decision.	Values play a role in determining priorities. For example, is the group more interested in taking the easiest route, or do they want to take a route that challenges them physically and tests their map and compass skills?
Experience: In simple decisions, little or no experience is necessary. As decisions become more complex, experience becomes more of an asset in predicting the outcome.	While the decision makers need to have basic map-reading skills, they don't need a large amount of experience.	The more experience the decision makers have in similar terrain, the better off they will probably be. Their experience will help determine whether an off-trail route is feasible given the abilities of the group.
Ownership: In simple decisions, group members feel little or no need to participate in the process or "own" the outcome. As decisions become more complex, group members frequently feel an increasingly greater need to participate in the process and commit themselves to the final outcome.	Ownership is not an issue because the group members do not see themselves as particularly threatened by the implications of any of the choices.	It is probably very important for group members to have input and ownership to the decision on the route they end up taking. If the route turns out to be more difficult than anticipated, it is helpful to have the entire group share ownership for the decision. In general, the more threatening the implications of the decision, the greater need for all members of the group to own the decision.

CHARACTERISTIC	SIMPLE SCENARIO	COMPLEX SCENARIO
Number of people desired for input: In simple decisions, one person can easily make or be empowered to make the decision. As decisions become more complex, it becomes increasingly preferable to have more minds exploring the decision. This is contingent upon the specific context or urgency of the decision.	Because of the simple nature of this decision, virtually any group member should be able to make it alone.	The more people you have, the more ideas, thoughts, and possible options will probably be available. Of course, involving additional minds takes considerably more time and adds complexity to the process.
Level of awareness or consciousness: In simple decisions, consciousness or reflection is usually at a very low level, and these decisions are made without even thinking about them. As decisions become more complex, it is important to make the process more overt and more conscious.	If enough thought was put into route selection before the trip, the group should be able to know which way to go almost automatically upon reaching the intersection.	The only implicit option would be a decision to take the trail. It would be foolhardy to take any of the off-trail routes without careful consideration of the consequences.
Control: In simple decisions, the control of the outcome is entirely in the hands of the decision makers. As decisions become more complex, external factors play a much larger role in the outcome.	In this case, the decision makers have full control over making the correct decision.	There are many variables out of control of the decision maker(s) that could play a role in whether the group meets its goals or not, including the weather, forest cover, and daylight.
Amount of judgment necessary: Simple decisions require little judgment. As decisions become more complex, it becomes increasingly important for decision makers to tap and then apply their repertoire of processed experience.	This decision needs a minimal amount of knowledge—skill in map interpretation and little else.	Judgment or "common sense" is essential in this scenario. For example, taking the most difficult route might be an example of using poor judgment if your group is made up of ten-year-olds.

Table 10.2. A CONTINUUM OF DECISION COMPLEXITY

CHARACTERISTIC	SIMPLE SCENARIO	COMPLEX SCENARIO
Predictability of the outcome	Certainty	Uncertainty
Information available	Readily available	Must "discover"
Time	Ample	Frequently limited
Options or choices	Obvious	Must be discovered
Analysis	Primarily objective	Largely subjective
Role of values	Little	Frequently large
Experience	Little needed	The more the merrier
Ownership	Little	Large
Number of people desired for input	Fewer	More
Level of awareness or consciousness needed	Low	High
Control	Large	Little
Amount of judgment necessary	Little	A lot

Instead, options are evaluated in terms of probability rather than certainty of success.

(2) Judgment is the accumulated wisdom we glean from past experience and apply to present problems. Judgment requires processing experience and adopting behaviors informed by that process. Decision makers with good judgment are able to increase the probability of making successful decisions because they understand how to draw upon their experience and apply it to the unique circumstances of each new challenge. Judgment gives one a broader per-

spective—a lens through which events are viewed in sharper focus and with greater clarity than would be the case otherwise.

B. The role of emotions in making quality decisions

1. Historically, Western culture has made a distinction between thought that is driven by reason and thought that is driven by emotion; i.e., the rational/emotional dichotomy. We continue in that tradition by advocating a decision-making process that is conscious, transparent, and teachable.

2. Recent brain-based research suggests that emotions cannot be separated from decision making. It is important that we recognize that emotions play a significant part in all of our thinking. Similarly, we need to accept that few of us have the ability to fully comprehend the role subconscious emotions play in our lives. Thus our challenge is to recognize the role of emotion in the decision-making process to the extent we are capable. To that end, we advocate following a ritualized process that includes an examination of our own motivations and emotions—recognizing that it will be incomplete—before reaching a final decision.

C. The role of intuition in making quality decisions

1. There are situations where some may feel that a decision maker should rely on intuition, simply follow his or her gut instinct, and ignore analytical thinking.

2. "Your decision can't be based just on facts, you must also consider *your subjective, intuitive or vague feeling-oriented reactions.* Do this by ruminating about each choice. Daydream about the likely outcomes for each alternative—how does each possible future feel to you? Some will feel 'right' and others 'wrong.' Some exciting and some scary. Ask yourself: What is the best that could happen if I make this choice? What is the worst that could happen? Are there ways to improve the 'wrong' alternatives or to overcome the fears?" (Tucker-Ladd 1996–2000).

3. While this may appear intuitive, we would argue that this is really just brainstorming and reflecting in a slightly different way. While there may be occasions that you simply go with your gut reaction, we would argue that is more the exception than the rule.

4. One purpose of many wilderness leadership courses is to teach judgment and make decision making as transparent as possible so people can learn from it. Since intuition is inexplicable and those who rely on it can't explain their rationale, it is almost impossible to learn from it or to teach it as part of a process that is transferable.

D. The transferable nature of decision making

1. Participants should understand that the decision-making process itself is a system of thought that can be applied in any situation, regardless of circumstance.
2. Participants should recognize that the process of decision making developed via wilderness leadership training has application outside of a wilderness setting. The decision-making process can readily be applied in nonwilderness situations, such as school, home, business, etc.
3. Experiences on the course should be interpreted as analogous to situations in other areas of life. For example, planning a off-trail day hike is really not much different from planning a family excursion for the day to Disney World. The accumulation of these analogous experiences and the ability to apply them appropriately is generally recognized as a defining characteristic of leaders possessing good judgment.
4. The leadership experiences encountered on a wilderness course will train participants in a pattern of behavior that is useful in other leadership situations. The responsibilities of a leader on a four-day expedition are essentially the same as those on a thirty-five-day expedition, and the leadership needed in the wilderness is not all that different from that needed in the business world.

Part 2. A Process for Making Decisions

A. Defining the decision-making process

1. The decision-making process is a series of conscious, ritualized steps followed to make a choice among options, for the purpose of realizing an objective.
   a) We emphasize the word *conscious* because decision makers need to be fully aware and focused on all aspects of decision making. The thinking behind the process should be as transparent/visible as possible.
   b) By using the word *ritualize,* we mean to suggest that decision makers should develop the meaningful habit of using a standardized procedure when confronted with choices.
   c) The process, as outlined below, is appropriate for almost any decision-making situation regardless of its complexity.
   d) The manner in which decision makers choose to engage the process will obviously depend upon the situation.

Decision at High Mountain

Early on the morning of Saturday, November 29th, Bob, Sue, and Mark headed into the High Mountain Wilderness Area of New York State's Adirondack Mountains on their third backpacking trip together. The weather was crisp and cool, with daytime highs in the thirties and the thermometer dipping into the teens at night. There were 2 inches of snow on the ground, with a possibility of additional accumulation over the weekend.

Bob and Sue, twenty-one and twenty-two respectively, were well dressed for the outing in wool pants and shirts, and they wore rubberized, insulated winter hiking boots. Both were well equipped with good quality, synthetic, insulated sleeping bags and insulated sleeping pads. Mark was not so well prepared, however. Although none of the hikers was highly experienced, Mark was eighteen, had only been backpacking on two previous occasions, and was not yet ready to spend the money necessary for the proper gear. Sitting in Bob's suburban New Jersey home, Sue and Bob had pleaded with Mark to outfit himself properly. Nonetheless, when they met early Saturday morning, Mark appeared decked in blue jeans, cotton thermal long johns, a hooded cotton sweatshirt, cotton tube socks, and leather work boots. He carried his gear in a borrowed, ill-fitted backpack and intended to sleep in a goose-down sleeping bag on an air mattress. The group would sleep together in Sue's three-person mountain tent.

Although the three had to be back at work early Monday, it was the last thing on their minds as they sped along the interstate highway on their six-hour drive. Bob casually shared with Sue that he forgot to tell his parents exactly where he was going, and Sue admitted she hadn't told her parents either. Mark spoke up, saying, "Don't worry! I told my parents we were going backpacking in the Adirondacks and, not to worry, we'd be back by 11:00 P.M. Sunday." The discussion turned to Mark's reluctance to acquire the proper clothing and equipment, creating a level of tension in the group that would last the weekend. The discussion ended as Bob pulled into the Complete Backpacker store to buy some new batteries for his flashlight before they reached the nearby trailhead.

The three hiked up the Lake Clear Trail that Saturday afternoon with the intention of staying overnight at the lake and returning to their car the next day. Although the trail to the lake was more than 4 miles long, the terrain was relatively easy, and the three friends reached their destination by early afternoon. After setting up camp and eating dinner, the three settled into their tent for a well-deserved rest. As the night sky darkened and the thermometer dipped, a gentle snow began to fall.

Bob was the first to awaken on Sunday morning to a trackless, white world covered by the accumulation of the previous evening's flurries. Finally emerging from their respective cocoons at about 8:30 A.M., the campers set to the task of preparing a hot breakfast of oatmeal and hot chocolate. Afterward, the three stayed in their sleeping bags, enjoying the warmth and friendly conversation. Around noon, they decided to have a hot lunch before heading back to their car. Much to their dismay, they found their otherwise dependable backpacking stove extremely difficult to light. Indeed, even after a frustrating hour of tinkering, the stove would only produce a very weak, short-lived flame. Finally, despairing of any progress, they gave up on the stove and munched on available prepackaged granola bars and gulped down some nearly frozen water.

By 1:30 P.M., all three were packed and ready to head back on the trail home. Talking excitedly about the beauty of the newly fallen snow and without paying any great heed to the few trail markers on the trees, the party moved out in what they thought was the direction from which they had come. After thirty minutes on the trail, Bob remarked how different everything

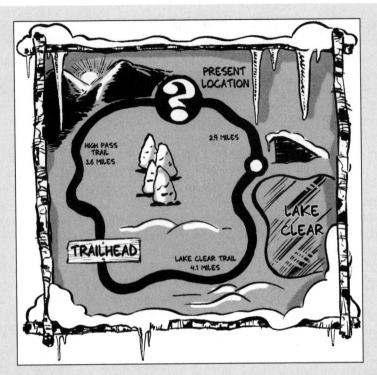

looked from the day before. Sue mentioned that they should be more attentive to the trail markers since they no longer had the footprints of earlier hikers to follow as they had the previous day. Mark said that he couldn't remember the last time he had seen a trail marker. Within another fifteen minutes, it became obvious to each of them that they were not on a trail and not exactly sure of their location.

Since Bob had the only map and compass in the group, he tried to figure out where they were. Though he had some elementary training in orienteering, it soon was obvious that his skills were not equal to the task at hand. Figuring that the trail had to be close by, they decided to spread out and look for markers. Within a few minutes, they discovered a marker of the appropriate color and headed down the trail with renewed confidence.

The three continued to hike for another forty-five minutes when Bob remarked that he could see a trail sign in the distance. Hustling over to the sign, to their great chagrin they read:

TRAILHEAD VIA HIGH PASS TRAIL 3.6 MILES

TRAILHEAD VIA LAKE CLEAR TRAIL 7 MILES

LAKE CLEAR LEAN-TO 2.9 MILES

Their hearts sank as they realized they had been walking in the wrong direction all this time. Now, at 3:30 P.M. on Sunday afternoon, with darkness only an hour away, they faced a decision. High Pass Trail was a direct route to the car, but a quick glance at the map revealed it involved a 500-foot gain in elevation. Returning to the trailhead by the route they had just traveled would take them past Lake Clear Lean-to on a familiar trail, but it would mean nearly 3½ more miles of trail.

What should they do?

2. Characteristics of the process

    a) Decision making always involves a choice and implies the consideration of more than one option. If only one course of action exists in a given situation, then no decision is required. In reality, there is virtually always more than one option; thus, we are in effect always making choices or decisions.

    b) The more complex the decision, the more it should be based on an explicit process as opposed to the exercise of preference. The logical steps taken to reach a decision should be easily understood to an independent observer.

        (1) For example, a simple decision, such as the choice between vanilla and chocolate pudding as the evening's dessert, is an exercise of preference. It does not necessarily have a basis in logic. Preference is an example of the most elementary form of a simple decision. The selection of a route to a given campsite should be a product of a more thorough process, the logic of which should include the consideration of time, terrain, physical condition of the group, and other factors. This is an example of a more complex decision.

        (2) The emphasis on rational thought in this process does not discount the role individual experience plays, nor preclude the use of hunches and "feelings" that may be based upon that experience. (See "the role of intuition in making quality decisions" on p. 151.)

        (3) Sometimes the likely consequences of particular choices are so similar that a lot of time and effort spent making those choices would seem a waste; a choice could just as well be made by the flip of a coin. There is no certainty, however, that this would be the case without following through the steps in the decision-making process, taking each possible choice into consideration.

        (4) Decision making implies action. The process of decision making is incomplete without an attempt to implement the decision.

        (5) The use of the decision-making process does not guarantee the outcome of a specific action. Consistent application of the process, however, tempered by the judgment that comes from experience, significantly increases the odds of meeting outcomes.

Reading the scenario Decision at High Mountain at this time, if you haven't yet, may be helpful.

B. Steps in the decision-making process

1. Recognize the context
    a) Decision making always takes place within a specific historical, physical, emotional/psychological, and cultural "context." Contributing factors might include:
        (1) Temperature, altitude, and topography of the area
        (2) Age, gender mix, and ethnicity of the group
        (3) Relationships among group members
        (4) Objectives of the individuals, group, or agency sponsoring the expedition
    b) The context for the Decision at High Mountain scenario includes the recognition that they are in a typical northeastern U.S. environment with all the associated traditions and customs found in this region of the world. The group members reflect their family ethnicity and culture as well as the culture that has been created as friends and acquaintances.

2. Identify and define the problem
    a) Three things must happen when identifying and defining the problem:
        (1) Recognition of an existing problem and the need for a decision to be made: Decision making starts when the group perceives a difference between what is and what is not desirable; i.e., a decision needs to be made.
        (2) Motivation to take action: The individual or group must desire to seek out and choose a course of action that will change the situation.
        (3) Goal setting: The individual or group must identify the objectives or goals so that everyone will be working toward a common end; i.e., the problem needs to be clearly identified.
    b) Defining the problem
        (1) The problem can be defined as the recognition of the difference between what exists and what is desirable.
        (2) The desire to meet some objective is always implied. Without some recognized objective, no decision is necessary or possible.
        (3) It is usually helpful to define the problem in terms of the situation you *are* in contrasted with the situation you would *like* to be in. The great American psychologist William James once said, "A problem well stated is half solved" (Adams n.d.).
        (4) In the Decision at High Mountain scenario, the process begins when the group recognizes that it has inadvertently gotten lost and is not proceeding along the trail in the direction they thought they

were going. Clearly, the group is motivated to improve their situation. The problem could be stated, "We are at the intersection of the High Pass Trail and the Lake Clear Trail and want to be safely at the trailhead as quickly as possible with as little risk as necessary."

(5) Failure to *define* the problem frequently leads to a wrong solution. English essayist, novelist, poet, and journalist Gilbert Keith Chesterton once wrote, "It isn't that they can't see the solution. It is that they can't see the problem" (Chesterton 1935).

(6) Examples of well-defined problems:

(a) I'm at the intersection of stream A and stream B on my way up Mt. Adams, and I want to find the safest, easiest, and fastest route to the top of the mountain.

(b) I'm at a small pond that is shaped like a horseshoe, but I don't know where I am. I want to figure out where I am and how to get back to camp.

(c) My tent partner is very disorganized with both our cooking gear and his personal gear, so I am left constantly having to pick up after him, which is driving me crazy. I would like him to keep himself organized (or I would like it so he doesn't drive me crazy).

(d) The group I am leading doesn't seem to be motivated at all. They mope around and don't seem to be enjoying themselves, and I would like them to get psyched about being outdoors.

(e) One of my campers just fell in a rapidly flowing river, and I need to safely get her out as quickly as possible.

(7) Sometimes it is helpful to write your more complex problems down. This will force you to give the problem proper thought and allow for you to clarify exactly what the problem is.

(8) Sometimes we define a problem too late for an easy solution. It is important to anticipate a problem before it becomes more complex. For example, leaders should recognize when the conditions for hypothermia exist and take steps to assure the safety of the group. Deciding that all group members should put on a hat and mittens is a simpler solution to implement than treating a hypothermia victim.

3. Clarify and analyze the problem

a) Clarification and analysis is a systematic consideration of all the factors that may bear on the situation.

(1) This stage of the decision-making process is analytic and reflective.
  (a) Some people find it easy, and others struggle with it.
  (b) The more complex the decision, the more effort should be put into this part of the decision-making process.
  (c) A Chinese proverb says, "To chop a tree quickly, spend twice the time sharpening the ax." Carpenters are frequently heard to say, "Measure twice, cut once." The essence of both quotes is that, by taking the time to analyze the situation, you will more often than not have a better result.
(2) This stage is characterized by asking, who, what, why, when, where, and how and the need to sort through facts, assumptions, constraints, values, and group dynamics.
b) Steps required to effectively clarify and analyze the problem:
(1) Gather facts: Collect information that can be confirmed by an independent observer to be true. In the Decision at High Mountain scenario, some of the facts are:
  (a) There are two trail routes out to the group's car.
  (b) Their clothing includes blue jeans, cotton hooded sweatshirts, wool clothing, and cold-weather Mickey Mouse boots.
  (c) Their equipment includes a mountain tent, sleeping bags, backpacking stove, one map, and one compass.
  (d) They are supposed to be back to work on Monday.
  (e) They have left vague emergency information.
(2) Examine and distinguish assumptions from facts
  (a) Explore information and/or beliefs that you or the group accepts as true but that cannot be proven or verified.
  (b) The challenge is to explore what you think *probably* exists or will *probably* happen. It is important to have a plausible explanation for your assumptions. Once a "fact" is revealed as an assumption, one can decide whether to change the weight one ascribes the assumption in the decision-making process.
  (c) In the Decision at High Mountain scenario, some of the assumptions might be:
    i) The weather will remain seasonably unpredictable.
    ii) It will be some time before anyone starts looking for them.

      iii) Their parents will worry if they don't come home on time.

      iv) They may be disciplined by employers for their absence.

(3) Recognize constraints

  (a) Recognize the limitations that the present circumstances impose on what you might do.

  (b) In the Decision at High Mountain scenario, some of the constraints that might be recognized are:

     i) Availability of food

     ii) Weather conditions

     iii) Time

     iv) Experience and expertise of group members

(4) Understand values

  (a) Try to understand the influence of those ideas, beliefs, and goals that are considered by the group to be most important to the group's success or survival.

  (b) Some considerations when reflecting on one's values include:

     i) "What is right is not always popular and what is popular is not always right" (Daniel Webster).

     ii) Resist peer pressure. Don't do it because someone else is doing it, but don't be afraid to use a role model and say something like, "What would Paul Petzoldt do in this situation?"

     iii) "If you have decided on a philosophy of life, most other decisions are made much easier" (Tucker-Ladd 1996–2000).

     iv) You reveal your priorities either consciously or unconsciously by how you spend your time.

     v) Some feel that "We are innately selfish, gregarious and just plain lazy . . . Don't allow your inherent selfishness to interfere with the final decision you make" (Hughes, Ginnett, and Curphy 1993).

  (c) In the Decision at High Mountain scenario, some of the values of the group might be:

     i) Sense of responsibility to employer

     ii) Consideration of family feelings and emotions

　　　　　iii) Loyalty to all the members of the party

　　　　　iv) Commitment to the survival of all party members

　　(5) Consider group dynamics

　　　　(a) Predict the impact that potential courses of action may have on individual morale and the ability of the group to function effectively as a unit.

　　　　(b) In the Decision at High Mountain scenario, some factors involving group dynamics might include:

　　　　　i) The least-experienced group member did not follow the advice of the more-experienced group members.

　　　　　ii) The individual who is least prepared is also the youngest.

　　　　　iii) There was tension within the group on the ride to the trailhead because of the aforementioned factors.

4. Generate options: In this stage of the process, ideas are first generated and subsequently narrowed down. Formulate options by using brainstorming to maximize your chances of generating as many solutions as possible. The goal is to consider a variety of possible solutions. It is a creative process.

　a) Brainstorming

　　(1) A technique in which an individual or group attempts to spontaneously create ideas that might provide a possible solution to an issue or problem.

　　　　(a) Brainstorming is used to maximize the chances of generating as many solutions as possible.

　　　　(b) This step of the process requires creativity and provides an opportunity to "think outside of the box."

　　　　(c) Brainstorming broadens the base of experience from which to draw constructive ideas. It improves the probability that all options will be thoroughly considered. In the context of group decision making, it encourages a sense of participant "ownership" of the final decision.

　　(2) Brainstorming "rules":

　　　　(a) One person should play the role of facilitator, encouraging the sharing of ideas and restraining the impulse to criticize or discount.

　　　　(b) Set a specific time frame for brainstorming. It is important to recognize that at some point you must move from brainstorming to decision making.

　　　　(c) Assign a recorder who will record ideas accurately without judging the quality of the ideas. Voicing opinions about ideas comes *after* brainstorming when you distill.

    (d) Only share your ideas if you are willing to let go of them. Once an idea is shared the group owns it, and its ultimate acceptance or rejection should not be taken personally.

    (e) Work for quantity, not quality. Judging the quality of the ideas also comes *after* brainstorming, during the weighing of options step of the decision-making process.

    (f) Do not criticize any of the ideas. All ideas must be afforded equal acceptance. To be effective, a brainstorming session must be governed by the attitude that "anything is possible." Again, evaluating the ideas comes *after* the brainstorming session.

    (g) Encourage the "piggybacking" of ideas. Let ideas trigger new ideas. What some may think are crazy ideas frequently help trigger good ideas.

b) Determining criteria for measuring success

    (1) We must have criteria for determining which of the options are preferable and to eventually know whether the decision has been successful or not.

    (2) In a wilderness setting the criteria might be:

        (a) Is everyone safe?

        (b) Is there minimum impact on the environment?

        (c) Are people able to remain relatively comfortable?

        (d) Are we able to meet predetermined individual and/or group goals?

        (e) Are there numerous attractive contingencies?

c) Distillation

    (1) Distillation is the narrowing down of options to the best two to four by holding the brainstormed ideas up for comparison against the established criteria for success.

    (2) Distillation comes *after* brainstorming. It is a distinctively different activity from brainstorming.

    (3) In the brainstorming stage we consciously refrain from critiquing options to encourage creativity. In the distillation stage we now must consciously evaluate and critique each option in order to bring focus and move toward a final choice.

d) Weighing options: Positive and negative outcomes

    (1) Now that we have narrowed down the infinite number of options

to a manageable number, we need to examine each of the remaining options more closely.

(2) One tool useful to accomplish this is the PMI (Plus, Minus, Interesting).

    (a) The PMI tool (see table 10.3) involves using a process that requires a chart with three columns, one each for Plus, Minus, and Interesting. An individual or group can easily look at an option and weigh its positive, negative, and interesting characteristics.

    (b) The PMI can be very helpful in providing a relatively objective analysis of each option.

See table 10.3, an abbreviated PMI, for some of the options in the Decision at High Mountain scenario.

  e) Contingencies

    (1) At this point in the decision-making process, it is appropriate to identify a contingency plan by outlining the "what ifs" (alternatives) of each option. For example, suppose a group is deciding whether or not to take a trailless hike to a marked trail that will lead to their campsite. Included in their decision-making process could be a plan (alternative) to answer the question, "What if we don't find the marked trail by dark?"

    (2) Often options that provide more or better contingencies are attractive because they provide more flexibility. In the Decision at High Mountain scenario, an option that has an attractive contingency is the option to walk out via the Lake Clear Trail. The contingency would be that if they had any problems, they could stay at the lean-to on the way out.

5. Make a decision

  a) Select a specific option.

  b) Making a decision means accepting responsibility for your choice. It also means accepting the possibility that you might be wrong or that you will make a less than optimal decision. The object is to make a good choice with the information and resources available at the time, not to make a perfect choice. You need to make the best decision possible *given your resources.*

  c) You may do one thing *if* you had more resources, more time, fewer constraints, etc., but your decision is what you *will* do in this particular situation.

Table 10.3. DECISION AT HIGH MOUNTAIN PMI			
OPTION	**PLUS (P)**	**MINUS (M)**	**INTERESTING (I)**
Return to and spend the night at Lake Clear lean-to	Will minimize travel after dark	Will have to spend another night; will not get home on time; family will worry	They will retrace their steps
Walk out to trailhead via High Pass Trail	They might get home that night	They might get lost due to unfamiliarity with the trail	They might have nice views from High Pass
Remain in place and set up camp	Will minimize risk of hypothermia or exhaustion	Will have to spend another night; will not get home on time; family will worry	They will experience camping in a non-established primitive campsite
Walk out to trailhead via Lake Clear Trail	Involves travel over familiar terrain	Involves longest route to travel	They will retrace their steps

    d) The entire decision-making process can be an individual or group process. The amount and level of input from group members may be based on the issue on hand, the experience of the group members, the complexity of the decision, or the level of "crisis." A leader sometimes has to ask, "Is this a problem/issue that warrants group decision making, or I am better off deciding it myself?" (See the "Group Decision Making" section on p. 165.)

6. Implement the decision: "A poor decision well executed is better than a good decision poorly executed" (Tucker-Ladd 1996–2000).

    a) Once a decision is made, its successful implementation is usually an issue of effective leadership.

    b) Considerations for effective implementation include:

        (1) Communication: Everyone must understand at all times what is to be done and why it is to be done.

        (2) Delegation: Everyone involved should have specific tasks for which they are personally responsible.

        (3) Monitoring: The leader needs to constantly monitor conditions and adjust his or her actions to the evolving situation.

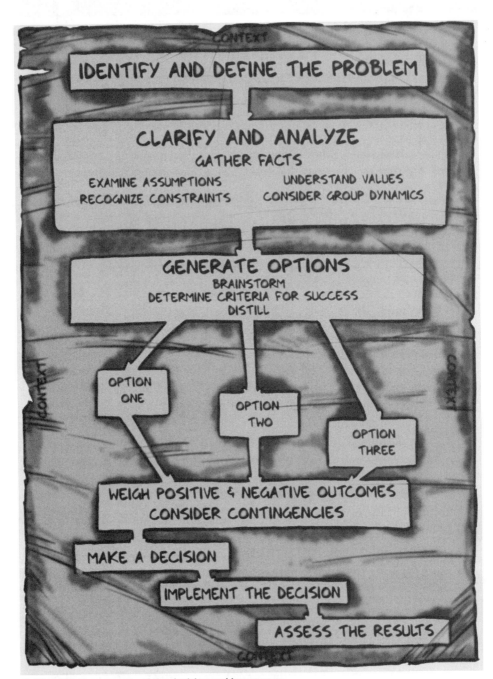

FIGURE 10.1. Components of the decision-making process

7. Assess the results
   a) In this step of the process, participants reflect on what has been learned from the decision-making experience.
   b) By incorporating these insights in their own future decisions, participants develop judgment.
      (1) This step in the process is critical to the development of good judgment; the decision-making process is not complete until it is reflected upon. (See the discussion of the experiential cycle in chapter 1, Teaching and Learning.)
      (2) The theme that runs throughout the entire process of leadership training is the explanation of why an action should be, is, or was taken; why it was performed in the way it was; and in what way the action might be improved now or for similar situations in the future (Cockrell 1991).

This is an appropriate time to discuss and assess the group's responses to the Decision at High Mountain scenario.

C. Special considerations for group decision making and building consensus

1. Group decision making
   a) In group decision making, all group members have input during the decision-making process. Research demonstrates and our experience supports the notion that "leaders could often improve group performance by using an optimal amount of participation in the decision-making process (Hughes, Ginnett, and Curphy 1993).
   b) The problem with group decision making is, who is going to take the blame or be responsible if things go haywire? Someone has to be responsible and accountable. It is important that there be a leader who accepts the ultimate responsibility for both the process (i.e., accepting group input) and implementing the decision.
   c) Given the above concern, we still feel that group decisions are extremely valuable because they have an opportunity to be:
      (1) More empowering, giving group members a sense of ownership and resulting in wider acceptance of the results of the decision
      (2) More creative as a result of more ideas and options being generated
2. Decision making by consensus
   a) When a high degree of ownership to the decision is desirable, decisions should be made by consensus whenever possible. The goal during consensus decision making is to have everyone find the decision acceptable.
   b) Consensus means that in coming to a decision, no one feels that his/her

position on the matter was misunderstood or that it wasn't given a proper hearing. The fundamental right of consensus is for all people to be able to express themselves in their own words and of their own will.

c) Consensus is not only about working to achieve better solutions, but also to promote the growth of community and trust.

d) Consensus is *not* voting. Voting is a win or lose model in which people are frequently more concerned with the numbers it takes to "win" than with the issue itself. Voting does not take into account individual feelings or needs. Voting is a quantitative, rather than qualitative, method of decision making.

e) A group that desires to use consensus decision making needs to recognize that other forms of decision making (e.g., individual, compromise, majority rules) may be, depending on the situation, necessary and appropriate.

f) Consensus cannot work unless people are responsible regarding their use of this power. For consensus to work effectively, we believe that a Full Value Contract is essential. (See chapter 1, Teaching and Learning.)

g) The thumb tool is a useful way to measure consensus in relatively small groups. (See chapter 1, Teaching and Learning.)

III. Instructional Strategies

A. Timing. Although the teaching of decision making starts on day one of a course and is reinforced daily with the activities listed below, the content of this chapter is usually taught once students have had an opportunity to experience the challenges of decision making on the trip. The activities below can be used in the classroom before the trip or within the first third of a trip.

B. Considerations

1. Teaching decision making: In teaching decision making, there are two important components: 1) Instructors need to make sure that students understand decision-making theory, and 2) Instructors must provide opportunities for students to make decisions and have students reflect on the decisions they and others around them make. A list of typical activities that need to take place on a wilderness course for students to be able to learn about decision making follows:

    a) Articulation of course outcomes: Participants need to understand the role and importance of decision making in relation to the course outcomes. Is it clearly communicated that decision making is an important learning outcome of the trip? Our experience dictates that this needs to be communicated at the beginning of a wilderness course and at least once more during the course.

b) Review of the assessment process: Participants also need to understand the role and importance of the assessment process as it relates to the assessment of one's decision-making ability. How will they receive feedback, when will they receive feedback, and what role will it play in grading, certification, or other forms of evaluation? As previously stated, this needs to be done at the beginning of a wilderness course and at least once more during the course.

c) Journals: Writing in journals encourages participants to formally identify and analyze decisions made by themselves and others during the course. The journals provide instructors with an opportunity to see into the student's mind and observe whether the student sees the decisions that are being made and whether the student is beginning to grasp how decisions are being made.

d) Leader of the Day (LOD): This provides opportunities for each student to make decisions within the leadership role.

e) Debriefings: Daily group debriefings give participants the opportunity to share and reflect on their analysis of decisions that have been made during the day. (See chapter 25, Group Processing and Debriefing, for more information on debriefing.)

f) Decision-making theory presentation: This presentation usually takes place well after students are already trying to recognize and analyze decisions, both their own and others being made around them. This allows the students to begin to understand the theoretical aspects of decision making and allow the students perspective on the decision-making process.

g) Opportunities for students to make decisions: These are the daily activities that take place naturally or are designed by the instructor that provide the grist of decision making for the mill of reflection. A list of typical activities that occur on a trip that provide such opportunities follows:

    (1) Student-led hikes: Trail and off-trail hikes, with and without instructor supervision, provide a multitude of opportunities for students to make decisions.

    (2) Reration/food drops: The numerous tasks associated with this activity provide numerous opportunities for decision making.

(3) Use of daily "camping skills": Finding a tent site, preparing meals, packing the pack, and most of the other camp skills also provide opportunities for making decisions.

(4) Designing lessons: As students design teaching lessons for a variety of learners, they also engage in the decision-making process.

2. Assessment: Observation and feedback

   a) Student decision making takes place within a framework of instructor observation and feedback. Instructor observations provide participants with feedback concerning their progress in mastering the decision-making process.

   b) Peer feedback affords participants additional input from the group concerning their decision-making performance.

C. Activities

1. The Adventure of Hair Worm Pass scenario

   a) Purpose:

      (1) To have individuals recognize the number, variety, and complexity of decisions made on a "typical" day in the wilderness

      (2) To have individuals consider the conscious and subconscious nature of decision making

      (3) To practice "defining the problem"

   b) The task: Have the students read the scenario, then, in small work groups, ask them to:

      (1) List all the decisions that they can find in the scenario.

      (2) Identify the decisions that were clearly conscious or subconscious.

      (3) Have each person select two fairly complex decisions found within the scenario. Each person defines the problems by first writing them down, then sharing them within their work group. Each work group then chooses at least two defined problems to share with the class.

2. The Decision at High Mountain scenario

   a) Purpose:

      (1) To identify the different components of the decision-making process as outlined in the text

      (2) To practice making a decision in a scenario situation

   b) The task: Have the students read the scenario, then, in small work groups, ask them to:

      (1) Describe the parts of the scenario as they pertain to the components of the decision-making process in figure 10.1.

(2) In their small groups, determine what their decision would be for the scenario. They should be able to describe how they arrived at their decision.
c) Instructors may also choose to use real-life situations in the field as a basis for discussion. Instructors should prepare their own analyses before class so that the students focus on the process, not the problem.
3. The How Complex Is This Decision Anyway? challenge (see the end of the chapter)
  a) Purpose:
    (1) To understand the characteristics in determining decision complexity
    (2) To practice the synthesis of ideas and information
    (3) To complete the task as described in the challenge

D. Materials

1. Scenarios from this chapter
2. Notebook
3. Pencil

Challenge

Knowledge Outcome

What do you want them to know?

Decision making: Participants understand the characteristics in determining decision complexity.

Title

How Complex Is This Decision Anyway?

Skill/Disposition Outcome

What skill/disposition do you want them to develop?

Leadership: synthesis of ideas and information

Essential Question or Key Issue:

How do the characteristics in determining decision complexity help us make decisions?

Description of Challenge/Task/Performance:

Using table 10.1 in chapter 10, Decision Making, get into small groups and create a scenario that includes as many of the characteristics as possible.

Be prepared to make an oral presentation of no more than fifteen minutes of your scenario to the entire group and explain how you incorporated the characteristics into your scenario. Feel free to use graphics, a skit, or other means of presentation to reinforce your points.

Criteria for Assessment and Feedback:

- The presentation is no more than fifteen minutes.
- The presentation is clear, concise, and free from confusion or ambiguity.
- The presentation is insightful in that it allows the audience to learn something new.
- The presentation makes clear connections between the scenario and the characteristics in determining decision complexity.

Developed by Leading EDGE, LLC for The Backcountry Classroom. *For more information log on to www.realworldlearning.info.*

Product Quality Checklist

Date: _____   Class Period: _____

Product Author(s):	Product Title/Name: How Complex Is This Decision Anyway?	Evaluator Name(s):

Observed	Standard/Criteria	Possible Points	Rating
	The presentation is no more than fifteen minutes.		
	The presentation is clear, concise, and free from confusion or ambiguity.		
	The presentation is insightful in that it allows the audience to learn something new.		
	The presentation makes clear connections between the scenario and the characteristics in determining decision complexity.		
	Total		

Observations:

Elements of Questionable Quality:	**Elements of Exceptional Quality:**

CHAPTER ELEVEN

Environmental Ethics

I. Outcomes

A. Outdoor leaders provide evidence of their *knowledge* and *understanding* by:

1. Describing how personal ethical orientation influences decision making in relationship to environmental conservation practices in the field
2. Describing the relationship between outdoor ethics and environmental ethics
3. Describing the impact of recreation users on the natural environment
4. Describing the concept of ethics as it relates to the natural environment and wilderness travel
5. Describing the seven "Leave No Trace" principles
6. Describing the consequences of individual and group behavior on the quality of the outdoor experience

B. Outdoor leaders provide evidence of their *skill* by:

1. Integrating "Leave No Trace" principles and practices into the daily routine of outdoor living

C. Outdoor leaders provide evidence of their *dispositions* by:

1. Modeling "Leave No Trace" principles and practices as the standard code of behavior while engaged in outdoor pursuits
2. Reflecting on how a personal environmental ethic can be transferred and applied to a broad spectrum of life situations and decisions

II. Content

A. Ethics

1. Definition of ethics

    A code of voluntary restrictions of individual freedom agreed upon by members of a society for the good of the community; conforming to the standards of conduct of a given profession.

    a) Ethics are socially derived. For instance, parents teach their children to be responsible, cooperative, and obedient in order to help maintain harmony within the family. Certain actions are considered "right," while others are condemned as "wrong" for the family. Children are taught that by giving up their immediate desire for complete freedom of action for themselves, they gain long-term security and the caring protection of the family environment for the benefit of all.

    b) Ethics are based on a common human understanding of the need for a specific standard of conduct, as well as a deeply felt desire to follow the standard. Ethics function as a system of strongly held values for groups or individuals.

2. Outdoor ethics

    Outdoor ethics is a holistic term that encompasses four distinct relationships that are affected by the behavior of the outdoor user (Matthews and Riley 1995). These relationships are closely linked to the concept of expedition behavior. Outdoor ethics guide behavior in four distinct areas (backpacking has been used here as the example activity to help define the relationships):

    a) Our behavior toward the environment: Does the backpacker hike down the middle of a muddy trail rather than widening it and causing additional damage to the natural environment?

    b) Our behavior toward the activity we are engaged in: What is the backpacker's attitude about the activity? Does the backpacker view it as only recreation for self-serving purposes such as boosting one's image to be "cool"? Or, does the backpacker balance self-pleasure with a sense of responsibility?

   c) Our behavior toward others: Does the backpacker observe rules of etiquette when encountering other users?

   d) Our behavior toward ourselves: Does the backpacker put personal safety at risk?

3. Environmental ethics

Environmental ethics form the fundamental building block in the creation of an individual's outdoor ethic. A user's ethical responsibility toward the natural world has significant ramifications. Outdoor recreation use in the United States has increased significantly based on the National Survey on Recreation and the Environment (NSRE). The 1994–95 NSRE is the latest in a series of national surveys that was started in 1960 by the Outdoor Recreation Resources Review Commission. Each time a survey is conducted, results show significant increases in outdoor recreation use. The 1994–95 "survey results show that 94.5 percent of Americans 16 years of age or older participated in at least one of the surveyed forms of outdoor recreation in the 12 months prior to being interviewed. That is almost 19 out of 20 people and approximately 189 million participants nationwide . . . Whether these activities were done for health reasons, as part of a vacation, as daily stress relief, or just for fun, it is apparent that demand for outdoor recreation is high . . ." (Cordell et al. 1999). Walking outdoors, bird-watching, sightseeing, and tent camping in established sites are examples of the most popular outdoor activities found in the survey. An increase in demand results in more impact on our natural environment. The user's ethical orientation has significant influence over the amount and type of user impact experienced by the environment.

   a) As the outdoor user develops and acts on her/his environmental ethic, it is important to understand the philosophical force that drives attitude and behavior. One or a combination of the following five approaches to environmental ethics helps explain the degree to which we value nature and why. They ultimately formulate the reasoning for the choices we make about the natural environment (Matthews and Riley 1995).

      (1) Anthropocentrism (human-centered): Nature must be maintained because it is necessary for humankind's survival. Objects in nature are valued because they benefit humans. The value placed on nature is human-centered, meaning that nature has only "extrinsic" value—value based only on the degree to which humans give it

value. Humans alone are the chosen species and are thus exempt in many ways from the laws of nature. Humans alone are "sacred," and nature is simply a context for survival and quality of survival.

Example 1: This river should be preserved for future generations.

Example 2: It is okay to hunt deer for recreation if the sport promotes healthy social interaction among friends and family.

(2) Theocentrism (God-centered): Our stewardship of and respect for nature is based on the degree to which we view nature and humans as "sacred" and a result of intelligent design by the Creator, regardless of whether one believes nature resulted from "creation," "evolution," or a combination of the two.

Example 1: The wilderness area should be protected because it is the will of the Creator.

Example 2: Wolves should be reintroduced because they are one of God's creatures that have been eradicated by humans.

(3) Sentientism (awareness of pain): Our duty toward natural objects is based on the degrees to which that object experiences pain or pleasure. Typically, the closer the natural object is to human evolution, the more we observe its rights.

Example 1: Hunting deer is cruel because it causes the animal great pain; therefore, it should not be allowed.

Example 2: Forests in the Pacific Northwest should not be cut because it destroys the homes of many sentient creatures.

(4) Biocentrism (life-centered): All living things have rights and deserve moral consideration regardless of their level of consciousness.

Example 1: The earth is a living organism, and altering or destroying nature is morally wrong.

Example 2: Hunting deer is justifiable only if used for subsistence.

(5) Holism (ecosystem-centered): This perspective places the greatest value on maintaining the entire ecosystem. The needs of the system come before the individual needs of any species. This was the perspective that Aldo Leopold took.

Example 1: Logging and fishing should be stopped until the steelhead salmon can recover and repopulate this river.

Example 2: Deer must be hunted to help maintain the natural balance since the natural predators have been eradicated.

4. Land ethic

The "land ethic" developed by Aldo Leopold is one of the most popular and influential environmental ethics of modern times.

  a) Those who value wilderness and the wilderness experience extend the notion of community to include the land and other life forms. The "land ethic" asserts "a thing is right when it tends to preserve the integrity, stability, and beauty of the biotic community. It is wrong when it tends to do otherwise" (Leopold 1966, p. 222). ". . . A land ethic changes the role of Homo sapiens from conqueror of the land community to plain member and citizen of it. It implies respect for his fellow-members, and also respect for the community as such" (Leopold 1966, p. 204).

  b) Implications of the "land ethic":

    (1) As professional wilderness education practitioners:

      (a) Professional ethics are a code of conduct governing the actions of those working in a particular field of employment. Professional ethics are designed to encourage a standard level of acceptable performance by practitioners.

      (b) Professional ethics benefit clients by providing them a standard by which to evaluate the performance of individual practitioners. They allow the public to have a general level of confidence in the integrity of the profession.

      (c) Professional ethics benefit practitioners by providing them with established standards that can serve as guidelines during times of difficult decision making. They help individual practitioners to know what other professionals in the field would do in a similar situation if faced with similar circumstances.

    (2) As members of our local community:

      (a) Does our behavior as individuals and as a family make a difference with regard to the quality of life in our community?

      (b) Should our belief in the "land ethic" influence our individual and family behavior in our home community?

      (c) Does our belief in the "land ethic" imply a responsibility to educate or influence others in our community to share our belief?

      (d) Does our belief in the "land ethic" imply a responsibility to influence community decision making insofar as it impacts upon the land?

(3) As members of our nations/states:
    (a) Does our behavior as citizens of our state or nation make a difference with regard to the quality of life in either?
    (b) Should our belief in the "land ethic" influence our behavior as citizens of our state and nation?
    (c) Does our belief in the "land ethic" imply a responsibility to act politically to influence state and national policies that have an impact on the land?

(4) As humans on this planet:
    (a) Does our behavior as human beings on this planet make a difference with regard to the quality of life on it?
    (b) Should our belief in the "land ethic" influence our behavior as it relates to all other living things on the planet?
    (c) As a result of this discussion, can students articulate their interpretation of universal principles?

5. Applying the "land ethic"

What are acceptable guidelines for contemporary uses of the natural environment?

a) Based on raised public awareness and a need for user education, codes of ethics have been developed by numerous professional organizations to provide a socially acceptable guideline of behavior for outdoor enthusiasts. Examples of ethical codes include:

(1) Mountain biking ethics developed by the International Mountain Biking Association
(2) Policy statements on climbing ethics developed by the Access Fund
(3) Caving ethics developed by the National Speleological Society
(4) International white-water safety ethics developed by the American Whitewater Affiliation
(5) Outdoor user ethics developed by Leave No Trace

6. Leave No Trace

a) A national code of outdoor ethics emerges.

One of the most popular and influential movements within recent years has been the development of the "Leave No Trace" ethic. Leave No Trace Center for Outdoor Ethics (LNT) is a nonprofit association located in Boulder, Colorado. Their mission is to promote and inspire responsible outdoor recreation through education, research, and partnerships. LNT was developed in the 1990s through a cooperative venture between the U.S.D.A. Forest Service and the National Outdoor Leadership School

(NOLS). The following code of ethics represents state-of-the-art knowledge and attitudes for all outdoor users to follow.

Keep in mind that these principles need to be adapted to various environments and activities. Contact Leave No Trace (www.lnt.org; 800-332-4100) for specific information about the environment and activities you participate in.

Applying the LNT ethics: Simply sharing the seven principles is the first step. However, outdoor leaders also need to understand the "whys" of each principle. For example, to know to camp 200 feet from water is not enough. Outdoor leaders must understand why this number was chosen and the biological and ecological principles that dictate the appropriate distance from a campsite to water. It is recommended that outdoor leaders become trained through LNT Trainer Programs and Master Trainer Courses.

b) Principles of Leave No Trace outdoor ethics
    (1) Plan ahead and prepare
        (a) Know the regulations and special concerns for the area you'll visit.
        (b) Prepare for extreme weather, hazards, and emergencies.
        (c) Schedule your trip to avoid times of high use.
        (d) Visit in small groups. Split larger parties into groups of four to six.
        (e) Repackage food to minimize waste.
        (f) Use a map and compass to eliminate the use of marking paint, rock cairns, or flagging.
    (2) Travel and camp on durable surfaces
        (a) Durable surfaces include established trails and campsites, rock, gravel, dry grasses or snow.
        (b) Protect riparian areas by camping at least 200 feet from lakes and streams.
        (c) Good campsites are found, not made. Altering a site is not necessary.
        (d) In popular areas:
            i) Concentrate use on existing trails and campsites
            ii) Walk single file in the middle of the trail, even when wet or muddy
            iii) Keep campsites small, focusing activity in areas where vegetation is absent

(e) In pristine areas:
- i) Disperse use to prevent the creation of campsites and trails
- ii) Avoid places where impacts are just beginning

(3) Dispose of waste properly
- (a) Pack it in, pack it out. Inspect your campsite and rest areas for trash or spilled foods. Pack out all trash, leftover food, and litter.
- (b) Deposit solid human waste in catholes dug 6 to 8 inches deep at least 200 feet from water, camp, and trails. Cover and disguise the cathole when finished.
- (c) Pack out toilet paper and hygiene products.
- (d) To wash yourself or your dishes, carry water 200 feet away from streams or lakes and use small amounts of biodegradable soap. Scatter strained dishwater.

(4) Leave what you find
- (a) Preserve the past: examine, but do not touch, cultural or historic structures and artifacts.
- (b) Leave rocks, plants, and other natural objects as you find them.
- (c) Avoid introducing or transporting nonnative species.
- (d) Do not build structures, furniture, or dig trenches.

(5) Minimize campfire impacts
- (a) Campfires can cause lasting impacts to the backcountry. Use a lightweight stove for cooking and enjoy a candle lantern for light.
- (b) Where fires are permitted, use established fire rings, fire pans, or mound fires.
- (c) Keep fires small. Only use sticks from the ground that can be broken by hand.
- (d) Burn all wood and coals to ash, put out campfires completely, and then scatter cool ashes.

(6) Respect wildlife
- (a) Observe wildlife from a distance. Do not follow or approach them.
- (b) Never feed animals. Feeding wildlife damages their health, alters natural behaviors, and exposes them to predators and other dangers.

(c) Protect wildlife and your food by storing rations and trash securely.

(d) Control pets at all times, or leave them at home.

(e) Avoid wildlife during sensitive times: mating, nesting, raising young, or winter.

(7) Be considerate of other visitors

(a) Respect other visitors and protect the quality of their experience.

(b) Be courteous. Yield to other users on the trail.

(c) Step to the downhill side of the trail when encountering pack stock.

(d) Take breaks and camp away from trails and other visitors.

(e) Let nature's sounds prevail. Avoid loud voices and noises.

B. Creating content during an educational experience to foster ethical development

The majority of content on outdoor and environmental ethics should be generated from participants reflecting on their wilderness experiences. The range of potential topics for discussion is endless. The following outline is therefore presented in a question/answer format designed to generate discussion. (See fig. 11.1 for a schematic representation of this approach.)

1. Observation/recognition

a) What kinds of backcountry conservation behavior have we observed while on this trip? Participants should be encouraged to note the full range of behavior they have seen.

b) Discussion leaders might use the following questions to guide discussion through various topics related to backcountry behavior:

(1) What evidence have we seen of human behavior while walking on the trail?

(a) Litter/waste

(b) Tree blazing

(c) Shortcutting of trails across switchbacks

(a) Trail erosion

(e) Trail widening

(f) Visual impact (e.g., large groups of people, bright clothing or equipment colors, lost equipment, etc.)

(g) Audio impact (e.g., groups yelling, radios, telephones)

(h) The absence of these signs

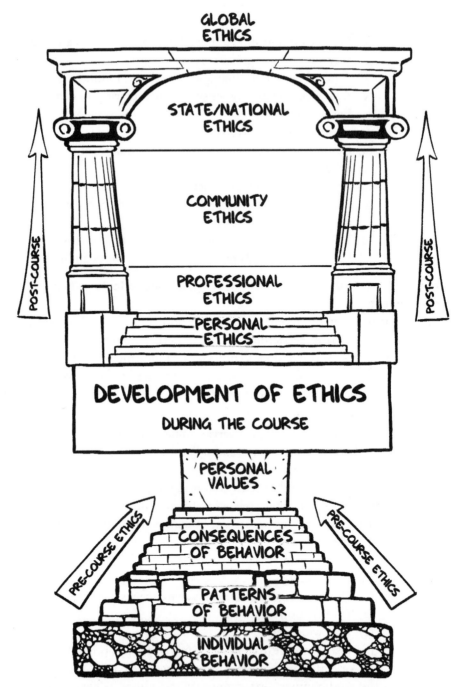

GLOBAL
ETHICS

STATE/NATIONAL
ETHICS

COMMUNITY
ETHICS

POST-COURSE

PROFESSIONAL
ETHICS

PERSONAL
ETHICS

DEVELOPMENT OF ETHICS

DURING THE COURSE

PERSONAL
VALUES

CONSEQUENCES
OF BEHAVIOR

PRE-COURSE ETHICS

PATTERNS
OF BEHAVIOR

INDIVIDUAL
BEHAVIOR

FIGURE 11.1. The lower portion represents development of ethics within oneself. The box containing the words *development of ethics* represents the content of this lesson and its application throughout a wilderness experience. Ideally, participants will start applying these ethics to the "outside" or larger world (i.e., to a broader context). The upper portion represents the application and synthesis of these newly developed ethics.

(2) What evidence have we seen of human behavior in selecting campsites?
   (a) Concentrated destruction of plants and soil surface
   (b) Sites located immediately adjacent to water
   (c) Sites on the trail or in the middle of scenic areas
   (d) Sites too close together
   (e) The absence of these signs
(3) What evidence have we seen of human behavior regarding the use
   of fire?
   (a) Indiscriminate tree cutting or broken branches
   (b) Scorched rocks, roots, and tree trunks
   (c) Multiple fire sites
   (d) Fire sites in inappropriate areas (e.g., summits, canoe
       landings, etc.)
   (e) Visual (e.g., huge bonfires built by others, smoke)
   (f) Fire rings littered with unburned garbage
   (g) The absence of these signs
(4) What evidence have we seen of behavior regarding personal and
   group sanitation and hygiene?
   (a) Toilet paper and human waste
   (b) Soap scum in water
   (c) Food waste on the ground or in the water
   (d) Presence of animals in campsites and on summits
       (looking for food handouts)
   (e) The absence of these signs
(5) What pre- and postexpeditionary behaviors impact the
   environment?
   (a) Intentionally selecting equipment and products for back-
       country expeditions that minimize environmental impact
       in their manufacture or use
   (b) Properly disposing of human waste that is carried out of
       the backcountry
   (b) Repacking food into disposable containers
   (d) Keeping group sizes small
2. Application/analysis
   a) Is there any pattern to the evidence of environmental behaviors that we
      have observed on this trip?
      (1) Yes. Clearly some people have chosen to behave in a way that leaves
          obvious evidence of their presence in the backcountry.

(2) No. Although we can't see the impact of their passing, it is prudent to assume that many people traveled through this area, leaving very little evidence behind.

b) Is the evidence of behaviors that we have observed strictly the result of individual action?

    (1) Yes. Someone either did or did not choose to act in a way that minimized their impact on the environment. Each individual contributes in his or her own way to the conditions we see in the backcountry and to the reputation of the group with which he/she traveled.

    (2) No. Because the collective attitude or behavior of the group is more than the sum of the attitudes or behaviors of its members, individuals will do things both good and bad as a member of a group that they would never think of doing as an individual. The influence of groups can have either positive or negative results for the environment.

c) What are the consequences of these patterns of behavior (i.e., minimizing versus ignoring one's impact on the environment)?

    (1) Behaviors that minimize impact on the environment may result in:

        (a) Preservation of the "natural" character or beauty of an area for an extended period of time or indefinitely (i.e., the aesthetic)

        (b) Preservation of the quality/purity of the natural resources of an area for an extended period of time (i.e., the biological)

        (c) Increase in the capacity of an area to support recreational use for an extended period of time (i.e., the carrying capacity)

    (2) Behaviors that contribute to impact on the environment of an area may result in:

        (a) Rapid deterioration of the "natural character" of an area over a short period of time (i.e., the aesthetic)

        (b) Rapid deterioration of the quality/purity of the natural resources of the area over a short period of time (i.e., the biological)

        (c) Decrease in the capacity of an area to support recreational use in a short period of time (i.e., the carrying capacity)

d) Types of impact actions

    (1) Illegal actions: Any action constituting a violation of regulations

that have been created to implement legislation that designates or protects wilderness lands

 Example: Motorized vehicle use in a wilderness area
(2) Careless actions: Any thoughtless actions that violate protective regulations

 Examples: Use of campfires where prohibited; exceeding party size limits
(3) Unskilled actions: Any harmful actions by wilderness users who lack skills or education

 Examples: Building a fire ring; washing dishes in or near water
(4) Uninformed actions: Any actions that could have been prevented with adequate transfer of information to visitors

 Example: Lack of accessible information about alternate trails and campsites contributes to overuse of some areas
(5) Unavoidable actions: Any impacts caused by human presence in wilderness that cannot be prevented by the utmost degree of carefulness

 Examples: Trail erosion; damage to vegetation in campsites
e) Impact actions and the roles of education and law enforcement:
(1) Illegal actions: Education is unlikely to have a significant positive effect on visitor behavior. People who knowingly do illegal things are rarely influenced by what is "right." These people are more likely to be influenced by the chance of being arrested for their actions. Law enforcement has the highest degree of effectiveness with this behavior.
(2) Careless actions: Education is likely to have some positive effect on visitor behavior. If people can be made aware of their careless actions, they can be influenced to be more careful. Some law enforcement may be necessary, but communication of expectations will usually provide sufficient motivation for most visitors.
(3) Unskilled actions: Education is likely to have a high degree of positive influence on visitor behavior. Once people have the "correct" skill, they are usually proud to exhibit it. Some law enforcement may be necessary, but education is most effective.
(4) Uninformed actions: Education is likely to have the highest degree of positive influence on visitor behavior. Once people are aware of other options and know what is "right," their behavior changes accordingly. Effective communication of information to visitors will likely eliminate the need for law enforcement.

(5) Unavoidable actions: Education is unlikely to have a significant positive effect on visitor behavior in this case. Something that is unavoidable can't be prevented. Limiting use is the most effective way to limit unavoidable impacts.

f) The role of ethics in protecting the natural environment:
(1) There needs to be a certain level of appreciation and concern for the "natural" environment.
(2) The belief in the outdoor ethic has to override the desire for comfort and convenience.
(3) Wilderness travelers need to be constantly aware of and sensitive to the impact of their actions on others.

g) Why do people adopt such patterns of behavior?
(1) Family background
(2) Education and training

h) What is the significance of these patterns?
(1) What can we recognize about those people who do not practice minimum-impact camping techniques?
(a) Some do not know about these techniques.
(b) Some do know of these techniques but will not use them because they are not convinced of their necessity.
(c) Some do know of these techniques but do not use them consistently for a variety of reasons. Many of these people do not consciously consider the consequences of their actions or do not believe that their individual behavior is significant.
(d) Some do not care. They may know that what they are doing is wrong but for various reasons don't care, and they may only change their behavior if they become concerned that they might "get caught."
(e) Some have not moved beyond the self-centered stage of moral development. Some argue that unless people move to an altruistic stage based on principles of justice, fairness, and self-respect, they will not have a motivation to implement ethical practices.
(2) Do the actions of these people tell us anything about their values?
(a) Yes. Their behavior reveals their values (i.e., the ideas, beliefs, or types of behavior that they consider to be most important in guiding their life decisions). These actions tell us that they do not value the wilderness or the wilder-

ness experience, or nature in general, as much as those who do practice minimum-impact techniques.

    (3) What can we know about those people who do practice minimum-impact camping techniques?

        (a) Since the practice of minimum-impact techniques requires a conscious effort, it is safe to assume that these people have chosen to use these techniques for specific reasons.

        (b) It is evident that people using minimum-impact techniques are aware of the consequences of their actions on the wilderness and the wilderness experience. Since their behavior is specifically intended to preserve wilderness and enhance the wilderness experience, it is safe to assume that they value both highly. It is their concern for wilderness that has caused them to consciously restrict their own freedom of action in the backcountry for the sake of preserving it for themselves and others.

III. Instructional Strategies

A. Timing. This topic should be incorporated into all aspects of an outdoor leadership curriculum. As such, it is impossible to deal with the total contents of this topic in the context of a traditional class. All of the issues embraced by this topic must be addressed on a daily basis as the course progresses.

B. Considerations

1. It is important to recognize that the objectives of this "lesson" go well beyond directing participants toward a specific set of backcountry conservation practices. By definition, the development of an environmental ethic suggests that participants will come to adopt a set of values that will be transferable to a variety of situations outside those of the immediate wilderness experience. To this end, instructors must be constantly aware of opportunities to help students recognize the broader implications of their backcountry behavior and assist them in understanding the need to establish a set of personal environmental standards that they can apply broadly to situations in later life.

2. The following sequence is suggested for creating opportunities for instruction/reflection on backcountry ethics and conservation practices:

a) Precourse instruction: Instructors should make a presentation at the opening orientation of the course that identifies specific procedures to be followed in the backcountry and sets the standard for acceptable environmental behavior during the course.

b) Teachable moments: Specific instruction concerning appropriate environmental behavior should be conducted as the opportunity or need arises throughout the course.

c) Modeling: Instructors must consistently model environmentally responsible behavior throughout the entire course.

d) Processing of decision-making experiences: During debriefings, campsite inspections, or in personal journals, participants should be encouraged to reflect upon those decision-making situations in which they have had to make choices regarding environmentally responsible conduct.

e) Formal class on environmental ethics and backcountry conservation practices: This formal class can be conducted using a "traditional" or SPEC (Student-centered, Problem-based, Experiential, Collaborative) approach during the latter third of the course after students have had the chance to experience situations and behaviors that reflect a range of environmental responsibility.

3. Assessment strategies

a) Once the concrete example has been examined, instructors should help participants "process" the experience. Instructors must establish a pattern of dialogue closely resembling that used during a debriefing. In essence, the instructor should strive to help participants move from a recognition of the significance of the specific behavior and its consequences through a discussion of the values that the behavior reveals to reach a general understanding of the need for a standard of environmental ethics. Once the participants understand the concept of personal environmental ethics, a discussion may ensue that explores the implications that such a code of ethics may have for one's behavior as a member of a local community, the state and nation, and, finally, as a citizen of the world.

   The instructor should observe to see that the transition from recognizing immediate circumstances to evaluating universal principles occurs at some point during the course. Instructors should be laying the groundwork for this transition from the very beginning of the trip so participants will have already discussed numerous incidents for the purpose of attaining a higher level of insight.

b) Utilize a personal trip journal to analyze decision making related to minimum-impact practices. Encourage students to analyze personal, peer, instructor, and group decisions on a daily basis. As the trip progresses, the instructor should witness a more sophisticated analysis based on experiences gained throughout the trip.

c) Pretest/posttest perception of attitude/behavior change: At the beginning of the trip, the instructor reads each of the outdoor-ethics principles to the participants in the form of a question:

    (1) Do you or would you take the time to learn the regulations and special concern for areas you visit?

    (2) Do you or would you adequately prepare for emergencies, hazards, and extreme weather?

    (3) Do you or would you schedule your trip to take place during low-use periods?

    (4) Do you or would you . . .

        Have the students record their "yes" or "no" answers in a personal journal. At the trip's end, reread the questions and have the students answer the same questions. Instruct the students to compare their results to the pretest and discuss.

C. Activities

1. An understanding of ethics requires that a participant see a link between individual human action and the broader system of personal values that the action represents. To achieve this understanding, it is often advisable for instructors to begin by directing participant attention to concrete examples of behavior that may bear fruitful examination. Following are a few strategies for initiating this process:

a) Ask participants to describe in detail some incident during the expedition that they think illustrated either a very good or very poor example of environmentally responsible behavior.

b) Ask participants to create a short skit to be shown to the group that illustrates a conflict between responsible and irresponsible environmental behavior.

c) Write up a few short scenarios that involve conflict or choices between practices of varying degrees of environmental responsibility.

d) Create and then read an open-ended story in which a choice must be made between responsible and irresponsible environmental behavior. Ask students to role-play a resolution to the problem in front of the group.

Example: A group of ten has backpacked all day in challenging terrain. It is about fifteen minutes before dark when they reach their intended destination. They find themselves in a small, pristine alpine meadow with steep slopes on all sides. A rainstorm seems to be blowing in, and the group is physically tired and hungry. A quick look at the map reveals a potentially more appropriate campsite 2 miles up the trail. What should they do?

e) Create an impact identification list for discussion. While in a heavy use area, divide the students into small groups. Instruct the groups to carefully survey the area and record all observable impacts caused by recreation users. Once the survey is complete, have students discuss their findings.

2. See the Leave No Trace Jingle challenge at the end of this chapter.

Challenge

Knowledge Outcome	Title	Skill/Disposition Outcome
What do you want them to know?		**What skill/disposition do you want them to develop?**
Environmental ethics: The participants can accurately describe and interpret Leave No Trace principles.	Leave No Trace Jingle	Decision making: brainstorms several different options

Essential Question or Key Issue:

How might the principles of the Leave No Trace (LNT) program be applied in a specific region/environment?

Description of Challenge/Task/Performance:

You have been hired by a Madison Avenue advertising firm to popularize the LNT message. They want you to develop a catchy and creative jingle that communicates the essence of the seven principles of the LNT approach as it applies to the area through which you are traveling. If they like your jingle, it will be broadcast across your radio listening region, and your entire group will receive a tuition waiver for next semester (only redeemable on February 30th!).

Be prepared to share your jingle with the other groups and explain how its contents reflect LNT principles. You will be expected to submit one legible copy of the jingle to your instructor. Please include the names of all group members on this copy.

You have _____ minutes to prepare your jingle.

Criteria for Assessment and Feedback:

Form criteria:
- The jingle is prepared within allotted time frame.
- A copy of the jingle with names of group members is submitted to the instructor.
- The jingle has lyrics that are easy to memorize.
- The jingle has a tune that can be hummed or whistled easily.
- The jingle is short: less than one minute in length.

Content criteria:
- The information communicated in the jingle is accurate.
- The jingle faithfully communicates the essence of the seven LNT principles.
- The information in the jingle is appropriate to a specific region.

Knowledge:
- Participants can accurately describe and interpret LNT principles.
- Team members can convincingly describe the connections between the message of the jingle and the LNT principles.

Skill: Decision making: Team members brainstorm several different options.
- Instructors hear group members discussing several possible versions of lyrics/tune for jingle.

Developed by Leading EDGE, LLC for **The Backcountry Classroom.** *For more information log on to www.realworldlearning.info.*

Product Quality Checklist

Date: _____   Class Period: _____

Product Author(s):	Product Title/Name: Leave No Trace Jingle	Evaluator Name(s):

Observed	Standard/Criteria	Possible Points	Rating
	The jingle is prepared within allotted time frame.		
	A copy of the jingle with names of group members is submitted to the instructor.		
	The jingle has lyrics that are easy to memorize.		
	The jingle has a tune that can be hummed or whistled easily.		
	The jingle is short: less than one minute in length.		
	The information communicated in the jingle is accurate.		
	The jingle faithfully communicates the essence of the seven LNT principles.		
	The information in the jingle is appropriate to a specific region.		
	Total		

Observations:

Elements of Questionable Quality:	**Elements of Exceptional Quality:**

CHAPTER TWELVE

Expedition Behavior

I: Outcomes

A. Outdoor leaders provide evidence of their *knowledge* and *understanding* by:

1. Describing the importance of good expedition behavior (EB)
2. Describing the relationship of expedition behavior to the success of an expedition
3. Explaining the interrelationships relevant to expedition behavior
4. Explaining how to communicate effectively to reduce or resolve conflicts
5. Describing the value of effective communication

B. Outdoor leaders provide evidence of their *skill* by:

1. Practicing good expedition behavior
2. Maintaining appropriate relations with all the stakeholders associated with backcountry travel
3. Setting the appropriate tone both prior to and during backcountry travel
4. Demonstrating good communication skills, including: appropriate body language, effective listening skills, empathy, giving and receiving of feedback, and effective management of conflict

C. Outdoor leaders provide evidence of their *dispositions* by:

1. Modeling appropriate expedition behavior
2. Being good listeners and communicators
3. Resolving conflicts in an effective manner

II. Content

A. Good expedition behavior is just one of four critical areas that lead to a successful expedition. The four critical areas are:

1. Proper pretrip planning
2. Good expedition behavior
3. Good leadership and quality decision-making skills
4. Competent, technical outdoor skills

B. Definition

1. "Good expedition behavior is an awareness of the relationships . . . which exist in the out-of-doors plus the motivation and character to be as concerned for others as one is for oneself" (Petzoldt 1984, p. 168).
2. Another definition of good expedition behavior comes from the *NOLS Wilderness Educator Notebook:* "Good EB means being a nice, helpful person; doing your share of the work; dealing with conflicts when they occur. The goal of good EB is to work well together, not to necessarily become good friends" (National Outdoor Leadership School 1999, p. 4-3).
3. Poor expedition behavior is characterized by "a breakdown in human relations caused by selfishness, rationalization, ignorance of personal faults, dodging blame or responsibility, physical weakness, and, in extreme cases, not being able to risk one's own survival to insure that of a companion" (Petzoldt 1984, p. 168).

C. Consequences of poor expedition behavior

1. Group members won't enjoy the expedition
2. Group objectives won't be met
3. Friendships may be lost
4. Individual or group safety may be compromised
5. The natural environment may be compromised

D. Promoting good expedition behavior

1. Setting the tone: Setting a tone before a trip starts is critical to the success of a trip.
   a) The key to setting a tone is communication. One must communicate many things, including those listed below. The following is adapted from correspondence received by members of a 1971 expedition up Mount McKinley (Petzoldt 1984):
      (1) The group objectives: There must be an understanding of and consensus on the group goals and objectives. It is important to agree

on the priorities and what will happen if the objectives cannot be met.

(2) Expectations: How group members can expect the trip to be conducted. These things might be considered "trip policy."
For example:

   (a) Hiking: Learn to hike using rhythmic breathing to prevent fatigue and exhaustion.

   (b) Short days: Everyone will go slowly to acclimatize and prevent exhaustion. Camp will be set up early to allow time for healthy, nutritious meals.

   (c) Eat well: Realize that diet affects attitude as well as strength.

   (d) Work load: Everyone does not have to do the same amount of work. Individuals should work to their capabilities. Work hard on good days, do less on others.

   (e) Sun: Watch out for the sun—it drains energy, and sunburn can be crippling.

   (f) Control body temperature: Try not to be too hot or too cold. Do what is necessary to keep the body temperature constant.

   (g) Water: Drink lots of liquids. Consequences arising from water loss can be extreme, and it must be replaced.

   (h) Sleep well: Being well rested contributes to getting along well with others.

(3) Additional policies or norms may need to be determined relating to things such as:

   (a) Feelings towards others

   (b) Respecting opinions

   (c) Proselytizing

   (d) Relations between participants

   (e) Relations between staff

   (f) Relations between staff and participants

   (g) Nudity

   (h) Sexist attitudes

2. Individual contributions to good expedition behavior: As individuals, we contribute to good expedition behavior by keeping the following in mind:

a) Be tolerant and considerate of others

b) Maintain good personal hygiene practices, important for:

   (1) Good health

      (2) Aesthetics (who wants to look at someone with granola and raisins in between their teeth?)

    c) Don't take offense

    d) Maintain a "cowlike" attitude—be laid back, have fun, don't let things become a hassle, etc.

    e) Switch tent partners if there is no way to get along

E. Expedition behavior interrelationships

1. Individual to individual: This relationship is personified by tent partners, but it exists between every individual in the group. Getting along with individuals can be accomplished by using the guidelines above.

2. Individual to group: The responsibility the individual has to be part of the group:

    a) Be organized but not compulsive

    b) Be reasonably clean and neat

    c) Be conscious of offensive and annoying habits

    d) Be cooperative

    e) Avoid dangerous activities

    f) Take part in group activities

    g) Be honest about personal needs (e.g., stop the group to take care of a blister)

3. Group to individual: The responsibility the group has to each individual. The group must accept each individual as a member of the group and keep from either ganging up on an individual or holding grudges against an individual.

4. Group to group

    a) Groups have a responsibility to respect each other. When encountering other groups, it is best to be courteous but leave the group to its own privacy. Except in an emergency, it is best not to impose on other groups (e.g., borrowing or using food or equipment).

    b) Be aware that your group is also made up of small groups (e.g., tent groups, cook groups, canoe pairs, rope teams). Be courteous of other groups within your larger group.

        Examples: Share food and equipment among cook groups as appropriate; share the ideal campsites instead of always trying to be the first into camp and scurrying to find the best site.

    c) When encountering uneducated campers who are doing unsafe or harmful things to the environment, one must use tact and a soft-sell educational approach. If an approach of aggressiveness or arrogance is used, the objective of changing their behavior may be negated; they may resent being told what to do by strangers.

5. Individual and group to multiple users: Understanding and accepting that everyone has a right to use the out-of-doors within the limitations of the law is an important concept. Just because a group does not like a certain outdoor activity does not mean that the activity shouldn't be allowed. Respect of all user groups will contribute to a better understanding of outdoor users and promote good public relations between groups.

6. Individual and group to administrative agencies: Understanding and respecting administrative agencies and their representatives contribute to good relations. Administrative representatives are generally hard-working professionals working for underfunded agencies. Their jobs are made easier when groups cooperate and work with them.
   a) Obey rules and regulations. Don't ask for special favors that must be denied.
   b) Be courteous and cooperative when encountering rangers and other administrative representatives in the field.
   c) Sign in and out at registration locations as appropriate.
   d) Do not expect field representatives to know everything about the out-of-doors or the areas for which they are responsible. Employees of administrative agencies may not be trained in the outdoors and are frequently transferred, providing little time to become experts in new geographic areas.

7. Individual and group to the local populace: Local residents of popular outdoor recreation areas often see visiting outdoor users as overeducated urban intruders. They sometimes feel politically threatened by these outsiders. Every effort should be made by outdoor users to understand their point of view and try to be cooperative and respectful.

F. Communication skills. Effective communication is essential for any successful expedition. The purpose of communication is to share, reach an understanding, resolve a conflict, or make a decision. It may be formal or informal, with short- or long-term goals (Brill 1998). Communication skills can be broken down into body language, listening skills, empathy, and prompts and probes (Egan 1990):

1. Body language
   a) Being aware of the message we convey with our body language and being able to read the body language of others is critical to effective communication.
   b) Research indicates that our body language and the tone of our voice

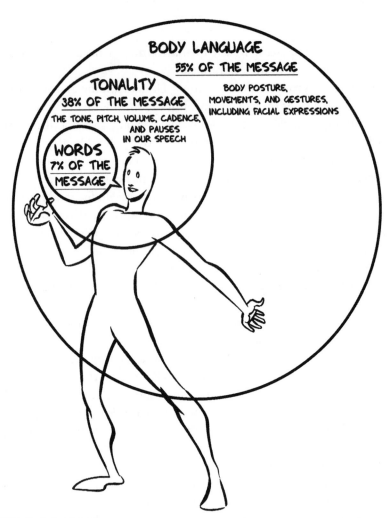

FIGURE 12.1. Body Language

contribute to approximately 93 percent of the understanding of the message we are attempting to communicate.

(1) Words: Although one might think that the words would make up the essence of our message, in reality they only make up 7 percent of what we are trying to say.

(2) Tonality: The tone, pitch, volume, cadence, and the pauses in our speech make up approximately 38 percent of our intended message.

(3) Body language: Our bodily postures, movements, and gestures, including facial expressions, make up approximately 55 percent of our intended message.

c) Using our body language effectively requires us to be sincere in our actions. Otherwise, these actions can be interpreted as "acting."

d) ROLES is an acronym for five specific behaviors:

    (1) Relaxed body posture without fidgeting

    (2) Open posture without crossed arms and legs

    (3) Lean toward the other person

    (4) Eye contact is important to maintain

    (5) Squarely face the person, as opposed to turning away

e) Other nonverbals include:

    (1) Bodily postures, movements, and gestures

    (2) Facial expressions, such as smiles or frowns

    (3) Voice tone, pitch, volume, cadence, and pauses

2. Listening skills

a) Good listeners find ways to confirm that they understand what the speaker is saying. Listeners subtly indicate this by their body language and confirm it by echoing or mirroring (paraphrasing) what they heard (e.g., "I think I understand you to be saying . . . Is that correct?").

b) Listening is an active process in which one attends to others, focuses on verbal and nonverbal messages, and asks questions or makes statements that are intended to clarify what others are saying. In this way, you can look for such things as:

    (1) The speaker's point of view

    (2) The main themes or points that the speaker is making

    (3) Any exaggerations, contradictions, or omissions in the speaker's story

c) Good listeners not only pay attention to their own nonverbal behavior, they are also aware of the speaker's behavior, which includes the items in the previous section, as well as:

    (1) Physiological responses of the speaker, including rapid breathing, blushing, paleness, and pupil dilation

    (2) Appearance, in terms of clothing, hygiene, etc.

    (3) Physical characteristics, including conditioning, stature, hair and eye color, etc.

d) Good listeners are attuned to what others say about their experiences, behaviors, thoughts, and feelings. For example, someone might say: "While we were on the trail this morning [experience], I began singing [behavior] as I experienced the grandeur [feeling] of the terrain. This kind of trip is really good for me [thought/belief]."

3. Empathy
   a) Empathy is a skill that lets us communicate our understanding of others.
      (1) It starts by listening to others.
      (2) It progresses by trying to understand the experiences, behaviors, feelings, and beliefs of others.
      (3) It is important to share your understanding with others.
      (4) It is not necessary for the listener to have the same experience in order to empathize. For example, an individual feels fear after a long white-water swim and is struggling to reenter the kayak. You have never taken a similar swim, but you can relate to the basic emotion of fear and the associated feelings.
   b) Empathic responding involves:
      (1) Sorting out the underlying message of the speaker by focusing on both the content of the message and the speaker's affect
      (2) Checking out the accuracy of your understanding by echoing or mirroring (paraphrasing or summarizing what you are hearing)
      (3) Asking questions to make sure you are on track
      (4) Using nods, eye contact, and other nonverbals to express understanding
4. Prompts and probes
   a) Prompts are verbal or nonverbal cues that encourage others to talk. For example, an interested look paired with silence might lead a speaker to continue talking about a subject.
   b) Probes are verbal questions that are used to elicit more specific information about others' experiences, beliefs, or feelings. An example of a probe during a debriefing of a morning's hike would be: "So, how were you feeling on the trail today?"
   c) Guidelines for the use of probes to help others open up (Egan 1990):
      (1) Don't overwhelm the speaker with too many questions
      (2) Ask questions that get at specific information that is useful
      (3) Ask open-ended questions
      (4) Focus your questions on the speaker, not others
      (5) When the speaker begins to talk, use empathy skills to keep the flow going

G. Feedback. A special form of communication concerns giving and receiving feedback. Being skilled at these is especially important for good expedition behavior since, on an expedition, our behavior inherently influences others and their behavior influences us.

1. Purpose of feedback
   a) Feedback provides recipients with information about the outcome of their behavior—how it affects us, how effective it has been to accomplish a certain goal, etc.
   b) Feedback can also motivate others by reinforcing selected behaviors and ignoring others.
   c) An effective model for giving and receiving feedback, commonly used in leadership development courses, occurs during a daily debriefing when there is a group discussion of individual leadership roles.
2. Giving feedback
   a) Make your comments specific. Talk about the person's behavior, not his or her motives or personality.
   b) Use the communication skills mentioned above, such as facing the recipient of your feedback and using good eye contact.
   c) First tell him what you like about what he did. This starts off your feedback on a positive note; to do otherwise may make receiving feedback an aversive experience.
   d) In doing so, start off your feedback using an "I" statement in which you use your experience and feelings as the basis for what you say. Speak for yourself, not others.
   e) Tell the person what you would like her to do—constructive criticism—rather than saying what you don't like. This form of feedback is easier to receive. Be honest, but try to be kind. Feedback should be given with a caring attitude.
   f) Do not overload the recipient with too much information.
   g) Timing: Give feedback when the person is in the "right frame of mind" and is ready to listen (e.g., at group debriefing).
3. Receiving feedback
   a) Receiving feedback is an active process, not a passive process of just listening.
   b) As with giving feedback, try to use good communication skills. Remember the verbal and nonverbal skills in section F.
   c) Try not to be defensive. Try to receive the feedback as a gift or an opportunity for growth.
   d) Try to limit your response to "thank you" rather than defending your actions. This allows time for the emotional impact of the feedback to subside so you can reflect on the feedback itself.
   e) Make sure that you understand the constructive feedback you are receiving. If you are not sure, use the prompts and probes discussed earlier to clarify the message.

f) Use your journal to summarize the feedback you received and to reflect on what, if anything, you plan to change.

g) After reflecting on the feedback, decide whether or not you want to make an action plan regarding what you want to change. Include a date when you will review your success in making changes.

h) Consider going back to a specific individual or the group at a later date to get feedback on how well you've made changes.

i) It is ultimately the right of the receiver to accept feedback. Keep in mind that the message is a matter of perception, and it might not always be accurate. Honesty with the self is key.

H. Conflict and its resolution. Conflict is a natural outgrowth of living with and having a relationship with others. How do you know when there is a problem that needs to be confronted? Often it is by identifying negative feelings that you have—for example, frustration, anger, or betrayal. It's best to resolve these conflicts as early as possible so that small problems don't escalate into big ones. You may know that you are overdue to confront conflict when you realize that, even if a confrontation provokes anger, you won't be any more miserable with the person being angry with you than you already are. Here is an outline of a general series of steps leading to the resolution of conflicts:

1. Identify your feelings. If they are negative, sort out the situation in which they are occurring. Then decide if this is a situation you can live with.

2. If you can't live comfortably with the situation, determine the other person(s) involved and talk to that person individually, separate from the group. The goal here is to keep this a private matter and nip the problem in the bud.

3. Apply strategies for giving and receiving feedback. In particular, start off your conversation with the other person using an "I" statement. A convenient aid to approaching others is to complete the following sentence: "I feel _____ when you _____. What I would like you to do is _____."

4. Apply effective communication skills as outlined above. Listen to what the other person is saying. If something is unclear, echoing or mirroring will help bring clarification.

5. Look for "win-win" solutions; that is, ways in which both people's needs are met.

6. Try to communicate your desire to cooperate and negotiate with openness to brainstorming.

7. If you can find a solution, make sure you both agree on the particulars of how the plan will be implemented.

8. Follow up this conversation at a later time to check in with the person, making sure that the conflict is resolved.
9. If you can't work out the issues directly with the other person, take the issue to the group discussion. Avoid talking behind the other person's back. A good way of taking issues to the group is, again, with an "I" statement.

III. Instructional Strategies

A. Timing. This class should be taught shortly after the group starts to meet and have discussions. The earlier this is done, the sooner the participants will practice effective communication skills, be aware of EB interrelationships, and better understand the essential role that good communication plays in successful expeditions.

It is important that the instructor integrate the skills into group debriefings by modeling and encouraging group members to use "I" statements, focus on behavior instead of personality, listen effectively, etc. By guiding the group through debriefing sessions (rewarding good technique and appropriately correcting poor technique), individuals will eventually integrate the skills as normal group behavior. It is particularly important that the instructor model the use of effective communication techniques.

B. Considerations. This class should be taught in a circular, group setting. It can be taught in one session or broken down into components to fit the time needs of the group.

1. Role playing is an excellent way to introduce the seven interrelationships of EB. Break the larger group into smaller groups and assign them each a role. The smaller groups create a scenario that portrays the relationship.
2. One way of teaching communication concepts is to formally go through the steps outlined above, but in an abbreviated fashion. For example, participants can provide feedback to each other (thereby practicing those skills) regarding the effectiveness of their nonverbals using the acronym ROLES.
3. Later, conflict-resolution skills can be solidified through a role play in which participants try to resolve common conflicts that are likely to occur. After the role play, a debriefing can include the following questions:
   a) Was the conflict introduced with an "I" statement of feelings?
   b) Did the person introducing the conflict statement do so in a nonthreatening way, in an atmosphere of openness and cooperation?
   c) Did the participants try to reach a "win-win" solution?
4. Assessment strategies: Communication is effective when each person has

been able to share feelings or thoughts with others. Assessing this component of communication can be accomplished by having participants get into groups of three where one person communicates a feeling, belief, or experience; another participant is the active listener; and the third, the observer. The listener should be able to accurately summarize what the speaker said, along with being able to identify the speaker's feelings and/or beliefs. The accuracy of this reflection is to be evaluated by the speaker.

The listener and observer are in the best position to provide feedback to the speaker regarding how well experiences, feelings, or beliefs were conveyed. The observer should note the use of nonverbals by both speaker and listeners, giving each one feedback about ROLES. Once this is accomplished, a new speaker, listener, and observer should be chosen within this triad. This process should continue until each person has been in all three positions.

At a more advanced level, this exercise can be altered so that the speaker and listener take a different position on the same topic (e.g., the best time for the group to break camp in the morning). The goal would be to resolve the conflict. In addition to the evaluation criteria listed above, this activity can be assessed by the extent to which the pair has been able to reach a mutually satisfying resolution.

C. Activities

1. See the Expedition Behavior: "Freeze Frame" challenge at the end of the chapter.

2. Moo Cow story: When preparing to discuss receiving feedback, we often tell the Moo Cow story to reinforce the idea that feedback is just information. The receiver of the information gets to determine the value of the information and whether he or she wants to act on the information. The story goes like this:

   When you see a cow out in a field, she is eating grass and nothing seems to be bothering her. The cow eating grass is like a person receiving feedback. She takes the grass in and it goes into the first stomach, and she gets nourishment from the grass that allows her to stay healthy, grow, and produce milk. Some of the grass then goes into the next stomach, where she gets additional nourishment for her health. This goes on with the third and fourth stomachs. People receive feedback and digest it like the cow digests the grass. Some of it is nourishing and allows us to grow and become a better person. But just as some of the grass is not nourishing to the cow and comes out leaving a "cow pie," some feedback is not nourishing, and we have to learn to discard it. Only the receiver of the feedback can determine whether it is nourishing or whether it is a "cow pie."

Challenge

Knowledge Outcome	Title	Skill/Disposition Outcome
What do you want them to know? The participants can describe the different relationships involving expedition behavior and list ways to promote positive behavior in each.	Expedition Behavior: "Freeze Frame"	**What skill/disposition do you want them to develop?** Leadership: creatively seeks alternative, original, and imaginative ideas/solutions

Essential Question or Key Issue:

How can we promote positive expedition behavior in each of the relationships important to the success of an expedition?

Description of Challenge/Task/Performance:

With the assistance of your teacher/instructor, brainstorm a list of situations (e.g., neat versus untidy tent partners, overbearing leadership style, crude or insensitive comments toward other multiple users, chauvinistic male behavior toward female environmental officer, etc.) encountered on a backcountry trip that typically lead to friction within each of the most important relationship areas. Create small teams. Each of the teams should select (or draw randomly) a different backcountry situation (such as those cited previously) to explore through a role play.

In your small team, create a role play of one or two minutes that reveals the evolution of a conflict within the context of the relationship and situation you've chosen/drawn. Perform the role play to the point where both the characteristics of the relationship and the specific issues of the conflict are obvious. Then "freeze frame" the role play. Engage the audience in a discussion wherein you:
- Clearly describe the characteristics of both parties in the relationship
- Analyze the process by which the parties came into conflict
- Suggest specific strategies for promoting positive expedition behavior within the relationship so that conflict does not arise so easily in the future

Following the discussion, the team that authored the role play may choose to act out a resolution to the conflict.

Criteria for Assessment and Feedback:

Form criteria:
- The role play has a story to tell. The plot line is obvious as it relates to the relationship and conflict depicted.
- The actors portray their characters convincingly.
- The actors stay in character throughout the skit.
- The actors "freeze frame" the role play when appropriate and conduct a discussion.

Content criteria:
- The role play accurately depicts the characteristics of the selected expeditionary relationship and conflict situation.
- The discussion focuses on the characteristics of each party in the relationship and how the conflict evolves between them.
- The discussion identifies some specific strategies for encouraging positive expedition behavior that may prevent future conflict.

Knowledge:
- Participants can describe/depict the characteristics of each of the expeditionary relationships.
- The audience and group members can accurately describe the characteristics of each party in the relationship and identify the circumstances that brought about conflict.

Skill: Leadership: creatively seeks alternative, original, and imaginative ideas/solutions
- During preparation for the role play, each group member offers at least one original idea for the plot of the role play.
- Each group member offers an idea different from others regarding ways to promote positive expedition behavior and thereby forestall conflict.

Product Quality Checklist

Date: _____   Class Period: _____

Product Author(s):	Product Title/Name:	Evaluator Name(s):
	Expedition Behavior: "Freeze Frame"	

Observed	Standard/Criteria	Possible Points	Rating
	The role play has a story to tell. The plot line is obvious as it relates to the relationship and conflict depicted.		
	The actors portray their characters convincingly.		
	The actors stay in character throughout the role play.		
	The actors "freeze frame" the role play when appropriate and conduct a discussion.		
	The role play accurately depicts the characteristics of the selected expeditionary relationship and conflict situation.		
	The discussion focuses on the characteristics of each party to the relationship and how the conflict evolves among them.		
	The discussion identifies some specific strategies for encouraging positive expedition behavior that may prevent future conflict.		
	Total		

Observations:

Elements of Questionable Quality:	Elements of Exceptional Quality:

CHAPTER THIRTEEN

Fire Site Preparation and Care

I. Outcomes

A. Outdoor leaders provide evidence of their *knowledge* and *understanding* by:

1. Describing considerations in determining whether to have a campfire or use a stove
2. Describing considerations in selecting a fire site
3. Comparing and critiquing various functions of fires
4. Describing soil types and their importance in selecting a fire site
5. Describing general fire safety considerations
6. Comparing and critiquing various sites used to build fires
7. Describing considerations in restoring a site to a natural condition

B. Outdoor leaders provide evidence of their *skill* by:

1. Selecting and creating a fire site with concern for safety and the environment
2. Restoring a fire site to a natural condition

C. Outdoor leaders provide evidence of their *dispositions* by:

1. Making decisions about the use of fires based on safety and environmental concerns rather than on the desire for a campfire
2. Using fires only when its clearly safe and environmentally acceptable

II. Content

A. Environmental considerations

1. Considerations in using a fire rather than a stove
   a) Fires should only be used when:
      (1) There is a safe location for a fire
      (2) There is little or no potential for adverse environmental impact
      (3) There is an ample supply of dead wood on the ground
      (4) Wood used will be naturally replenished within a reasonable time
      (5) No tools, such as an axe, hatchet, or saw, are necessary to acquire firewood
      (6) Group members have the skill to build a campfire that will meet outdoor-ethics guidelines
      (7) Rules and regulations permit them
   b) Except in an emergency, fires should be considered luxuries and not true necessities.
2. Site-selection considerations
   a) A site may be suitable if it:
      (1) Has an existing safe fireplace, in which case it should be used
      (2) Is pristine and shows little or no sign of human use
      (3) Has little chance of being used again before it has a chance to recover
      (4) Is heavily impacted and use will not appreciably impact it more
   b) Locations to avoid include:
      (1) Low-impact campsites that, with increased use, might become high-impact campsites
      (2) Biologically sensitive areas, such as those with many roots or easily damaged vegetation
      (3) Areas with waterlogged or large rocks that may explode or be blackened by the fire

B. Rationale for fires. Fires play a special role in the history of humans as well as the history of modern wilderness travel. Fires play a role in both function and aesthetics. Although the negative impacts of fire are numerous, fires can be used in many areas as long as good judgment prevails.

C. Functions of fires. These functions are listed by priority from highest to lowest. As environmental concerns increase, the function of the fire must be of a higher priority to justify its use.

1. Heat for emergency warmth and drying
    a) In an emergency situation, a fire could be a lifesaver.
    b) In most cases, however, proper clothing and equipment along with proper nutrition will provide adequate warmth and preclude the need for a fire.
2. Food preparation: This is a traditional and valid purpose for a fire, assuming environmental conditions permit.
3. Aesthetic/psychological appeal: This is another traditional purpose for a fire. Environmental concerns in many parts of North America negate justification for fires based purely on aesthetic grounds.
4. Heat for general warmth and drying
    a) Although heat is a pleasant by-product of a fire built for cooking or pleasure, it is difficult to justify it for warmth alone.
    b) For comfort and warmth when traveling in the backcountry, proper clothing, equipment, and good nutrition offer a sounder alternative to fires.

D. Soils. There are three basic layers of soil to recognize when selecting a site for a fire. (This is an oversimplification of soil types. Judgment should be used in choosing a fire site that minimizes impact.)

1. Litter
    a) Composed of leaves, twigs, and other natural organic matter
    b) Found on top of the ground
    c) Highly flammable—care must be taken not to build a fire on top of or next to litter
2. Duff
    a) Decomposing litter that may be compacted or compressed
    b) Generally found under the litter but sometimes found on the surface, particularly where an area has been heavily camped and the litter has been trampled or picked clean for fires
    c) Flammable and burns slowly, usually without flame—care must be taken not to build fires on duff, as duff fires can burn for days undetected until something more combustible is ignited
3. Mineral soil
    a) Inorganic material made up of sand, gravel, and stones
    b) Generally found under the duff, but sometimes found on or near the surface, particularly near streams and where trees have been uprooted

E. Safety considerations

1. General considerations: The Boy Scouts of America discuss three factors of fire safety:
   a) A safe location
   b) A safe fire
   c) Complete extinction of the fire
2. Specific considerations:
   a) Wind direction
   b) Tending the fire—never leave a fire unattended
   c) Distance from tents and other equipment
   d) Nearby combustible materials (roots, grasses, trees, duff)
   e) Available water
   f) Weather conditions (drought)

F. Sites

1. Established fireplaces: It's best to use an existing fire ring.
2. Existing informal fire rings
   a) In heavily camped areas, one or more fire rings may be found.
   b) If a fire ring exists, it should be used as long as it is safe. If the site is not safe, it is better not to have any fire than to create more impact within the area.
   c) If more than one fire ring exists in a campsite, it is advisable to leave a clean, well-placed one for others to use and then dismantle and reclaim the others. Always leave an existing fire ring in a high-impact site. Otherwise, one may be built again in a more undesirable location (Hampton and Cole 1988).
3. Mound fires
   a) Using a trowel or small shovel, a large stuff sack, and a ground cloth or plastic bag, collect soil, sand, or gravel from a natural source (e.g., the root hole of a fallen tree).
   b) Collect enough soil to spread at least 3 to 5 inches (8 to 12 centimeters) of soil over the ground cloth or garbage bag. The thickness of the soil is critical in preventing the heat generated by the fire from injuring plant or animal life in the soil below the ground cloth or plastic bag. If necessary, remove any natural litter or other readily combustible material from the site and save it for restoring the site later to a natural appearance.
   c) Ensure that the area is larger than the anticipated fire (approximately 2 feet square, or 60 centimeters).
   d) The site is now ready for building a fire.

4. Fire pans
   a) Use of a fire pan is a good alternative for fire building on a trip where weight is not a factor (e.g., canoeing, kayaking, or rafting).
   b) The pan should either be elevated off the ground or lined with mineral soil so the heat generated by the fire does not injure plant or animal life or scorch the ground.

G. Site restoration. This is the process of restoring the site to its natural condition before camp is broken to make it look as if there had been no fire there. Although this process applies to the entire campsite (e.g., tent sites, latrines, kitchen areas, meeting areas), we are concerned here with restoring fire sites to a natural appearance.

1. Considerations before restoring the site
   a) Be sure to burn the wood to ash and minimize large chunks of burnt wood. If large chunks remain, crush them to dust as thoroughly as possible.
   b) Put the fire out the night before breaking camp and cook on a stove the next morning.
2. Restoring the site
   a) Make sure the fire is completely out by dousing it with water and stirring until it is cool enough to touch with bare hands.
   b) Distribute the ashes randomly over a large area away from the campsite.
   c) If more wood than necessary was collected, scatter it through the woods.
   d) If a mound fire was used, replace the mineral soil in its original location.

III. Instructional Strategies

A. Timing. This lesson is best taught when fires are to be used. Whether fires are used or not, it is important to have a discussion about fires and their wise use.

B. Strategies. This lesson lends itself nicely to student instruction and works effectively if combined with chapter 14 (Fire Building) and chapter 19 (Food: Quick-Bread Baking).

C. Materials
1. A suitable site for building a fire
2. Shovel or trowel
3. Mound fire materials—large stuff bag, ground cloth, or plastic bag
4. Fire pan, if available

CHAPTER FOURTEEN

Fire Building

I. Outcomes

A. Outdoor leaders provide evidence of their *knowledge* and *understanding* by:

1. Describing safety considerations in fire construction
2. Describing environmental considerations in the selection of fuel and the construction, use, and care of the fire
3. Describing how to identify and select appropriate wood for the construction of a fire
4. Explaining the three components of fire and their role in fire building
5. Explaining the function of the common materials used in fire construction
6. Comparing and critiquing common methods of laying a fire
7. Describing considerations in starting a fire in both favorable and inclement weather conditions

B. Outdoor leaders provide evidence of their *skill* by:

1. Constructing, using, and caring for a fire with appropriate concern for safety and the environment
2. Identifying and selecting appropriate wood for the construction of a fire
3. Applying an understanding of the three components of fire in fire building and maintenance
4. Properly using the common materials for fire construction
5. Demonstrating a suitable technique for laying a fire
6. Starting a fire in favorable and inclement weather

C. Outdoor leaders provide evidence of their *dispositions* by:

1. Building and maintaining safe and environmentally sound fires

II. Content

A. Safety considerations

1. If necessary, review safety considerations from chapter 13, Fire Site Preparation and Care.
2. If necessary, review safety considerations from chapter 15, Food: Introduction to Cooking.
3. Some major safety considerations to reinforce are:
   a) Make sure there is a ready source of water available to put the fire out in the event of an emergency.
   b) Wear gloves around the fire to prevent burning and/or drying out hands.
   c) Never leave a fire unattended for more than a very short time.

B. Environmental considerations

1. If necessary, review environmental considerations in chapter 13, Fire Site Preparation and Care.
2. Some major considerations to reinforce are:
   a) If in doubt, use a stove.
   b) Only collect wood that is already down on the ground.

C. Identifying and selecting firewood

1. As a general rule, you should not use firewood:
   a) Any larger than what you can readily break by hand (about 3 inches in diameter)
   b) That requires use of an axe, hatchet, or saw
2. The selection of firewood is generally a function of availability and adherence to local rules and regulations. In most regions of the country, there isn't a lot of choice. Ideally, one would select firewood based on the following considerations:
   a) Softwoods (e.g., pine, spruce, and cedar) are convenient for use as tinder and kindling. They ignite readily and burn hot.
   b) Hardwoods (e.g., maple, yellow birch, and black cherry) are excellent for obtaining hot, long-lasting coals, providing a steady temperature for cooking and baking.
3. Firewood selection should be based on the following considerations:
   a) Only collect wood that is already down. In very rainy weather when it's been determined that a fire is necessary, one might make an exception and pick the fine, dead tinder that is still attached in the undergrowth

of a conifer. This won't be necessary if you keep a "twiggy bag" (see p. 218) available.

b) Collect enough wood to maintain the fire (usually twice as much as originally estimated). Few things are as frustrating as having to run off and collect firewood once the fire is started.

c) Collect wood of different sizes (from less than the size of a matchstick to up to 3 inches in diameter) and stack the wood according to size. This provides convenient access to wood as the fire is being started.

D. Three components of fire. There must be a balance of fuel, heat, and oxygen to have a successful fire. When having difficulty starting a fire, it is often helpful to determine which component is out of balance and try to establish the proper balance.

1. Fuel: Wood provides the fuel in campfires. The key is to have the correct size fuel for the amount of heat present. For example, if you have fuel the size of 4-inch logs, heat generated from fuel the size of matchsticks won't be sufficient to ignite it.

2. Heat: Heat ignites the fuel and must be balanced with it. Large fuel will not ignite until the heat of the fire rises to a suitable temperature to thoroughly heat the wood. Water vapor is often profuse next to the ground and will inhibit combustion. The fire should be ignited a few inches above ground level.

3. Oxygen: There must be room for oxygen. Allow for ample air circulation and arrange the fuel so that oxygen can get to the fire.

E. Materials in fire construction

1. Tinder
   a) Definition: Fine, flammable material that will ignite from the heat of a match.
   b) Examples: Birch bark (collected from the ground), pine, or spruce pitch, and fine twigs (twiggies).
   c) Observations: If the group must depend on fires, it is important to have a plastic bag of these materials set aside for a rainy day.
   d) Homemade fire starters:
      (1) Jelly balls: Cotton balls soaked in petroleum jelly and stored in a film canister.
      (2) Egg-carton starter: Fill an egg carton with wood shavings and/or dryer lint; pour melted wax over the top. When dried, each egg section can be broken off to create "eggs" of fire starters.

2. Kindling
   a) Definition: Small-diameter branches (¾ inch or less) or split wood that ignites from the heat of the burning tinder and, in turn, provides the heat to ignite the larger fuel.
   b) Examples: Softwoods such as pine, spruce, cedar, and fir are very suitable for kindling. They ignite readily and give off plenty of heat to ignite larger fuels.
3. Fuel
   a) Definition: Firewood that provides coals and uniform heat for cooking.
   b) Examples: Hardwoods such as maple, hickory, and apple do an admirable job of providing good coals for cooking.

F. Laying the fire
   1. Everyone has a favorite way to lay a fire. How it is laid is not as important as how well it functions. Does the lay of the fire allow for the proper balance of the three elements necessary for a good fire?
   2. When using a mound fire, or if the ground is particularly cold or moist, it is helpful to lay a row of logs, bark, or other material on the ground before the fire is laid. This insulates the fire from cold and moisture and allows the heat to be used for combustion rather than be absorbed by the ground.
   3. Pile the tinder (the most combustible material) at the bottom. As the heat rises, it will ignite the larger wood (kindling) laid on top of it. Finish laying the fire using one of the methods below before igniting the tinder and kindling.
   4. Types of fires:
      a) Lean-to (see fig. 14.1)
         (1) Provide a bed of tinder, and then lean tinder and kindling against a "lean-to support" or larger piece of kindling.
         (2) An efficient fire can often be quickly built using this method.
      b) Tepee (see fig. 14.2)
         (1) By building a tepee of kindling around an abundant supply of tinder, a healthy fire can eventually grow by gradually increasing the size of the outermost wood.
         (2) At some point, the tepee will collapse from its own weight. The challenge is not to let it collapse until the fire is large enough to sustain itself.
         (3) A tepee fire is one of the most effective lays in rainy weather as it allows the outer wood to dry while the inner tinder and kindling is burning.

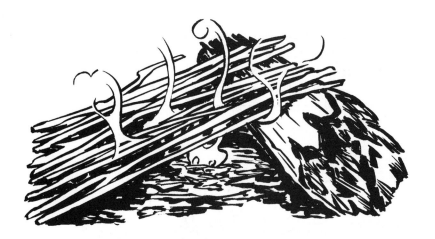

FIGURE 14.1. Lean-to fire

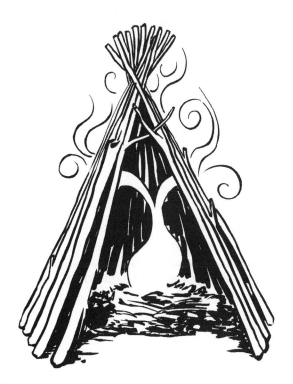

FIGURE 14.2. Tepee fire

(4) To keep the tepee going until the outer wood ignites, continue to carefully replace tinder and kindling as it burns.

c) Log cabin (see fig. 14.3)

(1) A series of logs are crisscrossed log-cabin style, allowing for plenty of oxygen and a place to carefully set cooking pots.

(2) It generally takes much more time and effort to successfully use this method.

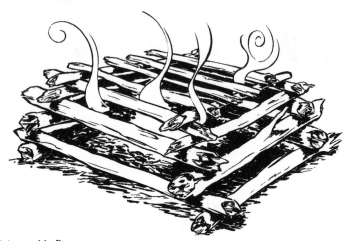

FIGURE 14.3. Log cabin fire

G. Inclement-weather suggestions

1. Make a twiggy bag (i.e., a bag of twiggies, birch bark, pitch, and other tinder collected and saved for a rainy day) on a dry day.
2. Use homemade fire starters as described above (see tinder).
3. Oozing pitch from coniferous trees ignites under the most adverse conditions. Carefully scrape pitch from the tree, trying not to injure the bark.
4. Look for dry tinder under logs, boulders, at the base of large trees, and other dry areas.
5. Carve dry wood out of the core of wet kindling.
6. Build a tepee fire, being sure to keep the center well stoked.

H. Lighting the fire

1. Don't be afraid to use paper if it's available.
2. When striking a match, remember that heat rises, and try to hold the lit end

of the match lower than the rest of the match. This will allow the match to stay lit and burn hotter.

3. Light the fire upwind so the heat generated will be blown toward the fire and not away from it.

4. Homemade or commercial fire starters can be carried for lighting fires in extremely damp or emergency conditions.

III. Instructional Strategies

A. Timing. Depending on whether stoves are used extensively or not, this class can be taught as needed and in conjunction with chapter 13, Fire Site Preparation and Care. Whether fires are used or not, it is important to have a discussion about fires and their wise use.

B. Strategies

1. This class lends itself nicely to student teaching.
2. Many instructors use a lecture/demonstration format followed by participant practice of the skill.

C. Materials

1. Fuel
2. Matches
3. Cotton gloves
4. Shovel
5. Water
6. Twiggy bag
7. Examples of homemade fire starters

CHAPTER FIFTEEN

Food: Introduction to Cooking

I. Outcomes

A. Outdoor leaders provide evidence of their *knowledge* and *understanding* by:

1. Describing general safety principles and considerations in organizing a kitchen in an outdoor setting
2. Describing basic cooking principles, tools, and utensils
3. Describing environmentally sound dishwashing practices

B. Outdoor leaders provide evidence of their *skill* by:

1. Establishing a safe, organized kitchen
2. Properly using the basic cooking utensils employed in cooking
3. Sterilizing utensils prior to eating
4. Incorporating basic cooking principles to consistently prepare well-balanced meals
5. Demonstrating use of environmentally sound dishwashing practices

C. Outdoor leaders provide evidence of their *dispositions* by:

1. Consistently modeling safety and organization when cooking in the outdoors
2. Sterilizing utensils prior to eating
3. Consistently modeling concern for minimizing the amount of food waste

II. Content

A. Safety in the cooking area

1. If cooking fires are used, they should be located downwind (at least 50 feet) and well away from nylon tents, backpacks, sleeping bags, and other combustible items. Cooking areas using stoves should be about 15 feet from the tent site to keep the cooking area organized and uncluttered.

   a) Whether a stove or cooking fire is used, a circular "safe" area about 4 to 5 feet in diameter should be created around it.

      (1) No one should walk through, reach over, or engage in horseplay near the fire or stove in the "safe" area.

      (2) Only those directly involved with cooking food should work in the "safe" area.

      (3) The cooking area should be located in an area free from natural hazards that may trip, poke, or otherwise hinder the cook from working safely.

      (4) The cook should designate a comfortable spot to sit near the fire or stove so that he or she may work without constantly shifting around the flames.

      (5) After the stove has been filled, the fuel bottle should be closed securely and removed from the cooking area.

   b) Sterilize cooking and eating utensils before using them.

      (1) Sterilizing utensils minimizes the chance of intestinal illness due to bacterial growth that may occur between uses. Although cleaning cooking and eating utensils is important after eating in order to prevent bacterial growth, sterilizing is senseless after meals because utensils become contaminated when packed.

      (2) To conserve fuel when cooking on stoves, you can designate one or two cook groups as "sterilization stations."

      (3) If cooking on a fire, each fire pit can have a sterilization pot.

   c) Use gloves and/or pot grips when handling hot items.

   d) Hot liquids and hot grease should be given special consideration as potential safety hazards.

      (1) When pouring from a pot or fry pan, the pouring motion should be directed away from the pourer.

      (2) Do not pour hot liquids into a handheld container. Instead, place containers on a flat, stable platform or on the ground.

   e) Before stirring, it is advisable to remove pots with hot or boiling food from the stove or fire to prevent accidentally dumping dinner or scalding the cook.

f) It is advisable to remove pots from the fire before adding food. This prevents plastic bags from burning and minimizes the chance of scalding arms and hands.

g) Do not pass hot items over another person. We have seen severe burns to the ankles and feet when items are spilled under these circumstances.

h) When cooking over a fire, a full water bottle, large pot, or billy can should be kept handy for dousing flames or watering the fringes of the fire site.

i) When using a stove, an empty pot or billy can should be handy for inverting over the stove to smother a "flare-up."

j) Cooks must be particularly aware of potential dangers, such as loose clothing or long hair that may ignite around fires or stoves.
   (1) Long sleeves should be rolled up.
   (2) Nylon wind pants or wind jackets should be removed or protected from heat and sparks.
   (3) Long hair should be tied back and kept out of the face and away from flames.

k) Use a hard surface to cut bread, cheese, pepperoni, or other items rather than cutting on your leg.

l) When using a knife, cut away from you.

2. Food preparation in bear country

a) Bears have an acute sense of smell and may be attracted to the smell of food or any other strong odors (except human scent).

b) Cook and eat early, because bears are most active at dusk.

c) Prepare and cook food close to an existing fire ring, if possible.

d) Never eat or store food in a tent. The odor will remain even after the food is gone.

e) Do not use sleeping pads, jackets, etc., as tablecloths in bear country; make sure these items are cleaned or laundered before a trip in bear country to eliminate food odors from previous trips.

f) Store containers that hold or have held food, drink mix, or fuel away from the tent at night.

g) Don't sleep in clothing that has been soiled with food, stored with food, or worn while cooking.

h) To avoid having food smells on clothing, try not to wipe your hands on your face or clothing. It may be advisable to cook in your wind gear, and then place the wind gear in the food bag when you hang it.

B. Cooking tools and utensils. Participants should be introduced to each of the following cooking tools and utensils commonly issued:

1. Cooking pots: Two nesting pots can be used for all boiling. Pots also serve as mixing bowls and as useful vessels for carrying water to the cooking area, washing clothes and body, or smothering flames on a "flared-up" stove.

2. Pot grips: Useful for gripping hot cooking pots.

3. Fry pan
    a) Used for frying food.
    b) With a lid, it can be turned into a Dutch oven.

4. Stovetop oven/Bundt pan and stabilizing tin
    a) The stovetop oven is used for baking on top of the stove.
    b) The stabilizing tin is a circular piece of aluminum flashing material with a hole in the middle. This 8-inch-diameter tin is placed on top of the stove to help stabilize the ring pan oven while baking.
    c) The stabilizing tin also serves to distribute heat more evenly when doing stovetop baking.

5. Metal or heat-resistant serving spoon

6. Metal or heat-resistant spatula

7. Collapsible plastic water jug or nylon water sack
    a) Used for carrying and storing water at the campsite
    b) Usually holds two to three gallons of water

8. Metal or heat-resistant (Lexan) cup, bowl, and spoon
    a) Issued as personal eating gear, but may also be used for mixing sauces, pastes, etc.
    b) Should be submersed in boiling water daily for sterilization.

9. Wide-mouth plastic (Lexan) quart bottle
    a) Should be leakproof and able to withstand immersion in boiling water for sterilization
    b) Holds drinking water for the trail, but may also be used in food preparation
    c) Can also be used to rehydrate food items

10. Cotton gloves: Serve as potholders and also protect hands from excessive drying and cracking when working with fires or stoves.

11. Storage bags: Cotton/polyester bags can be used for storing stoves, pots, pans, billy cans, or utensils. They are particularly helpful in keeping pack contents clean once pots and pans become covered in soot.

C. Organization of the kitchen area

1. The kitchen area should be used exclusively for preparing food. It should be separated from the cooking area by at least a few feet in order to minimize traffic around the stove or fire.
2. All utensils, pots, and pans required for cooking a meal should be organized and laid out in an orderly fashion in the cooking area.
   a) Sleeping pads, jackets, or stuff sacks such as the cooking equipment storage bags can be laid on the ground to serve as "tablecloths," helping keep utensils clean and organized. (Do not do this in bear country, however.)
   b) Cooks should be encouraged to put all utensils back in place after each use. This helps avoid confusion while cooking and prevents the loss of equipment. Pot grips and spoons, in particular, have a tendency to easily get lost.
3. All ingredients required for preparing a meal can be organized in the "kitchen" area.
   a) Ingredients used in meal preparation can be removed from the food bag and arranged on the "tablecloth."
   b) All food bags that will be used for preparing a meal should be opened beforehand to allow easy access.
   c) Some cooks like to arrange ingredients in the order that they will be needed and replace each item in the food bag after use. This maintains organization and helps prevent the accidental doubling of ingredients in the pot.
4. All advance preparation for the meal should be complete before lighting the stove. This will conserve fuel and prevent the need for hasty scrambling at the last minute around a lighted stove.

D. Dish washing

1. Utensils and cookware should be cleaned well away from water sources.
2. Properly dispose of food waste (see chapter 17, Food: Waste Disposal).
3. If abrasives are necessary, use dead pine needles, spruce twigs, or other natural litter as scouring pads, which can be burned or packed out after use.
4. Pots with stuck or burnt food on the inside can be soaked overnight. By morning, the food residue will have softened up and will be easier to remove. In bear country, clean pots immediately after use.
5. Rinse water must be carefully disposed of using practices appropriate for the area (see chapter 17, Food: Waste Disposal).

6. The use of soap is discouraged because it is not necessary and can lead to intestinal illness. Most dish soaps are designed for hot water and do not rinse well in cold water.
7. In marine environments:
   a) Wastewater from cooking should be drained into the ocean.
   b) Wash your dishes at the ocean's edge, using soapless saltwater and sand as a scouring pad.
   c) When in doubt about proper practices, consult rangers and land managers in the area of travel.

III. Instructional Strategies

A. Timing. This class is best taught within the first few days or in a precourse shakedown to give participants the ability to develop their organizational skills.

B. Considerations. This class is often taught in lecture/discussion format, although it can also be taught in conjunction with Food: Granola Preparation (chapter 16), Food: Quick-Bread Baking (chapter 19), or Food: Yeast Baking (chapter 20).

C. Materials
1. A good kitchen area
2. A safe cooking area with stove or fire
3. Cooking pots
4. Pot grips
5. Fry pan with lid
6. Stovetop oven/Bundt pan and stabilizing tin
7. Serving spoon
8. Spatula
9. Water jug or sack
10. Cup, bowl, and spoon
11. Water bottle
12. Cotton gloves
13. Storage bags for utensils and pots
14. Food bags

CHAPTER SIXTEEN

Food: Granola Preparation

Why granola? Granola preparation is a good choice for an initial introduction to chapter 15 (Food: Introduction to Cooking) and chapter 42 (Stove Operation). This lesson can be taught on the first morning of a course or trip, and participants can then immediately apply the lesson by preparing their own breakfast. Instructors can easily monitor stove use for safety and stove-operation problems without having to wander from one campsite to another. A variety of ingredients are needed for granola preparation, and others are optional, allowing participants to experience the flexibility and creativity of the Total Food Planning method (explained in chapter 21, Food: Nutrition, Rations Planning, and Packaging). Granola can be served with milk, providing a nutritious breakfast at the outset of an experience when stress levels may be high. The volume of food prepared by participants is less critical; any extra granola prepared can be consumed later as a snack.

I. Outcomes

A. Outdoor leaders provide evidence of their *knowledge* and *understanding* by:

1. Properly identifying the cooking equipment and utensils necessary for food preparation
2. Listing the correct ingredients for food preparation

B. Outdoor leaders provide evidence of their *skill* by:

1. Preparing a batch of granola suitable for consumption

C. Outdoor leaders provide evidence of their *dispositions* by:

1. Modeling safety, organization, and use of basic cooking principles when preparing meals

II. Content

A. Cooking tools and utensils. For granola preparation introduce cooking tools and utensils of the type issued to participants as expedition gear.

1. Frying pan with lid.
   a) Usually 8 to 10 inches in diameter.
   b) A nonstick coating helps eliminate the problem of food sticking to the pan while frying and greatly aids in ease of cleanup.
2. Pot grips should be used to safely hold pans over the stove or fire or remove pans.
3. Metal or heat-resistant serving spoon.
4. Metal or heat-resistant spatula.
5. Collapsible plastic water jug or nylon water sack.
6. Metal or Lexan plastic cup, bowl, and spoon (issued as personal eating gear, but may also be used for mixing sauces, pastes, etc.).
7. Cotton gloves: Used to protect hands from excessive drying and cracking when working with fire. They also serve well as pot holders.
8. Storage bags: Cotton/polyester bags used for storing pots, pans, or utensils. Particularly helpful in keeping pack contents clean once pots and pans become covered in soot.

B. Granola preparation

1. Assemble all ingredients and utensils required for granola preparation prior to lighting the stove.
   a) Tools and utensils:
      (1) Stove, fuel, matches
      (2) Frying pan
      (3) Spatula
      (4) Pot grips
      (5) Cotton gloves
      (6) Cup, bowl, spoon
   b) Ingredients:
      (1) Rolled oats
      (2) Fruits of choice, chopped into bite-size pieces: raisins, dates, apricots, coconut, etc.
      (3) Nuts and seeds of choice: almonds, peanuts, sunflower seeds, cashews, etc.
      (4) Sweeteners of choice: honey, brown sugar, white sugar
      (5) Margarine

(6) Salt

(7) Peanut butter (optional)

(8) M&M's (optional)

(9) Powdered milk: Mix with water to serve with granola

2. Start stove (see chapter 42, Stove Operation)

3. Sterilize utensils (see chapter 15, Food: Introduction to Cooking)—*be sure to have sterilized your utensils beforehand*

4. Cooking procedure:

   a) Melt 3 to 4 tablespoons of margarine in frying pan

   b) Add oats, stir, and brown

   c) Add a pinch of salt

   d) Add nuts and continue to brown mixture

   e) Add sweeteners to taste; allow sugars to melt and mix with other ingredients

   f) Add fruits

   g) Continue to fry until mixture is browned and toasted to preference

5. Can be served warm or cool, as a cereal with milk; can also be allowed to cool, then bagged and eaten as a trail snack.

III. Instructional Strategies

A. Timing. This class is usually taught on the first morning as a preparatory lesson for the first breakfast.

B. Considerations

1. This class is often taught in conjunction with the class on stove operation (see chapter 42).

2. This is effectively taught in a lecture/demonstration format. After the instructor finishes the lesson, participants can then immediately go and prepare their own granola for breakfast. Instructors should visit each kitchen/cooking area to assist.

3. If a large enough central area is available, this class can be taught in a step-by-step approach, and participants can actually prepare their meal with the instructor as the lesson is taught. One instructor can teach while another circulates among cook groups, offering assistance.

C. Materials

1. Cooking tools and utensils:

   a) Stove, fuel, matches

b) Frying pan and/or tote oven

c) Pot grips

d) Serving spoon

e) Spatula

f) Water jug or sack

g) Cup, bowl, and spoon

h) Water bottle

i) Cotton gloves

j) Storage sacks

2. Ingredients:

a) Oats

b) Dried fruits of choice (raisins, dates, apricots, coconut, etc.)

c) Nuts and seeds of choice (almonds, peanuts, sunflower seeds, cashews, etc.)

d) Sweeteners of choice (honey, white sugar, brown sugar)

e) Margarine

f) Salt

g) Peanut butter

h) M&M's

i) Powdered milk

CHAPTER SEVENTEEN

Food: Waste Disposal

I. Outcomes

A. Outdoor leaders provide evidence of their *knowledge* and *understanding* by:

1. Explaining the importance of proper food and wastewater disposal
2. Comparing and critiquing appropriate methods of food and wastewater disposal
3. Describing the limitations of using a fire for disposal of food waste
4. Explaining why the best option for food waste disposal is packing it back to "civilization" and disposing of it appropriately
5. Explaining the importance of cooking no more food than can be eaten

B. Outdoor leaders provide evidence of their *skill* by:

1. Using proper food waste disposal practices in the backcountry
2. Packing food waste back to "civilization" and disposing of it appropriately
3. Cooking no more food than can be eaten

C. Outdoor leaders provide evidence of their *dispositions* by:

1. Modeling proper food waste disposal practices
2. Cooking only the amount of food that will be eaten and thereby minimizing food waste
3. Minimizing the physical and aesthetic impact of food waste on wildlife and the environment

II. Content

A. Why show concern about how we dispose of food waste?

1. To prevent contamination of the water supply
   a) Eutrophication (see chapter 4, Bathing and Washing)
   b) Aesthetics: Who wants to see food waste on the bottom of a lake or stream, in a fireplace, or anywhere in the backcountry?
   c) Illegality: It is illegal to randomly dispose of food waste on land or in the water in virtually all of the federal and state wilderness areas.
2. To minimize alteration of wildlife feeding and migration habits
3. To minimize wildlife (e.g., squirrels, chipmunks, raccoons, bears, insects) feeding on human food waste
4. To minimize negative impact on the aesthetics of a campsite and cooking area
5. To increase the social carrying capacity; i.e., the number of people that can use the area before it seems too crowded

B. Disposal of wastewater and food particles

1. Wastewater should be strained to remove as much food as possible from the water.
   a) Strain the wastewater using a strainer, nylon or wire screen, a bandanna, or other suitable material.
   b) In the absence of a strainer or screen, a makeshift strainer can be constructed. Pack some forest litter inside a plastic bag and puncture small holes in the bottom of the bag. After straining the water, you need to pack out the strained food waste, the litter, and the plastic bag.
2. Food waste and the strained particles should be bagged and packed out. In rare cases, you may be able to completely burn food waste in a hot fire (see C. below).
3. After straining food particles, properly dispose of wastewater by dispersing/broadcasting the water over a wide area at least 200 feet from the nearest water source, campsite, or trail.

C. Fires for food waste disposal

1. Some waste, such as paper, will burn nicely in fires (first make sure that paper food wrappers are not lined with foil). Unfortunately, food waste rarely burns well.

2. If you think you have a hot enough fire to burn food waste completely, then try it, but be sure to scrape through the ashes once the fire is out to remove any remaining food waste for packing out.
3. We do not recommend putting any wastewater into fires.

D. Packing food out

1. If in doubt, pack food out
2. Try to minimize the amount of food waste that must be packed out by not cooking more food than you can eat

E. Food disposal in bear country

1. Never bury leftover food
2. Only burn leftover food in extremely hot fires where it will burn completely
3. Only cook what you will eat—leftovers are difficult to store and protect from bears (because the food is often wet, and because leftover food usually produces a stronger, thus more attractive, odor)
4. Put all garbage and any uneaten food in plastic bags and hang them in a bear bag

III. Instructional Strategies

A. Timing. This information can be taught using the teachable moment on the first day in the field.

B. Activities

1. As the group enters a campsite, ask participants what type of food disposal might be most appropriate and why.
2. Depending on the age level and motivation, instructors may have to monitor the group closely to insure compliance with proper food disposal techniques.

C. Materials

1. Shovel
2. Firepit or fireplace
3. Food waste
4. Wire or nylon screen, strainer, or makeshift strainer
5. "Natural" screen of litter in a perforated plastic bag

CHAPTER EIGHTEEN

Food: Identification, Organization, and Preparation Tips

I. Outcomes

A. Outdoor leaders provide evidence of their *knowledge* and *understanding* by:

1. Describing how to identify bulk foods used in the Total Food Planning method and the importance of proper identification
2. Describing considerations in food care and organization
3. Describing food preparation tips and ideas

B. Outdoor leaders provide evidence of their *skill* by:

1. Identifying food items
2. Consistently demonstrating good organization of food items
3. Using cooking tips appropriately

C. Outdoor leaders provide evidence of their *dispositions* by:

1. Modeling proper care and organization of food items

II. Content

A. Food identification. Go through the food bags, identifying each food item and giving preparation ideas (see the food list at the end of this chapter).

B. Food care and organization

1. Organizing food bags
   a) Foods can be sorted and organized alphabetically, by meals, by color, or by any other preferred method.
   b) Once foods are organized, they can be packed in food bags in a consistent, organized fashion so they can be found easily next time they are needed.

2. Keeping food bags clean
   a) If a bag breaks, rebag the food item and clean up as soon as possible.
   b) As garbage accumulates, keep it in one plastic bag.

3. Plastic bags
   a) We recommend packing food in plastic bags and using overhand knots to close them. Keep the knots loose. If knots get tight, twist the working end and push it back through the knot to untie it.
   b) Lift the bags from below the knot or from the bottom of the bag (so knots don't tighten).
   c) Double-bag food items when a leak or puncture would cause disastrous consequences (i.e., spaghetti, sugar, and flour).

4. Plastic containers
   a) They may not be leakproof; if in doubt, store them in plastic bags. Messy or sticky items such as honey should be bagged to prevent soiling other items in the food bag.
   b) Handle containers with care—wide-mouthed container lids sometimes crack.

5. Food preservation
   a) Food items that will not easily spoil should be chosen for a trip.
   b) In hot environments or conditions, care should be taken to keep items such as cheese, margarine, and meats cool by keeping them in the shade and packing them toward the center of the pack. This will:
      (1) Provide for easier handling
      (2) Discourage mold growth
      (3) Prevent deterioration of taste (although nutritional quality generally remains the same)

C. General food preparation ideas

1. Fruits, vegetables, and TVP (textured vegetable protein) should be rehydrated in hot water before adding to the meal.
2. Flour makes a good thickener. A good white sauce can be made with flour, water, margarine, salt, pepper, and other spices of choice.
3. Vegetable oil, margarine, and powdered milk should be added to most dinners for the nutritional gain.

III. Instructional Strategies

A. Timing

1. This unit is designed to help students through the maze of plastic bags, identifying food items and providing general ideas on how to prepare food.
2. It is best taught on the second or third day in a relaxed setting.
3. It can be prefaced by the Food: Introduction to Cooking chapter (chapter 15) so students can cook their first meals. (Some outdoor programs teach granola preparation [chapter 16] on the first morning and food identification [chapter 18] on the second or third day.)
4. This class may be followed with specific classes on quick-bread baking (chapter 19), yeast baking (chapter 20), and nutrition, rations planning, and food packaging (chapter 21). Cooking techniques can also be shared on an individual basis using teachable moments. Regardless of how the topic is taught, it is important to encourage creativity and experimentation. Have a *NOLS Cookery* or similar publication available for participants to use for ideas.

B. Considerations

1. As the instructor identifies each item, participants can identify food from their own bags. This allows participants to become familiar with each food item in their provisions.
2. See the list of suggested food items and preparation tips at the end of the chapter.

C. Activities

1. Food ID Jeopardy: A fun activity for learning to identify food is to play a Jeopardy game with food items.
   a) Hold up an item such as pancake mix and provide an answer such as "This item is usually used to create a breakfast." Students have to respond with the question, "What is pancake mix?" You can then have a

brief discussion on how to differentiate it from flour, how to use it, etc.

b) Take the time to create the answers ahead of time.

c) Make it fun and provide prizes (e.g., candy bars, "sleep-in" permission slips, invitations to dinner). Ham up the role of Alex Trebek and make sure students frame their responses in the form of a question.

2. Identification of food can be done in any combination of the following ways:

a) Pull foods out randomly and pass them around. Comment on how to identify them and provide preparation ideas.

b) Sort foods by similar color and point out the subtle differences between foods.

c) Go through foods by meal groups: dinners, breakfasts, and lunches.

d) Go through a "master food list" alphabetically (see table 21.1 in chapter 21).

D. Materials

1. All participant food bags
2. *NOLS Cookery* (see References and Recommended Reading) or similar publication

Suggested Food Items and Preparation Tips

Apples (dried): Add to hot cereal, eat raw, or rehydrate for baking.

Apricots (dried): Add to hot cereal, eat raw, or rehydrate for baking.

Baking powder

Beef base: Start with less than a teaspoon, as it is very salty. Add base to water.

Brownie mix: Mix : water = 8 : 1.

Bulgur: Prepare the same way as rice. Can be used with or instead of rice, or combined with veggies to make a tabbouleh salad.

Candy

Cashews

Cheese: Cheddar, mozzarella, muenster, and colby.

Cheesecake mix: Add to already-mixed milk, stir, and let set. Mix : milk = 1 : 1.

Chicken base: Start with less than a teaspoon, as it is very salty. Add base to water.

Chili base: Mix with water to taste.

Cocoa: Mix with water and/or milk.

Coconut: Add to granola or use for baking.

Cornmeal: Add to pancake mix, breads, tortillas, etc.

Cream of Wheat: Water : Cream of Wheat = 4 : 1.

Dates: Add to hot cereal, eat raw, or rehydrate for baking.

Egg noodles: Bring water to a boil, and then add noodles and about a tablespoon of oil (to keep noodles from sticking together).

Fruit drink: Orange, lemon, fruit.

Flour (unbleached and whole wheat): Whole wheat flour can be mixed with unbleached flour. Use between a 2 : 1 and 1 : 1 ratio (unbleached : whole wheat).

Gingerbread mix: Add enough water to form a thick, runny consistency.

Honey: Use in addition to or instead of other sweeteners.

Jell-O: Use as a high-energy hot drink. (It is difficult to make Jell-O gel in the field.)

Macaroni: Bring water to a boil, and then add noodles and about a tablespoon of oil (to keep pasta from sticking together).

Margarine: Add a little to every dinner for a good source of energy.

Milk (powdered): Mixes best when cold. Water : milk = 2 : 1.

Mushroom soup base: Add water to base, to taste.

Nuts (mixed)

Oatmeal (rolled, not instant): Cooks in ten to twelve minutes. Water : oatmeal = 2 : 1.

Onions (dried): Rehydrate twelve to fifteen minutes in hot water.

Pancake mix: Add water.

Peanut butter

Peanuts

Pepper (dried): Rehydrate twelve to fifteen minutes in hot water.

Pepperoni: Can be cut up in dinners or used for lunch.

Popcorn

Potatoes (powdered): Good as a thickener, in potato pancakes, or just as potatoes.

Potatoes (sliced): Rehydrate by covering with water in a fry pan. Let sit for ten to fifteen minutes (don't stir or turn over).

Prunes: Add to hot cereal, eat raw, or rehydrate for baking.

Pudding (instant chocolate or vanilla): Add milk, stir, and let set. Milk : pudding = 4 : 1.

Raisins (regular and golden): Add to hot cereal, eat raw, or rehydrate for baking.

Rice: Add to water, and then boil for fifteen to twenty minutes. Water : rice = 2 : 1.

Salt

Soy sauce

Spaghetti: Bring water to a boil, and then add pasta and about a tablespoon of oil (to keep pasta from sticking together).

Sugar (white and brown): Use in addition to or instead of other sweeteners.

Sunflower seeds

Tea (regular and herbal)

Tomato base: Add water to base.

Trail mix

TVP (textured vegetable protein): An inexpensive meat substitute. It has meat texture but very little taste and no fat. Best if rehydrated in hot water for fifteen to twenty minutes.

Vanilla

Vegetable oil: Add to dinners; use for popcorn, pancakes, etc.

Vegetables (dried, mixed): Rehydrate twelve to fifteen minutes in hot water.

Vinegar

Walnuts

Wheatena: Water : Wheatena = 4 : 1.

Yeast

CHAPTER NINETEEN

Food: Quick-Bread Baking

I. Outcomes

A. Outdoor leaders provide evidence of their *knowledge* and *understanding* by:

1. Identifying basic baking ingredients and describing general baking principles
2. Describing basic quick-bread recipes and explaining cooking procedures

B. Outdoor leaders provide evidence of their *skill* by:

1. Correctly using the major tools, utensils, ingredients, and procedures employed in baking
2. Building an oven platform and fire suitable for baking
3. Using ingredients effectively and successfully baking on both a stove and fire

C. Outdoor leaders provide evidence of their *dispositions* by:

1. Using baking as a means of promoting social interaction
2. Creating well-balanced meals that include baked goods
3. Modeling creativity while baking diverse, nutritional foods in the backcountry

II. Content

A. The joys of baking. Preparing nutritious and tasty baked goods can directly contribute to the success of any backcountry expedition.

1. Baking and the diet
   a) Baked goods can add variety to the common backcountry menu. Biscuits, rolls, and bread all greatly enhance the sense of creativity associated with good cooking.
   b) Baked goods can add courses to a meal that otherwise would be missing (e.g., appetizers, desserts, etc.).
   c) Baked goods provide a good source of protein and carbohydrates.
2. Baking and group morale/expedition behavior
   a) Sharing baked goods at the end of a tough day can renew group enthusiasm and spirit.
   b) Baking allows individuals in the group to demonstrate skills and creativity in a noncompetitive way.
   c) Baking for the group and sharing with others can serve as a means of showing appreciation.
   d) Baking in small groups provides an opportunity for group members to share a relaxing, productive, and social occasion that fosters communication, mutual cooperation, and understanding.

B. General baking principles. Baked products add variety to the menu while using few ingredients.

1. Common ingredients include flour, sugar, shortening, eggs, water or milk, and leavening agents.
   a) Flours: Classified as strong or weak depending on their protein content. Strong flours are high in protein, and weak flours are low in protein. Strong flours are used for making bread products. All-purpose and wheat are examples of strong flours.
   b) Shortening: Any fat used in baking is called a shortening.
   c) Eggs: Powdered eggs and egg whites, as well as egg substitutes, can be found and purchased with a little effort.
      (1) Powdered whole eggs: Typically 1 cup of powdered whole egg + 1 cup of water = 6 eggs
      (2) Powdered egg whites: Dried egg white (albumen) can be reconstituted: 2 tsp. of powdered egg white + 2 Tbsp. of warm water = 1 egg white
      (3) Egg substitutes: There are a number of commercial and homemade egg substitutes.

(a) Ener-G Egg Replacer: 1 tsp. of powder + 2 Tbsp. of water = 1 whole egg

(b) Flax seed

 i) To use flax seed, combine ⅛ cup of water and 3 to 4 tsp. of flax seed. Bring to a boil, and then simmer for five to seven minutes. A thickened gel will form. Strain the flax seed. This recipe makes enough for one egg.

 ii) It will bind the ingredients, but it will not serve as a leavening agent.

(c) 2 Tbsp. of water + 1 Tbsp. of oil + 2 tsp. of baking powder = 1 egg

d) Leavening agents: Baking soda and baking powder are chemical leavening agents that release gases produced by chemical reactions. (For baking using yeast, see chapter 20, Food: Yeast Baking.)

C. Baking tools and recipes

1. Baking tools and utensils

a) Backpacking stove, fuel, and matches. Baking on a good stove is a joy since temperature levels can be maintained over long periods of time.

b) Cooking pot (as a mixing bowl).

c) Large serving spoon.

d) Pot grips.

e) The fry-pan oven.

 (1) The fry-pan oven is usually a nonstick 10-inch fry pan and an aluminum 10-inch lid.

 (2) The fry-pan oven is designed to bake dough with a moderate level of consistent heat from both below and above.

 (3) The fry pan can be placed directly on a bed of coals or a very low flame from a stove. Heat from above is supplied by placing hot coals (and/or a twiggy fire) on the fry-pan lid.

 (4) Depending upon the recipe, the fry-pan oven can work with bottom heat only by turning the product over halfway through the baking process. (For best results the stove must be used on the lowest heat setting, and the lid must fit tightly so that the heat is held in.)

 (5) When using a fire, the fry pan must be placed on a completely level and stable platform of coals. Caution must be exercised in setting the pan on two or more sticks above the coals since the sticks may burn through and tip the pan into the fire.

     (6) Exercise caution with plastic-handled fry pans by keeping the handle away from excessive heat.

2. Quick bread

  a) As suggested, quick breads are a breeze to make if you adhere to a few golden rules:

    (1) Measure ingredients accurately.

    (2) Avoid overmixing the batter/dough. When you add the liquid, stir until the dry ingredients are just moistened. The batter/dough will be lumpy.

    (3) If your bread has a bitter or soapy aftertaste, there's probably too much leavening (baking powder or baking soda) in it.

  b) Dough mixtures for quick breads are generally of two types:

    (1) Soft doughs are used for biscuit-type products. These products are rolled out and cut into desired shapes.

    (2) Batters may be either pour batters, which are liquid enough to pour (pancakes), or drop batters, which are thicker and will drop from a spoon (quick bread).

3. Basic biscuits

  a) Recipe

    (1) 2 cups all-purpose flour

    (2) 1 Tbsp. baking powder

    (3) 1 tsp. salt

    (4) ¼ cup butter/margarine

    (5) ¾ cup milk

  b) Directions

    (1) Mix the dry ingredients thoroughly.

    (2) Cut in the butter/margarine. Using a mixing spoon or clean hands, mix until it resembles coarse cornmeal.

    (3) Add liquid and mix just until the ingredients are combined and a soft dough is formed.

    (4) Do not overmix!

    (5) Place the dough on a clean surface and knead lightly by pressing it out and folding it in half. If the dough is sticky, add a small amount of flour.

    (6) Form dough into desired shape for baking and place in baking pan.

6. Basic quick bread

  a) Recipe

(1) 1½ cups all-purpose flour

(2) ½ cup sugar

(3) 1½ tsp. baking powder

(4) ¼ tsp. of salt

(5) ¼ tsp. of baking soda

(6) ¾ cup of milk

(7) ⅛ cup of cooking oil

(8) ¾ cup of nuts, fruits, or combination of both

b) Directions

(1) Mix dry ingredients thoroughly

(2) Mix liquid ingredients

(3) Make a well in the center of the dry ingredients and add wet ingredients

(4) Mix just until moistened

(5) Spoon batter into the baking pan

5. Fry breads

a) Fry breads are another type of quick bread popular on the trail. Fry breads are prepared using the basic quick-bread recipe.

b) Directions

(1) Once the dough is prepared, small handfuls are flattened into round shapes and fried.

(2) If desired, these "palm breads" can then be filled with ingredients such as cheese, pepperoni, fruit, etc.; rolled into a ball; and fried.

(3) Vegetable oil works best for fry breads, although margarine will also work. Make sure that the oil is hot enough before starting to fry (a drop of water will sizzle when dropped into the correct-temperature oil).

(4) Generally, smaller fry breads cook more thoroughly than larger, thick ones.

(5) Fry breads should be evenly browned on all sides, cooled, and served.

(6) Plain fry breads rolled in sugar and cinnamon make excellent doughnutlike snacks.

III. Instructional Strategies

A. Timing

1. This class should be conducted early in the expedition so that students can add variety and substance to their meals.

2. Classes in stove operation (chapter 42) and introductory cooking (chapter 15) are obvious prerequisites.

B. Considerations

1. This class is most commonly taught as a group discussion/demonstration.
2. An efficient timeline for this particular lesson might be:
    a) Introduce all baking tools and utensils
    b) Discuss leavening agents
    c) Conclude with a taste test and discuss recipe variations
3. This class is frequently taught before lunch or dinner so that students can put their new knowledge to immediate use.
4. For additional recipes and ideas, see *NOLS Cookery* (see References and Recommended Reading) or a similar publication.

C. Materials

1. Fry pan and lid
2. Stovetop oven
3. Stove
4. Pot grips
5. Bowl
6. Water
7. Pot (for mixing)
8. Large serving spoon
9. Ingredients

CHAPTER TWENTY

Food: Yeast Baking

I. Outcomes

A. Outdoor leaders provide evidence of their *knowledge* and *understanding* by:

1. Identifying basic baking ingredients for baking with yeast and describing how yeast works as a leavening agent
2. Describing a basic yeast dough recipe and variations, and explaining cooking procedures

B. Outdoor leaders provide evidence of their *skill* by:

1. Correctly using tools, utensils, ingredients, and cooking procedures to bake with yeast
2. Building an oven platform and fire suitable for baking
3. Using ingredients effectively and successfully baking on both a stove and fire

C. Outdoor leaders provide evidence of their *dispositions* by:

1. Using baking as a means of promoting social interaction
2. Creating well-balanced meals that include baked goods
3. Modeling creativity while baking diverse, nutritious foods in the backcountry

II. Content

A. The joys of yeast baking. The flavor and texture that yeast adds to bread products is a welcome addition to any meal in the backcountry. Yeast offers the opportunity to take baking to a higher level.

1. Baking and the diet
   a) Yeast breads can add variety to the common backcountry menu. Good yeast bread, buns, cinnamon rolls, etc., are always a welcome addition to the menu.
   b) Yeast breads provide a good source of protein and carbohydrates.
2. Baking and group morale/expedition behavior
   a) Baking with yeast can be an extremely relaxing, satisfying, and productive activity for the individual and the entire group.
   b) The slow, patient pace associated with rising dough and baking bread allows for moments of contemplative solitude or quiet group conversation unhurried by the demands of the daily itinerary.
   c) Baking with yeast allows individuals in the group to demonstrate skills in a creative and noncompetitive way.
   d) Baking for the group and sharing with others can serve as a means of showing appreciation.

B. The science of yeast baking

1. Yeast are one-celled organisms that come alive and metabolize if given the proper environment—warm water and a food source of sugar or starch.
   a) Water temperature must not be too hot or too cool. Optimum temperature for yeast growth is 110°F or water slightly hot to the touch. Temperatures 140°F and higher will kill yeast.
   b) Fermentation is the process by which yeast acts on carbohydrates (flour and sugar) and changes them into carbon dioxide gas and alcohol. This release of gas produces the leavening action in yeast products.
2. In order to make bread that rises well, flour with high protein content should be used (see the "general baking principles" section in chapter 19).

C. Yeast baking tools and recipes

1. Baking tools and utensils
   a) Backpacking stove, fuel, and matches. Yeast baking on a good stove is a joy since temperature levels can be maintained at a constant level over long periods of time.
   b) Cooking pot (as a mixing bowl).
   c) Large serving spoon.

d) Pot grips.

e) Fry-pan oven (see chapter 19, Food: Quick-Bread Baking, for a description of the fry-pan oven and its use).

2. Basic yeast dough

a) Recipe

(1) 3 to 4 cups flour (half wheat and half white is fine)

(2) 2 tsp. salt (a small spice cap equals about 1 tsp.)

(3) 2 Tbsp. sugar

(4) 1 Tbsp. butter or oil

(5) 1¾ cup warm water

(6) 1 Tbsp. yeast

b) Directions

(1) Organize the kitchen area and ingredients. Be sure everything is readily accessible.

(2) Heat water on the stove. Pour into a cup or bowl and let it cool until it is warm to the touch. Add the yeast and 1 tsp. of sugar and stir gently. Allow this yeast solution to stand for about five minutes. The solution should show gas-bubble formations within a few minutes and become frothy if the yeast is fresh and properly metabolizing. (Remember, the yeast will die if the water is too hot.)

(3) If there are no signs of gas activity, you will need to start over.

(4) Mix half of the flour with the salt, remaining sugar, and butter or oil in a mixing pot.

(5) Add the yeast mixture to the dry ingredients and mix thoroughly to develop gluten. The batter should become stringy.

(6) Add the remaining flour and continue to mix until the dough is thick.

(7) Remove the dough from the mixing pot and place on a flat, clean surface where you can knead the dough.

(8) Knead the dough by using the palms of your hands. Press the dough out and fold it in half. If the dough is sticky, add a small amount of flour.

(9) The dough will be smooth and springy when done.

(10) Shape the dough into a loaf and place in a well-oiled fry pan. Cover the pan with a plastic bag or a moist bandanna and let it rise for one hour or until it doubles in size. If it is a cold day, place the pan on top of a pot of boiling water.

(11) Once the dough has risen, bake the bread for thirty to fifty minutes. It can be baked any number of ways, including:

(a) The "flip method": Where the heat source comes only from the bottom (e.g., a fire or a stove), and when one side is cooked, you flip the bread over to cook the opposite side.

(b) "Twiggy fire": Where the bread is not cooked on either a fire or a stove, but rather on a "twiggy" fire—a fire made with very small sticks—so the bread is heated from the top as well as the bottom.

(c) Stovetop oven: A baking device designed to work specifically on stoves where the heat is designed to radiate around the pan and provide heat to all sides of the bread.

(12) The bread is done when the surface is golden brown, crisp, and sounds hollow when thumped with a finger. Cool for five to ten minutes before cutting and serving.

3. Leading EDGE sweet dough

a) Recipe

(1) 1 Tbsp. yeast

(2) 1 tsp. sugar

(3) ½ cup warm water (110°F)

(4) ½ cup powdered milk solution (powdered milk and water)

(5) 1½ Tbsp. margarine

(6) 2 Tbsp. cooking oil

(7) ½ Tbsp. salt

(8) ¾ cup honey

(9) ½ cup hot water

(10) 1 egg (optional)

(11) 2 cups wheat flour

(12) 2 to 3 cups white flour

b) Directions

(1) Organize the kitchen area and ingredients. Be sure everything is readily accessible.

(2) Heat water on the stove. Pour into a cup or bowl and let it cool until it is warm to the touch. Add the yeast and sugar and stir gently. Allow this yeast solution to stand for about five minutes. The solution should show gas-bubble formations within a few minutes and become frothy if the yeast is fresh and properly metabolizing. (Remember, the yeast will die if the water is too hot.)

(3) If there are no signs of gas activity, you will need to start over.

(4) Mix half of the flour and the remaining ingredients in a mixing pot.

(5) Add the yeast mixture to the dry ingredients and mix thoroughly to develop gluten. The batter will become stringy.

(6) Add the remaining flour and continue to mix until the dough is thick.

(7) Remove the dough from the mixing pot and place on a flat, clean surface where you can knead the dough.

(8) Knead the dough by using the palms of your hands. Press the dough out and fold it in half. If the dough is sticky, add a small amount of flour.

(9) The dough will be smooth and springy when done.

(10) Shape the dough into desired shapes, such as rolls, loaves, or sticks, and place in a well-oiled fry pan. Cover the pan with a plastic bag or a moist bandanna and let it rise for one hour or until it doubles in size. If it is a cold day, place the pan on top of a pot of boiling water.

(11) Once the dough has risen, bake the bread for thirty to fifty minutes using the flip method, a twiggy fire on the fry-pan lid with the stove on low heat, or on a fire (see chapter 19, Food: Quick-Bread Baking, for baking techniques using stoves and fires). The bread is done when the surface is golden brown, crisp, and sounds hollow when thumped with a finger.

(12) Cool for five to ten minutes before cutting and serving.

III. Instructional Strategies

A. Timing

1. This class should follow the quick-bread baking lesson (chapter 19) after students have gained experience baking quick breads and fry breads.
2. Classes in stove operation (chapter 42) and introductory cooking (chapter 15) are obvious prerequisites.

B. Considerations

1. This class is most commonly taught as a group discussion/demonstration.
2. An efficient timeline for this particular lesson might be:
   a) Introduce all baking tools and utensils
   b) Discuss yeast as a leavening agent
      (1) Prepare dough and let it rise
      (2) While the dough is rising, the class can break into small groups, prepare dough, and let it rise

(3) Once the instructor's dough has finished rising, bring the class together and demonstrate how to bake the dough

    c) Conclude with a taste test and discuss recipe variations

3. This class is frequently taught before lunch or dinner so that students can put their new knowledge to immediate use.

4. For additional recipes and ideas, see *NOLS Cookery* (see References and Recommended Reading) or a similar publication.

C. Materials

1. Fry pan and lid
2. Stovetop oven
3. Stove
4. Pot grips
5. Bowl
6. Water
7. Pot (for mixing)
8. Large serving spoon
9. Ingredients

CHAPTER TWENTY-ONE

Food: Nutrition, Rations Planning, and Packaging

I. Outcomes

A. Outdoor leaders provide evidence of their *knowledge* and *understanding* by:

1. Describing the importance of good nutrition in wilderness travel
2. Explaining the body's nutritional needs
3. Describing various considerations in food planning
4. Describing and explaining the "Total Food Planning" philosophy of ration planning for backcountry trips
5. Explaining the role computers can play in food planning
6. Describe considerations in purchasing and packaging food for backcountry travel

B. Outdoor leaders provide evidence of their *skill* by:

1. Maintaining good physical, mental, and emotional health by proper food planning that meets nutritional needs
2. Using the "Total Food Planning" method to plan food for an extended backcountry expedition
3. Practicing proper food packaging techniques

C. Outdoor leaders provide evidence of their *dispositions* by:

1. Modeling creativity while baking diverse, nutritious foods in the backcountry
2. Preparing and eating healthy meals

II. Content

A. Food plays important roles in:

1. Staying healthy: Keeping well nourished plays an instrumental role in fighting illness and disease.
2. Building and repairing body tissue.
3. Attitude: Without good nutrition, disposition and attitude deteriorate rapidly.
4. Energy: Food provides the energy that allows us to take part in physical activities.
5. Mental alertness: Thought processes and decision-making abilities deteriorate without good nutrition.

B. Specific nutritional needs

1. Calories
   a) A calorie is a unit of heat used to measure the energy value of food. It takes 1 calorie to raise 1 gram of water 1°C.
   b) Individual daily caloric needs range from approximately 1,800 per day for a sedentary individual to more than 6,500 for an expedition member in some severe environments.
   c) In general, individual daily caloric needs for wilderness travelers range between:
      (1) 2,500 and 4,000 in summer
      (2) 3,500 and 6,000 in winter
2. Carbohydrates
   a) Provide short-term energy
   b) Should make up approximately 60 percent of an individual's diet
   c) Are found in starches and sugars such as:
      (1) Pastas (macaroni, noodles, spaghetti)
      (2) Rice
      (3) Potatoes
      (4) Drink mixes
      (5) Candy
      (6) Fruit
3. Fats
   a) Provide long-term energy.
   b) Transport fat-soluble vitamins (A, D, E, and K).
   c) Are major flavor enhancers of food.
   d) Convert to fat tissue in the body. Fat tissue:

(1) Protects internal organs

(2) Insulates our bodies

e) Should make up approximately 20 to 25 percent of an individual's diet.

f) Are found in:

(1) Cheese

(2) Nuts

(3) Vegetable oil

(4) Meats

(5) Margarine

4. Proteins

a) Provide for the building of cells and tissue, such as skin and muscles.

b) Keep the immune system running well.

c) Deliver oxygen and nutrients to muscles.

d) Should make up approximately 15 to 20 percent of an individual's diet.

e) Are made up of twenty-two amino acids. Of these twenty-two, all but eight are produced in our bodies. The other eight must be obtained through proteins in food.

f) Complete proteins versus incomplete proteins

(1) Complete proteins: These include all eight of the essential amino acids that the body cannot produce. Therefore, they provide a full complement of protein. Examples include:

(a) Meats

(b) Fish

(c) Soy products

(2) Incomplete proteins: These include some, but not all, of the eight essential amino acids. Therefore, they do not provide a full complement of protein. Examples of incomplete proteins include:

(a) Cereals

(b) Vegetables and fruit

(c) Legumes (e.g., beans, peanuts, lentils)

(3) Incomplete proteins can be made complete by combining two or more foods (e.g., beans and vegetables) together in the same meal. Although this usually happens naturally, it is helpful to be aware of this to insure that complete proteins are consumed regularly. Research shows that complementary proteins do not need to be ingested at the same time, but they should be consumed within the same day for maximum protein benefit.

5. Vitamins and minerals

a) Are essential for the effective functioning of all body processes.

b) Are ingested in adequate amounts if participants consume a variety of foods and the recommended high number of calories. Supplemental vitamins and minerals are usually unnecessary.

6. Water: a critical nutritional element
   a) Water is necessary to:
      (1) Aid digestion
      (2) Keep cells healthy
      (2) Regulate body temperature
      (3) Help eliminate bodily wastes
   b) Dehydration
      (1) Backcountry activities increase the danger of dehydration. Dehydration is more likely:
         (a) During strenuous activity (water is lost through perspiration)
         (b) At higher altitudes (water is lost through increased respiration in drier air)
         (c) In cold weather (water is lost through respiration and perspiration)
      (2) A minimum of two to four quarts in summer and three to five quarts in winter may be needed each day to prevent dehydration.

C. Food-planning considerations. Depending on the objectives and length of the trip, the following criteria should be considered:

1. Energy content: How many calories does the food item supply in relation to its bulk and weight?
2. Nutritional balance: What nutritional requirements does it meet?
3. Bulk and weight: How much space does it require, and how much does it weigh?
4. Spoilage: What is the chance of a food item spoiling before it is consumed?
5. Expense and availability: Is it available, and if so, can the group afford it?
6. Ease of packaging and handling
   a) Packaging: Is it packaged, or can it be repackaged in an environmentally friendly manner?
   b) Ease of handling: How easily may it be handled without spilling, making a mess, etc.?
7. Variety: Is there a great enough variety to meet the group's goals?
   a) The longer the trip, the more important this becomes as a morale booster.
   b) The more variety, the better the chance of appealing to everyone's food tastes. Few people want to eat the same thing day after day.

8. Preparation time: Can it be prepared in a reasonable amount of time?
9. Supplementary wild foods:
   a) Are they available?
   b) Can they be harvested legally?
   c) Are participants knowledgeable enough to prevent accidental poisoning?
   d) Can they be harvested without impacting the environment (e.g., plants chosen will be naturally replenished within a reasonable time)?

D. Rations planning

1. "Total Food Planning": This process is based on determining caloric needs and ensuring that the group has enough food to meet those needs while staying within weight and budget constraints.
   a) The advantages of "Total Food Planning" are:
      (1) A large variety of foods can be used to make an endless variety of meals.
      (2) It allows spontaneity and creativity in cooking and eating.
      (3) It does away with the need to plan specific meals. Individuals can meet caloric needs yet eat what they want when they want, within reason.
      (4) The financial savings are generally substantial when use of prepackaged meals is minimized by "cooking from scratch."
   b) Planning criteria
      (1) Caloric needs: During summer months, between 3,200 and 3,750 calories are planned per person per day, depending on activity level and weather.
      (2) Weight needs: Approximately two pounds of food per person per day are required during summer months.
      (3) Budget needs: Nutritious meals can be provided while meeting virtually any budget constraints.
2. How "Total Food Planning" works (see table 21.1)
   a) Calories: Multiply the number of people (P) going on the trip times the number of days (D) of the trip times the minimum number of calories (C) to be brought per person per day. This is the minimum number of calories needed for the trip (e.g., 12[P] x 33[D] x 3,500[C] = 1,386,000). (See "total calories needed" at the bottom of table 21.1.)
   b) Weight: Multiply the number of people (P) going on the trip times the number of days (D) of the trip times the maximum number of pounds (P) to be brought per person per day. This is the maximum number of pounds of food to be brought on the trip (e.g., 12[P] x 33[D] x 2[P] =

792). (See "total pounds needed" at the bottom of table 21.1.)

    c) Cost: Multiply the number of people (P) going on the trip times the number of days (D) of the trip times the maximum amount of money ($) to be spent per person per day. This is the maximum amount of money to be spent on food for the trip (e.g., 12[P] x 33[D] x $5.00 = $1,980.00). (See "total budget" at the bottom of table 21.1.)

    d) Working with the results: Use these figures and the planning considerations to develop a food list that meets calorie, weight, and cost criteria.

E. Computers and the food-planning process. Spreadsheet software can be used to save time and anguish, making food planning easier.

    1. A shopping list can be created that meets the minimum caloric needs and the maximum pound and cost parameters. Once the database is established, at the press of a button the computer will do all the computations and generate food lists.

    2. A nutritional analysis of the food selected for the trip can be done.

F. Purchasing food for backcountry trips. Food items can be purchased at:

    1. Wholesale food stores (e.g., Sam's Club, Costco)

    2. Food co-ops

    3. Wholesale food distributors

    4. Local grocery stores

    5. Specialty stores (for items such as freeze-dried foods)

G. Packaging food for backcountry trips

    1. Plastic containers and plastic bags are:

        a) Lightweight compared to glass, tin cans, and aluminum foil

        b) Safer than glass (because glass breaks)

        c) Easy to pack and carry out

        d) A good "environmental" choice when reusable (e.g., film canisters for spices, plastic jars with lids for peanut butter and honey)

    2. Use overhand knots instead of twist ties

        a) Twist ties can puncture holes in other bags.

        b) Twist ties can be easily lost, creating litter.

        c) Zippered plastic bags are useful for short trips, but "zippers" sometimes become plugged with food and function poorly.

    3. Wrapping cheese: In hot and humid weather it is sometimes advisable to wrap cheese in freezer wrap or cheesecloth. This helps absorb oils and will delay formation of mold.

III. Instructional Strategies

A. Timing. Depending on how the course is designed, this lesson can be taught as part of the shakedown (i.e., a short trip at the beginning of a course designed to provide an intense philosophical orientation and skills preparation) or near the end of the course.

1. On some courses, students plan their own rations as part of the shakedown exercise. In this case, this lesson should be taught the first day.
2. Some outdoor programs preplan food for a trip and involve participants in food planning at a later point. In this case, this lesson becomes a lower priority and is taught later in the course, using the trip as an example.

B. Activities

1. Rations-planning activity: Have participants develop a rations plan and use it during a trip. Keep good records of what is brought and what is returned so caloric consumption can be tracked. It is much easier and more practical for this exercise to be done by tent groups rather than individually. This requires cooperation and is more practical than having participants compile separate lists and then combine food with their tent partners.

C. Materials. See the master food list (table 21.1)

Table 21.1. MASTER FOOD LIST

Names:

Total number of people: 12

Total number of days: 33

	Pounds ordered	Calories per pound	Total calories	Cost per pound	Total cost
Apples (dried)	10	1,102	10,563	$1.52	$14.57
Apricots (dried)	14	1,081	15,081	$1.59	$22.18
Bacon pieces	0	2,836	0	$1.99	$0.00
Bagels	0	1,800	0	$1.24	$0.00
Baking powder	3	585	1,883	$0.80	$2.58
Beef base	3	1,082	3,484	$2.32	$7.47
Bread	0	1,102	0	$1.05	$0.00
Brownie mix	8	1,828	13,732	$1.33	$9.99
Bulgur	3	1,621	5,219	$0.32	$1.03
Candy (hard)	11	1,751	18,535	$1.76	$18.63
Cashews	0	2,604	0	$2.09	$0.00
Cheese					
Cheddar	23	1,826	41,152	$1.94	$43.72
Colby	33	1,786	59,417	$1.75	$58.22
Mozzarella	21	1,270	27,259	$1.72	$36.92
Muenster	41	1,671	68,144	$1.66	$67.70
Cheesecake mix	5	3,500	18,524	$2.23	$11.80
Chicken base	2	1,117	2,397	$2.32	$4.98
Chili base	1	1,450	1,556	$2.55	$2.74
Chocolate bars	0	1,650	0	$3.38	$0.00
Cocoa with milk	26	1,628	41,931	$1.99	$51.25
Coconut	3	2,468	7,765	$0.93	$2.93
Cornmeal	0	1,610	0	$0.21	$0.00
Crackers	0	1,828	0	$2.35	$0.00
Cream of Wheat	0	1,658	0	$1.12	$0.00
Dates	6	1,243	8,004	$1.12	$7.21
Egg noodles	9	1,760	15,110	$0.61	$5.24
Eggs, freeze-dried (1 lb = 32 eggs)	0	2,697	0	$6.83	$0.00
Flour					
Unbleached	50	1,650	82,500	$0.19	$9.50
Whole wheat	20	1,651	33,020	$0.31	$6.20
Fruit drink					
Fruit flavor	0	1,950	0	$0.99	$0.00
Lemon	0	1,950	0	$0.99	$0.00
Orange	52	1,950	100,449	$0.99	$51.00
Tang	0	1,950	0	$1.65	$0.00
Gingerbread mix	12	1,928	22,760	$1.47	$17.35
Granola	0	2,211	0	$1.30	$0.00
Ham (cooked)	0	1,800	0	$3.00	$0.00

	Pounds ordered	Calories per pound	Total calories	Cost per pound	Total cost
Honey	18	1,379	25,158	$0.78	$14.23
Hot cereal (Wheatena)	5	1,618	8,682	$0.96	$5.15
Jell-O	4	1,683	7,225	$1.84	$7.90
M&M's	9	2,100	18,029	$2.39	$20.52
Macaroni	18	1,674	30,540	$0.61	$11.13
Margarine	40	3,387	134,489	$0.57	$22.63
Mighty Mush	5	1,750	9,390	$0.80	$4.29
Milk (powdered)	23	1,650	37,950	$1.47	$33.81
Mushroom soup base	2	2,000	4,293	$3.44	$7.38
Nuts (mixed)	3	2,694	8,673	$2.49	$8.02
Oatmeal	29	1,672	48,447	$0.29	$8.40
Onions (dried)	3	1,465	4,717	$2.32	$7.47
Pancake mix	19	1,615	31,197	$0.70	$13.52
Pancake syrup	4	1,600	6,868	$0.79	$3.39
Peanut butter	20	2,682	54,687	$1.04	$21.21
Peanuts	14	2,558	35,687	$1.17	$16.32
Pepperoni	13	2,255	29,040	$4.40	$56.66
Peppers (dried)	1	1,000	1,073	$17.80	$19.10
Popcorn	2	1,642	3,524	$0.27	$0.58
Potatoes					
Powdered	3	1,650	5,312	$1.15	$3.70
Sliced	4	1,624	6,971	$2.56	$10.99
Prunes	6	1,018	6,555	$0.87	$5.60
Pudding					
Chocolate	3	1,637	5,270	$2.05	$6.60
Vanilla	2	1,637	3,514	$2.05	$4.40
Raisins					
Golden	0	1,368	0	$0.88	$0.00
Regular	25	1,359	33,544	$0.88	$21.72
Rice	12	1,647	19,443	$0.42	$4.96
Salami	0	2,041	0	$4.40	$0.00
Salt	0	0	0	$0.16	$0.00
Sloppy Joe base	1	1,400	1,502	$2.22	$2.38
Soup blend with dried vegetables	8	1,600	12,020	$5.60	$42.07
Sour cream	2	1,600	3,434	$5.09	$10.92
Soy nuts	8	1,800	13,522	$0.76	$5.71
Spaghetti	17	1,674	28,744	$0.61	$10.47
Sugar					
Brown	17	1,700	29,190	$0.70	$12.02
White	8	1,700	12,771	$0.36	$2.70
Sunflower seeds	9	2,550	21,893	$0.55	$4.72
Tea bags ($/bag)					
Regular	0	0	0	$0.01	$0.00
Spice	0	0	0	$0.07	$0.00

	Pounds ordered	Calories per pound	Total calories	Cost per pound	Total cost
Tomato base	9	1,350	11,590	$6.58	$56.49
Trail mix	11	2,000	21,463	$1.74	$18.67
TVP					
Beef	4	1,500	6,439	$2.96	$12.71
Chicken	4	1,500	6,439	$2.96	$12.71
Ham	4	1,500	6,439	$2.96	$12.71
Vanilla	0	0	0	$14.16	$0.00
Vegetable oil	13	4,000	51,512	$0.80	$10.30
Vinegar	0	54	0	$0.49	$0.00
Walnuts	5	2,950	15,829	$2.57	$13.79
Yeast	0	1,250	0	$1.21	$0.00
TOTAL:	764		1,421,396		$1,020.60
	Total pounds needed (summer): 792		**Total calories needed:** 1,386,000		**Total budget:** $1,287

Please note that these are only sample food costs, which may not represent the actual cost of food in your area.

CHAPTER TWENTY-TWO

Food: Protection

I. Outcomes

A. Outdoor leaders provide evidence of their *knowledge* and *understanding* by:

1. Explaining general principles of protecting food from wildlife
2. Describing, comparing, and critiquing various methods of food protection

B. Outdoor leaders provide evidence of their *skill* by:

1. Appropriately protecting food from wildlife

C. Outdoor leaders provide evidence of their *dispositions* by:

1. Modeling adequate protection of food from animals

II. Content

A. The need for food protection

1. Some of the consequences of animals accessing food are obvious:
   a) Campers may lose some or all of their food.
   b) Food bags and other equipment may be damaged or destroyed.
   c) In some areas there is a potential for campers to be injured or, in rare cases, even killed from animals coming into camp in search of food.
2. Examples of animals known to ransack food bags and pilfer the food:
   a) Insects
   b) Mice—particularly common in heavily camped areas
   c) Chipmunks
   d) Squirrels, which can readily chew through nylon and run up, down, or across nearly any hanging line; considered by many to be the most ruthless animal encountered in the outdoors

e) Raccoons—creative, intelligent, and dexterous

f) Bears—creative, intelligent, inquisitive, opportunistic, and potentially dangerous

3. Ethical considerations: Although it might be cute to feed chipmunks or other critters, feeding wildlife frequently has detrimental and sometimes fatal consequences.

   a) It may cause wildlife to lose their fear of humans. When humans become a source of food, animals risk losing their food-finding skills.

   b) Attracting animals may cause additional risks, such as safety problems for both the animals and people (e.g., rabid animals, bears), sanitation problems (e.g., eating from a pot that a raccoon has licked), and damaged equipment (e.g., mice or squirrels eating food bags or packs).

   c) Even the slightest trace of human food has the potential to influence animal behavior. Habituated bears—and other animals in some cases—lose their natural desire to forage. Human food and trash can also make animals sick. Wilderness travelers can help break the cycle by not feeding wild animals and adequately protecting food when traveling in the backcountry.

   d) Considerations when traveling in bear country: Bears that rely on human food are more likely to become aggressive and be considered a nuisance. Forest managers are more likely to have to kill these bears when they are determined to be a risk to human safety. Studies have shown that bears that rely on human food are more likely to be overweight, are generally less active, and delay finding a den as early as naturally foraging bears. This has the potential to make them more susceptible to hunters and road mortality.

      (1) Be on the lookout for bear sign (tracks, scat, claw marks on trees/stumps); try to avoid surprising bears (be noisy and sing/talk)

      (2) The kitchen/sleeping/food storage triangle: Choose separate locations for cooking, sleeping, and hanging food that form the points of a roughly unilateral triangle, taking into consideration the following:

         (a) Locate your kitchen/cooking area on a sandbar if near a river, or in an open meadow with good visibility

         (b) Locate your tent upwind and uphill of the cooking area to help prevent cooking smells from reaching your tent site

         (c) Hang food bags downwind of your tent site

      (3) Food storage in bear country

         (a) Never store food in your tent (a good policy anywhere)

(b) Hang food and other scented items, such as soaps, tooth-paste, lip balm, sunscreen, toothbrushes, insect repellent, unused film cartridges, and first-aid kits

(c) Hang food and all scented items during the day if the group leaves camp

B. Considerations in determining whether to protect food or not. Although we recommend always protecting food, factors such as the amount of use a campsite receives and the pristine nature of a site help determine whether to protect food or not. The following guidelines will help when using good judgment in protecting food.

1. If in doubt, protect food.
2. When traveling in remote areas where animals have not experienced human use, protecting food may not be necessary.
3. If you are unfamiliar with an area, ask a forest ranger or other resource management professional what practices are recommended.

C. Means of food protection. Food protection can range from hanging it from a tree limb in a bag or pack 4 feet off the ground to keep mice and squirrels away to high-powered electric fences designed to keep mountain lions and grizzly bears away. Here we will discuss the two most common means of food protection: hanging food bags and animal-proof food canisters.

1. Hanging food bags
   a) Look for a site and make all preparations to hang food during daylight hours.
   b) Find a site that meets the following requirements:
      (1) For small mammals it should be at least 4 feet (1½ meters) off the ground and 4 feet from the nearest tree.
      (2) For bears it should be at least 12 feet (4 meters) off the ground and 6 feet (2 meters) from the nearest tree.
   c) Select a method that will work best for the chosen site (see fig. 22.1):
      (1) Two-tree method: Ideal, most secure method
      (2) Single-tree method: Works well in many instances, particularly for protection from small mammals
      (3) Single-branch method: Works best with a lightweight food bag and a strong branch
2. Bear-resistant food canisters
   a) Food canisters are durable, odor-tight, plastic cylinders that slide into a backpack or strap to the outside.
   b) Canisters are about the size of a small sleeping bag, are 10 to 14 inches

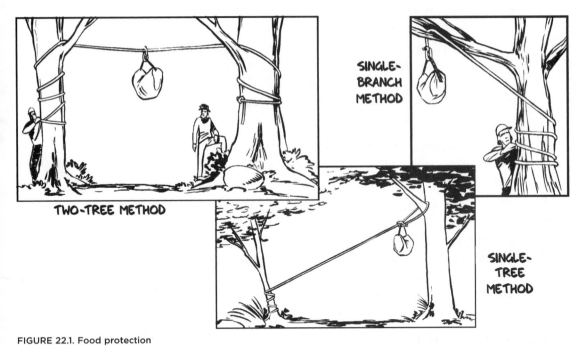

TWO-TREE METHOD

SINGLE-BRANCH METHOD

SINGLE-TREE METHOD

FIGURE 22.1. Food protection

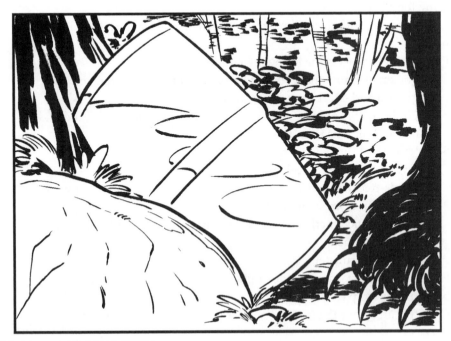

FIGURE 22.2. A bear-resistant food canister

in length and 8 to 9 inches in diameter, and weigh approximately two to three pounds.

c) The specially designed lids resemble childproof medicine bottle caps and are designed so bears cannot open or break them.

d) Most hold three days' worth of food for two people. You can save room by keeping out your first day's lunch and dinner.

e) These canisters have been proven to be the most effective means to protect food and have been tested against grizzly bears; their use is required in many national parks.

f) Do not hang a canister from a tree. Simply conceal it at least 50 feet from tent or sleeping area under a bush or tree. If the outside is kept clean, bears may not even show an interest.

g) Using food canisters gives your group the freedom to camp anywhere and eliminates the need to search for a suitable tree from which to hang food.

III. Instructional Strategies

A. Timing. This class can be taught using the teachable moment at the beginning of a course and before problems develop. Depending on the animals found in the region, it could be followed up with a more formal class as time permits or circumstances demand.

B. Considerations

1. This class lends itself nicely to student instruction. It is a relatively simple class, yet provides an opportunity for the demonstration of many elements essential to good teaching.

2. Many instructors use a lecture/demonstration approach followed by student practice of the skill.

C. Materials

1. Rope: At least 40 feet (13 meters) of ¼-inch (0.5 centimeter) diameter nylon cord

2. Food bags

3. Carabiner(s): one or two (optional)

4. Small pulley (optional)

CHAPTER TWENTY-THREE

Group Development

I. Outcomes

A. Outdoor leaders provide evidence of their *knowledge* and *understanding* by:

1. Describing the stages of group development
2. Describing leader behaviors and considerations for each stage of group development
3. Describing the task versus process dimensions of group development
4. Describing emotional factors that influence group development
5. Describing various roles that group members take on while in a group
6. Comparing leader behaviors within each stage of group development
7. Comparing process versus task functions
8. Critiquing the effectiveness of personal roles as a group member
9. Critiquing leader behaviors during each stage of group development

B. Outdoor leaders provide evidence of their *skill* by:

1. Identifying the stages of group development using the Jones or Tuckman models
2. Identifying task versus process behaviors
3. Exhibiting the appropriate behaviors during each stage of group development
4. Identifying various individual roles in a group
5. Identifying emotional behaviors that influence group development

C. Outdoor leaders provide evidence of their *dispositions* by:

1. Consistently monitoring stages of group development
2. Showing appreciation for group development theory as a tool for deeper understanding of groups

3. Demonstrating awareness of and making decisions based on the needs of the group
4. Celebrating the diversity of group members and what they contribute toward the success of group goals

II. Content

A. Participants and assigned leaders make up the group. All group members have needs, expectations, skills, and emotions.

1. Groups have both task functions (i.e., content, things to do) and process functions, sometimes known as maintenance functions (i.e., ways to keep in working order, interpersonal relations) to perform.
2. The nature of the task and the experience of the group dictate the balance between task and process functions.
3. The leadership style used by the assigned leader in any stage or in any situation will affect the task/process balance.
4. Group members will assume a variety of roles and behaviors to accommodate task and process functions.
5. As roles and behaviors emerge from the group and are accepted, the group begins to take on a unique personality.
6. The process that moves a group from a collection of individuals to a productive, interactive group follows a pattern.

B. Theories of group development

1. Two theories are frequently used by outdoor leaders to analyze the group dynamics of outdoor education experiences, developed by Tuckman (in 1965) and Jones (in 1973). These models are similar, yet each provides unique insight into the growth and development of effective groups. Being familiar with both models will help enhance the leader's understanding of group dynamics. These stages can be identified and tracked by outdoor leaders.

   a) Jones's model will be looked at first (see table 23.1). Use the figure to interpret the four stages of group development as well as the accompanying task and process behaviors at each stage. Groups may advance at different rates along the task and process dimensions. For a group to become effective, it must balance task and process functions. The following points may help the leader interpret table 23.1.

      (1) There are four stages to the Jones group development model.

Table 23.1. THE JONES THEORY OF GROUP DEVELOPMENT

Stages of Group Development	Overall Stage Description	Phases of Task Behavior at Each Stage	Task Behavior Characteristics at Each Stage	Phases of Process Behaviors at Each Stage	Task Process Characteristics at Each Stage
Stage I: Immature Group	• Group dependent upon leader • Group attempts to learn leader and program expectations • Group learns tasks and standards • Members may be eager but show concerns for task and others	**Orientation**	• Group must learn what tasks are; how work is done; learn standards • Members must learn what is expected of group by leaders, program, and/or organization	**Dependency**	• Members are dependent on leader for structure, direction, assurance, and protection • Members who have problems with leader authority may block growth • Members who experience significant personal changes may block development
Stage II: Fractional Group	• Stage of general dissatisfaction • Members argue, communicate poorly, struggle for leadership, personalize issues • Members experience internal conflict between initial expectations and reality • Members experience low morale, conflict, dissatisfaction with dependence on leader	**Organization**	• Group chooses how to organize work to accomplish tasks • Group strives to agree on procedures for problem solving, decision making, leadership concerns, and conflict management	**Conflict**	• Differences in points of view and personality emerge • Internal struggles for informal leadership, influence, power, and visibility occur • Open or hidden (behind-the-scenes) conflict occurs • Members withhold support for one another
Stage III: Sharing Group	• Trust and respect grow in group • Leader expresses satisfaction in group accomplishments • Self-esteem among members increases • Appropriate end-state for some growth-oriented groups • Not appropriate end-state for groups with task productivity responsibilities • Members may not want to "rock the boat," so maximum effectiveness and efficiency are not achieved	**Open Data Flow**	• Information exchanged freely among members relevant to tasks • Information such as opinions, facts, intuition, and other data shared among group members	**Cohesion**	• Group must face internal conflicts to reach this stage • Members are open about feelings and reactions to others' behaviors • Negotiation occurs to deal with interpersonal struggles • Members experience feelings of group cohesion
Stage IV: Effective Team	• High productivity • Members move beyond own comfort level—willing to "rock the boat" • High problem-solving and decision-making ability • Members feel pride and want to be part of successful experience • Task effectiveness and efficiency carried out at increasing levels • Focus on realizing team goals	**Problem Solving**	• Group has achieved sufficient level of information sharing and openness in order to move to higher level of problem solving • Group uses information to diagnose barriers to goal attainment and decision making • Group is able to implement corrective measures to attain goals	**Interdependence**	• Members recognize true need for one another • Group can org͏ itself in • Group can ͏ highly flexibl͏ • Group can ͏ team or in͏ • Member͏ trust ar͏ • Memb͏ ideas͏ tech͏ flir͏

The information contained in this table was compiled from Group Development Assessment Facilitator Guide, J. E. Jones and W. L. Bearley. King

(2) Separate task and process functions correspond with the four stages. Task and process behaviors advance at each stage as a group becomes more functional.

(3) The model is not linear, although most groups experience more than one stage. Groups can get stuck in a stage if the process and task functions are not balanced.

(4) Note the difference between the sharing group and the effective team. Many groups and leaders confuse these stages in the field. Sharing groups feel cohesion and work together well but do not want to upset the "status quo" by introducing more conflict. Effective teams are not afraid to express differences and do it in a productive manner. Effective teams truly recognize and appreciate the diversity of individual members. Problem solving and productivity are maximized.

(5) Jones and Bearley (1994) have developed an assessment tool for the developmental levels (growth) of groups. Ewert and Heywood (1991) used the assessment to look at group development on Outward Bound courses. Results suggested that experiential programs like Outward Bound do promote group development. They also found that long courses (nine days or more) were not more effective than short courses.

b) Tuckman (1965) developed one of the most popular models of group development. Tuckman reviewed group development literature, discovering distinct patterns and creating four stages of development. A fifth stage has been added to explain the process of ending a group. The following represents a brief description of each stage (Schoel, Prouty, and Radcliffe 1988).

(1) Forming: This stage is ambiguous for the participants. They may search for structure and test the leader. At this stage, the group can be described as a collection of individuals. The group is dependent on the leader. Members may exhibit the following behaviors: nervousness, withdrawal, awkwardness, acting out, hyperactivity, or excitement.

(2) Storming: Members are trying to organize themselves into roles. Members may show impatience with each other, especially less skilled or "different" members. Members may interrupt or disagree over plans or ideas. They are vying for attention and leadership within the group. Open power struggles emerge. The leaders may be attacked or blamed for problems. Testing of group norms

occurs. Members may exhibit confusion or anger, or they may experience disillusionment.

(3) Norming: This is a period of reconciliation when members listen and seek consensus, begin to accept differences, and are willing to compromise and work together to accomplish tasks. Individuals are defining their roles within the group. Standards for behavior are agreed upon and are followed more consistently.

(4) Performing: The group is functional and interpersonal relationships are strong. The group is capable of working together to efficiently and effectively accomplish tasks. Members may experience open communication, pride as a group member, feelings of cohesion, and group identity.

(5) Transforming/termination: This is when a group ends. Members are satisfied and unwilling to reassess norms or to introduce new ideas for consideration. Apathy and a slower progress toward reaching new goals may occur. The group may reminisce about past group experiences as they prepare to separate. Some individuals may withdraw. Members may revert back to old ways. Members may celebrate based on feelings of success and pride. Characteristics of the transforming stage may also occur when there are major changes such as course transitions or when members leave due to sickness or injury. The group may revert back to the forming stage as a way of adjusting to new changes. Change in leadership may cause a group to transition, i.e., an old instructor leaves and a new skills instructor enters the group. (Fig. 23.1 graphically combines the Jones and Tuckman models.)

C. Leadership considerations and behaviors. What should the leader consider at each stage in order to promote group development? What are appropriate behaviors to promote development? See table 23.2 for specific suggestions based on the Jones and Tuckman models. It should be noted that this is not a recipe, but only a general guideline. Outdoor leaders must use their judgment and weigh all factors when considering actions to influence group dynamics. The following are general leadership skills that enhance group development:

1. Set a tone early. Encourage consistent behaviors (i.e., respect, tolerance, etc.) and open communication.
2. Communicate through listening, feedback, and constructive criticism.
3. Empower the group by allowing participants to make decisions as their ability to do so becomes apparent.

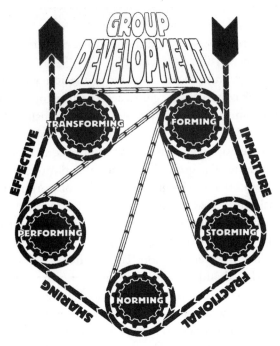

FIGURE 23.1. The Jones and Tuckman models of group development

4. Use conflict-resolution techniques.
5. Explain group dynamics within the framework of expedition behavior.
6. Use an appropriate leadership style for the developmental phase of the group.
7. Allow for group maintenance (e.g., clarify ideas, evaluate suggestions, diagnose problems, etc.).

D. Emotional factors

1. Emotional factors may affect the ability of the group to move from one stage to another.
2. Shutz (1966) developed a theory that includes three emotional phases or levels that the group experiences. The emotional or psychological phases are cyclical and continuous, and emotional needs in each phase must be satisfied before moving on. The phases coincide with the group's development and the degree to which members feel part of the group.
   a) Inclusion: People wonder if they fit in and have appropriate skills to help the group meet goals, or if they will be accepted. This is an early issue that may reoccur with each new situation.
      (1) Signs of when inclusion is adequate:
         (a) Individual needs are recognized and accepted.

Table 23.2. LEADER BEHAVIORS TO PROMOTE GROUP DEVELOPMENT

Jones's Stages of Group Development	Leader Considerations and Behaviors	Tuckman's Stages of Group Development	Leader Considerations and Behaviors
Stage I: Immature Group	• Provide structure • Help establish effective group norms • Make tasks clear • Provide proper perspective • Be sensitive to dependency needs of members for direction, support, and inspiration	**Stage 1: Forming**	• Be nurturing and accepting • Be relaxed, clear, open, and honest • Be energetic, smile, and use humor • Explain purposes and goals • Describe leader's role • Give information equally to all members
Stage II: Fractional Group	• Task behaviors restricted because group is organizing itself • Process behaviors jeopardized by conflict • Leaders must expose conflict and assist in resolving conflicts • Leaders help group work toward coexistence, managing conflicts and making decisions	**Stage 2: Storming**	• Do not panic or become disappointed with the group • Do not become authoritarian • Do not solve problems • Be supportive and validate struggle • Teach conflict-resolution skills and help group understand that conflict is a natural and healthy part of the process • Do not become defensive if attacked
Stage III: Sharing Group	• Leader's role and style changes significantly • Leader supports group efforts to move toward a higher stage • Group may not want to move to higher stage due to feelings of comfort • If leader's focus is on group harmony, she/he may get stuck with the group and lose momentum • Leader must push group toward interdependence	**Stage 3: Norming**	• Continue to support and praise positive behaviors • Reinforce the development of group norms by providing positive feedback and perspective to the process • Involve the group in decisions and let consequences occur without compromising safety • Reinforce attempts to resolve conflict and help group refine conflict-management skills • Revisit and adjust initial behavioral contracts if appropriate
Stage IV: Effective Team	• Leader's role changes to participant, consultant, and inspirer • Leader becomes involved with task only as needed • Leader and group share influence • Leader provides group with vision • Leader challenges group to move to excellence and works with group to achieve synergy	**Stage 4: Performing**	• Group has achieved sufficient level of information sharing and openness in order to move to higher level of problem solving • Group uses information to diagnose barriers to goal attainment and decision making • Group is able to implement corrective measures to attain goals
		Stage 5: Transforming	• Affirm, celebrate, and support • Prepare students for leaving and reentry—discuss transition • Provide ceremony, awards, certificates, T-shirts to validate the experience • Talk about feelings and emotions associated with change—these may appear well before the trip ends • Share feelings and learning • Help members make sense of the experience • Spend time one on one with students to sort out personal issues if appropriate

    (b) Participation is evenly distributed among members.

    (c) There is good interaction.

    (d) The group can articulate goals and is committed to its goals.

  (2) Signs of when inclusion is inadequate:

    (a) Members may be late to meetings.

    (b) Some members may physically stand back or remove themselves from the group.

    (c) There is little or excessive interaction so that participation is unevenly distributed.

    (d) An overall lack of confidence is observable in the group.

    (e) There is a lack of cooperation.

    (f) Individual (versus group) behaviors and decisions are evident.

b) Control: These are feelings among group members about roles and their associated responsibility and power—who has it, and who wants it. Control issues reflect each person's feelings of where power is in a group. They also reflect one's own feeling of competence in any given circumstance.

  (1) Signs of when control is adequate:

    (a) The decision-making process is clear.

    (b) Conflict is accepted and dealt with.

    (c) There is shared leadership and power.

    (d) There is bargaining within the group.

    (e) The group is productive at both task and group-maintenance functions.

  (2) Signs of when control is inadequate:

    (a) The group uses poor decision-making processes.

    (b) There are power struggles.

    (c) There is a lack of leadership.

    (d) There is criticism and competitiveness within the group.

    (e) The instructor may resort to using a more definite structure and imposing decisions.

c) Affection: These are feelings of liking others and being liked.

  (1) Signs of when affection is adequate:

    (a) Communication is open and honest.

    (b) Feelings are expressed.

    (c) Group members feel free to be different and still be accepted.

    (d) Group members are receptive to new ideas.

(e) Group members feel close to one another.

(2) Signs of when affection is inadequate:

(a) There is limited communication.

(b) Members withhold feedback.

(c) There is a lack of trust in others.

(d) There is dissatisfaction with the group.

3. As the cyclical stages are repeated, ideas and feelings are also repeated and deepened.

4. Everyone, including instructors, experiences emotional stages of feeling adequate, liked, and competent, as well as converse feelings. It is important to give enough information and enough responsibility for the group to establish bonds to keep it functioning.

E. Group roles

1. Group members tend to take on roles to achieve or impede group goals (Jordan 1996). Identifying and understanding group roles provides another tool for the leader and group members to analyze the group process. Individuals can be given specific feedback based on the roles they portray. Roles tend to either hinder or promote group effectiveness.

2. Positive group roles: Group members take on positive roles to enhance group morale and to achieve group goals. Positive group roles contribute to the balance of task and process dimensions of group development. Jordan (1996) identifies and describes the following as positive member roles.

a) Clarifier: The member who seeks clarification and helps others see more clearly.

b) Compromiser: The member who works to find the middle ground so that everyone can find agreement in difficult situations.

c) Consensus seeker: The member who ensures that everyone participates equally in all group activities and discussions.

d) Encourager: The supportive member who encourages others to do their best. This person acts as a cheerleader.

e) Gatekeeper: The member who keeps the group on task while ensuring that everyone is included.

f) Harmonizer: The morale booster who helps others deal with conflict by identifying similarities shared.

g) Initiator: The member who gets things started by initiating both process and task functions.

h) Opinion/information giver: The member who shares his/her own opinion and knowledge appropriately during group activities.

i) Opinion/information seeker: The member who solicits opinions and information from group members who may be quiet or uncomfortable.

j) Problem solver: The member who accurately identifies problems and helps the group solve issues and resolve conflicts.

k) Summarizer: The member who adds perspective to the process by summarizing the issues and problems at hand.

l) Timekeeper: The member who keeps track of time and assists the group in moving toward the goal in a timely manner.

3. Negative group roles: Negative group roles hinder group functioning, both process and task functions. Any role taken to an extreme can be negative. Individuals may not be aware of negative role behavior. It is important for a leader to be able to identify these behaviors and address them appropriately so the group will continue to develop. Jordan (1996) identifies and describes the following as negative member roles.

a) Blocker: This person disagrees with others beyond reason and may use statements such as, "we have never done it this way" or "it will never work like this, there are better ways to do it." This person stops forward movement.

b) Clown/entertainer: This member disrupts group functioning through inappropriate or untimely humor or attention-seeking behavior.

c) Digressor: This member takes the group from tangent to tangent so that the group finds it difficult to stay on task. This behavior may be intentional or unintentional.

d) Disassociator: This member disengages from the group process by daydreaming or by physically removing himself or herself.

e) Instigator: This member upsets others by getting them involved in issues other than the task at hand.

f) Scapegoating: This is where a group member or the whole group targets one group member as the cause of problems.

III. Instructional Strategies

A. Timing

1. An appropriate time to address group development is when the group has reached a storming stage. To assist the group in managing conflict, the leader should share a model of group development. This will help the group to understand that its problems are part of a natural process. This type of intervention turns theory into application.

2. Group development can be taught after the group has had enough time

together to experience several stages. By using past history, real examples of behavior can be identified to bring the models to life.

B. Considerations. Using the following activities, the instructor may assess an individual's ability to identify stages of group development based on actual experience.

C. Activities

1. Have students reflect on a past group experience and describe their memories and perceptions of group development. The students should be able to identify specific behaviors.
2. "Freeze Frame Assessment": After group development has been introduced, tell the group that the leader will intervene during group problem-solving situations. For example, the group may be deciding what the hiking route will be for the next few days. During the group discussion, the leader will yell "freeze!" Everyone must freeze by not moving and becoming silent. The leader will then ask the group to identify the various task and process functions being exhibited in the moment. This is a powerful way to enhance the understanding of task versus process functions.
3. Have students incorporate the developmental progression in their journals. The leaders should wait until the group has had enough time together to experience several stages. After presenting a group development model, have students identify stages by recording corresponding behaviors.
4. Have students divide into four or five small groups. Each small group will be assigned a stage of development. Groups must reflect back over the trip thus far, identifying specific occasions when various stages were reached and explaining why. This may be used as the stage to brainstorm strategies to move to more advanced stages, if applicable.
5. During periods of conflict, the leader may give a brief explanation of barriers. Shutz's emotional phases can be addressed to help explain member needs. Journaling or small group discussions may be used to identify specific signs. This information can be processed through journaling or through a group meeting.
6. Role identification exercise: Have group members create a list of all potential roles a group member might exhibit. Names are then placed by a corresponding role based on observed behaviors. Then a master chart is compiled or lists are simply passed around a circle for everyone to read and discuss. This self-awareness exercise allows individuals to see how their peers perceive them. Warning: Instructors must be ready to intervene and guide the group as negative roles are discussed.

CHAPTER TWENTY-FOUR

Group Orienting and Monitoring

Orienting and monitoring groups are important leadership functions. To properly orient a group and monitor the group's progress throughout an expedition is an essential duty. The time taken to do a quality job at this task separates a quality, intentional leader from the mediocre, reactive leader. Orienting a group will have significant ramifications on the quality of the experience, safety, and care for the environment. Orienting and monitoring cannot be overlooked or underemphasized. (See fig. 24.1 for an overview of the factors involved in properly orienting a group for a wilderness expedition.)

I. Outcomes

A. Outdoor leaders provide evidence of their *knowledge* and *understanding* by:

1. Describing the process of setting the overall tone for an outdoor experience
2. Describing the process of goal setting
3. Describing the process of establishing positive group norms, both static and dynamic
4. Describing important logistical tasks to be accomplished before a trip
5. Describing how to monitor group and individual dynamics
6. Describing how to monitor safety and environmental impact during a trip
7. Comparing effective versus ineffective group dynamics while monitoring a group
8. Comparing effective versus ineffective individual dynamics while monitoring a group
9. Critiquing group goals and the processes of goal setting and setting a tone during the orientation period

B. Outdoor leaders provide evidence of their *skill* by:

1. Setting the overall tone for an outdoor experience
2. Facilitating goal setting for a group
3. Establishing positive group norms
4. Accomplishing critical logistical tasks before a trip
5. Monitoring group and individual dynamics during a trip
6. Monitoring safety and environmental impact during a trip

C. Outdoor leaders provide evidence of their *dispositions* by:

1. Consciously setting the tone for a group at the beginning of a trip
2. Spending an appropriate amount of time establishing goals
3. Role modeling behavior to help develop positive group norms
4. Carefully accomplishing important logistical tasks at trip start
5. Consistently monitoring group and individual dynamics during a trip
6. Consistently monitoring safety and environmental impact during a trip

II. Content

A. Orienting a group. In order to ensure success, a leader must know how to orient a group. The following four factors typically define a successful expedition: (1) goal accomplishment, (2) having a safe experience, (3) having an enjoyable (fun) experience, and (4) protecting the natural environment. (See fig. 24.1 for a summary of the orienting process.)

1. There are four steps that a leader should follow in the orientation process of a wilderness experience:
   a) Setting the tone: Creating an atmosphere of trust and mutual respect
   b) Establishing goals: Creating a common vision and purpose
   c) Establishing group structure and group norms: Creating acceptable standards of group behavior (frequently called a Full Value Contract)
   d) Logistical tasks: Ensuring that participants are properly prepared to go into the field
2. The first element of an orientation: Setting the tone. It is the leader's job to establish a positive tone when corresponding with the group via mail, e-mail, or telephone, and when a group eventually comes together. When individuals come together for a common purpose, the initial stage of group development must be taken into consideration (see chapter 23, Group Development)—the leader can use the developmental characteristics of a newly formed group to set the tone.

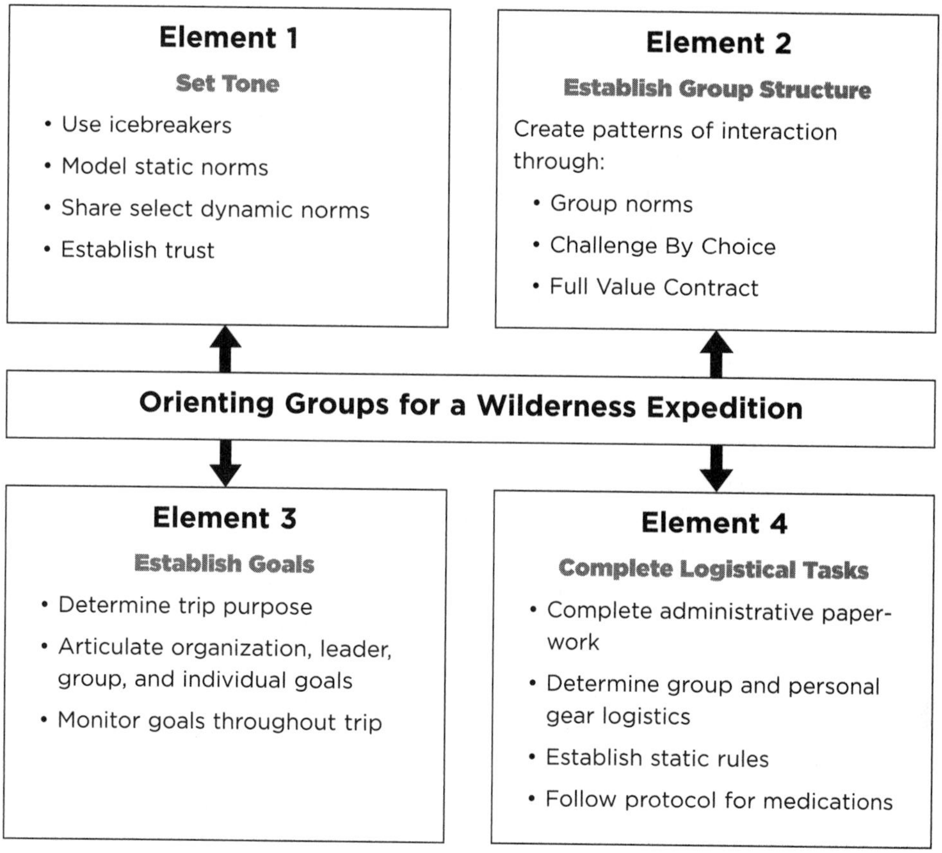

| **Element 1** | **Element 2** |
| Set Tone | Establish Group Structure |

Element 1

Set Tone

- Use icebreakers
- Model static norms
- Share select dynamic norms
- Establish trust

Element 2

Establish Group Structure

Create patterns of interaction through:

- Group norms
- Challenge By Choice
- Full Value Contract

Orienting Groups for a Wilderness Expedition

Element 3

Establish Goals

- Determine trip purpose
- Articulate organization, leader, group, and individual goals
- Monitor goals throughout trip

Element 4

Complete Logistical Tasks

- Complete administrative paperwork
- Determine group and personal gear logistics
- Establish static rules
- Follow protocol for medications

FIGURE 24.1. Orienting groups

a) Characteristics of a new group may include:
   (1) Participants feeling anxious, uncomfortable, or shy
   (2) Participants acting out and being loud and animated to gain attention or to show excitement
   (3) Participants questioning their roles in the group
   (4) Participants questioning how they should or should not act
   (5) Participants wanting to be accepted into the group
   (6) Participants wanting to know what is going to happen and when (they may have many questions)
   (7) Participants being curious about the leader as a person and what the leader's expectations are
   (8) Participants seeking guidance and approval from the leader
b) Keeping the above characteristics in mind, how can a leader establish a positive tone?

(1) Initiate icebreakers to relieve tension and to foster enjoyment from the beginning. Examples: Name games, tag games, or simple problem-solving activities.

(2) Establish and model static norms; i.e., expected behaviors that remain constant. Activities such as role modeling, and promoting appropriate behaviors such as listening, respect, organization, etc.

(3) Dynamic norms are policies, rules, or regulations that change as needed. An extensive laundry list of rules and regulations should be avoided. Keep it short and simple! (This will be discussed in more detail later in the chapter.)

(4) Establish trust: Elements of trust are openness and sharing, and also acceptance and support.

    (a) "The key to building and maintaining trust is being trustworthy." The more accepting and supportive the leaders can be, the more participants will disclose their thoughts, feelings, reactions, and ideas with you. The more trustworthy a leader is, the more a member will share with you on a personal level (Johnson and Johnson 2000, p. 134). Group participants are taking personal risks when they disclose feelings and ideas. Being able to openly share is critical for setting a healthy tone. Good judgment should be used as to what is appropriate to share with a group. A leader who is trusted will be well informed of all issues within the group.

    (b) "Acceptance is probably the first and deepest concern to arise in a group. Acceptance is the key to reducing anxiety and fears about being vulnerable" (Johnson and Johnson 2000, p. 134). One of the main things a leader should do is to publicly praise others when they see appropriate trust-building behaviors (i.e., when you see individuals helping one another or giving compliments to one another). This reinforces appropriate behaviors. The leader should also confront inappropriate behaviors in a positive, supportive way by making suggestions for more appropriate ways to interact. Referring back to the norms that were set is a good strategy.

(5) Violating trust: Once trust is lost, it can be extremely difficult to reestablish. Rejection, ridicule, or disrespect toward a group member's openness will destroy trust. Also, the leader has to be open

and disclose appropriate information and feelings. Group participants may react in a negative fashion to a leader who is not open and who withholds information as a form of power. If a mistake is made, don't be afraid to apologize to the group. The apology must be sincere and immediate. Your actions must correspond to your words in order to be credible.

3. The second element of an orientation: Establishing goals and objectives. Goal setting is a critical but often overlooked task. For most people the goals of a wilderness trip seem apparent and therefore receive little attention. The lack of attention to goals can be a big mistake. Lack of goals or unclear goals will result in a poor experience that negatively affects safety, enjoyment, and the natural environment. Therefore, all groups preparing to go into the wilderness must first clarify their goals.

a) The first step: Determine the primary purpose of the trip. People engage in a wide variety of wilderness trips for a multitude of reasons. Each type of experience will dictate the types of goals needed to guide the experience. The following represents possible trip types:

(1) Service trips: A volunteer experience designed to help people or the environment

(2) Developmental trips: A wilderness experience where group participants are working on specific skills to enhance interpersonal and/or intrapersonal skills (i.e., a corporate development group works on skills to develop a more cohesive, effective team)

(3) Recreational trips: A wilderness experience for leisure to promote social interaction and enjoyment of the great outdoors

(4) Skills-based trips: A wilderness experience where the primary focus is on developing technical outdoor skills, such as mountaineering, rock climbing, white-water canoeing, or coastal sea kayaking

(5) Destination trips: A wilderness experience where the primary goal is to climb a specific peak or paddle the length of a wilderness river

(6) Therapeutic trips: A wilderness experience used as a therapeutic tool to assist individuals with psychological or physical problems to become more functional members of society (e.g., youth-at-risk wilderness programs)

(7) Spiritual trips: A wilderness experience used to explore spiritual development

(8) Multipurpose trip: A wilderness experience where any of the above trip types are combined

b) After the trip type is determined, trip goals must be articulated before the trip starts and during the early portion of the trip. It is frequently wise to revisit goals throughout the trip. This is not a simple task because there are diverse agendas. All agendas should be clarified to reduce misunderstandings. One of the most common sources of conflict during a wilderness expedition is a result of goal incongruity. The following represents the diverse sources of goals for a single trip:

(1) Organizational goals: This might include a brief overview of organizational history, mission, and program goals. During orientation, the leader or an appropriate administrator should share overall organizational goals.

(2) Leader goals: The leader will have personal goals and expectations that should be articulated and made clear to all participants, such as how participants should act, what will be accomplished, how the environment will be treated, rules for safety, etc. These are also considered the static norms. They remain constant. The leader should also be specific about his or her role—and how that role will be played out. The leader might give specific examples of the type of leadership style that will be used and why. The leader should also share his or her expectations of how the group will interact and accomplish daily tasks, etc.

(3) Participant goals: Each participant will have individual goals, such as to have fun, to fish a lot, to eat certain foods, to "hang out" with certain groups of people, to engage in favorite activities, etc. During orientation the leaders should allow each individual to express personal goals (desires and expectations). An effective format to accomplish this is to arrange the group in a circle and have each individual share his/her goals. Participant goals must be congruent with the organizational and leader's goals. If they are not, these issues must be resolved if a trip is to be successful.

(4) Group goals: The group as a whole will have goals, such as what activities will be accomplished, how far it will travel, how participants will interact, who will take on certain roles in camp and on the trail, etc. These are considered the dynamic norms. They are flexible and can change. Like the participant goals, group goals must be congruent with the organizational and leader's goals. If they are not, these issues must be resolved if a trip is to be successful.

c) Revisiting goals: After about the second or third day of a multiday trip, review the goals during a daily group debriefing session. This simple step is often overlooked. Once in the field, perspectives change and individuals tend to lose sight of the larger goals because there is a tendency to become self-involved and focus on individual goals.

(1) Throughout the trip, group participants and leaders should revisit the goals when major decisions have to be made. Higher-quality decisions will be made with all goals taken into consideration. This is particularly true when difficult decisions have to be made, such as turning back or altering preplanned activities. It may be appropriate to revisit goals when the group experiences conflict. Goal clarification can assist in conflict management.

(2) Finally, at the trip's end, feelings of success and accomplishment will be magnified if the leader takes participants through this process. Goal clarification provides the direction and purpose individuals need to reach a specific outcome. A successful trip outcome is accomplished when the individual, leader, group, and organizational goals are met. This is a time to celebrate.

4. The third element of an orientation: Establishing group structure and group norms. The third element is broken down into three sections: (1) First, patterns of interaction are discussed, as well as the definition of group norms; (2) next, the concept of "Challenge By Choice" is discussed as a tool to establish norms and to help set a positive tone; and (3) finally, a tool called the "Full Value Contract" is introduced as a way to provide structure and to develop healthy norms.

a) Patterns of interaction: "The way a leader structures a group will determine how productive it will be" (Johnson and Johnson 2000, p. 22). Group structure "is a stable pattern of interaction among participants" (Johnson and Johnson 2000, p. 26). Patterns of interaction include two key concepts:

(1) Group roles: Participants take on formal and informal roles that affect group structure. Roles revolve around responsibility of each group member.

(a) Formal roles: May be assigned, such as logistician, patrol leader, etc.

(b) Informal roles: May be voluntarily taken on by participants with particular interests or skills, such as cook, lead climber, naturalist, etc. Of course, these roles may change periodically if the leader has structured the sharing of duties (tasks).

(c) "Once roles are assumed, participants expect individuals to conform, behave a certain way, and to fulfill role requirements" (Johnson and Johnson 2000, p. 26).

(d) Role conflicts occur when role obligations are not fulfilled or are not properly identified. Participants come to expect roles to be fulfilled. If a member does not fulfill his or her role, this affects others and creates a role conflict.

(2) Group norms: ". . . common beliefs regarding appropriate behavior, attitudes, and perceptions of members" (Johnson and Johnson 2000, p. 28).

(a) Group norms form the standards of behavior within a group. Norms can be established formally and informally.

(b) If a member wishes to stay in the group and maintain the acceptance of others, he/she must conform to the group norms. Norms can be positive or negative.

(c) Examples of negative informal norms:

  i) Older participants tease younger, less experienced participants.

  ii) Cliques form among popular participants, excluding others from conversations, jokes, and activities. This is an example of a fractionalized group. The group is not unified toward group goals.

(d) Examples of positive informal norms:

  i) Participants allow everyone to speak when making a group decision and ensure that no one is left out.

  ii) Participants respect each other's differences and don't make fun of or tell insulting jokes behind each other's backs. This is an example of a group that is unified toward meeting the group goals.

b) Challenge By Choice (CBC): The purpose of using CBC is to give the participants control over the amount of risk and challenge they are willing to take. In other words, the leader lets the participants decide at what level they will participate. This is an effective way to empower participants. Participants will experience varying levels of fear, doubt, or hesitation when faced with an adventure challenge, such as rock climbing or white-water canoeing. A leader must recognize the benefit of letting participants make participation choices for themselves. There are many ethical issues that arise from forcing an individual to participate. Forcing individuals to do something gives them no control over their personal or physical well-being. Therefore, it is the leader's task to challenge and encourage each group member to take growth-producing risks. Peer pressure to participate can also force participation. A leader can use CBC as a mechanism to set a positive tone for group interaction and to help control negative peer pressure. CBC should not be used as an excuse not to participate. During the orientation, leaders should explain that CBC should be used to decide at what level one will participate. Schoel, Prouty, and Radcliff (1988) describe CBC like this:

(1) A chance to try a potentially difficult or frightening challenge in an atmosphere of support and challenge

(2) The opportunity to "back off" when performance pressures or self-doubt become too strong, knowing that an opportunity for a future attempt may be available

(3) A chance to try difficult tasks, recognizing that the attempt is more significant than performance results

(4) Respect for individual ideas and choices (Schoel, Prouty, and Radcliff 1988, p. 131)

c) Full Value Contract (FVC): Creating a Full Value Contract is one of the most important things to do when orienting a group. Its creation allows the group to develop dynamic group norms; i.e., rules for the group to live by. (See the SPEC Teacher's Tool Bucket in chapter 1 for more on the Full Value Contract.)

(1) The FVC addresses the following issues:

(a) The FVC helps establish group structure that is conducive to success (goals, tasks, and interpersonal dynamics).

(b) If used correctly, the FVC addresses fears that a group member may have before a wilderness experience. It is not uncommon for individuals to wonder if they are capable of completing the expedition, if they will be accepted by others, if they will fit into the group, and what is expected of them as a group member. This begins to establish a safe learning structure that builds trust among participants.

(c) The FVC can be used to set expectations for a high level of participation in order to reduce participant passivity (low motivation).

(d) The FVC helps set a tone of respect—self-respect and respect for others. Individuals sometimes have a tendency to discount themselves due to lack of self-confidence or negative messages from others that they are not capable.

Participants sometimes have a tendency to discount others in the group for various reasons. It is usually because someone else is different in some way; e.g., belief system, culture, physical ability, etc.

(2) Schoel, Prouty, and Radcliff (1988) describe the Full Value Contract as an agreement to:
  (a) Work together as a group toward individual and group goals.
  (b) Adhere to certain safety and group behavior guidelines.
  (c) Give and receive feedback, both positive and negative, and to work toward changing behavior when it is appropriate (p. 95).

(3) The leader has the option to present the contract in verbal or written form. An effective way to present the Full Value Contract is to engage the group in the development of the contract. After agreeing to the content of the contract, participants should verbally agree to or sign the contract. A written contract allows for a visual reference tool that can be introduced when the FVC needs to be reviewed. It adds to the accountability of participants. The contract can be revisited throughout the expedition and restructured as necessary. It takes practice for a leader to use this tool effectively, but, if used correctly, the FVC can make expeditions more enjoyable and safer for all.

(4) The following outline contains suggestions for the formulation of an FVC:
  (a) Present the concept and purpose of the contract. Sometimes it is helpful to have some key questions for the group to respond to that will help define the Full Value Contract.
  (b) For example, what will it look like during our trip if we:
    i) Play and work fair?
    ii) Play and work hard?
    iii) Play and work physically safe?
    iv) Play and work emotionally safe?

(5) It is important for the FVC to be written in language the students understand and described by behaviors they can see or hear.

(6) Have someone in the group be a recorder to write the contract down as the group agrees on its content.

(7) State that there are two main aspects to the contract:

(a) To respect yourself: Treat others as you would like to be treated. Do not discount yourself and try your best. The idea is to try every activity to the best of your ability.

(b) To fully respect others in the group:

    i) Be helpful to others: Be selfless, not selfish.

    ii) Don't put other people down: No name calling; use appropriate language.

    iii) Support others by giving them praise when they do something for the good of the group or the environment.

    iv) Keep safety at the forefront of all decisions. For example, there may be general safety rules that everyone must follow. It is tempting to do your own thing, but it may be at the expense of others. Example: You are camping with your group in a remote wilderness area, and you go alone to a "hot" fishing spot before everyone wakes up when you were supposed to travel in groups of three when not in the campsite. You fall and get hurt, which puts everyone at risk.

    v) The FVC could represent the overall trip goals and the commitment to those goals. (Many other behaviors or values could be integrated into the contract. It is up to the leader and participants to develop the contract to suit their needs.)

5. The fourth element of an orientation: Logistical tasks. During the orientation process, the leader must also address the logistical considerations to properly prepare the group. Because situations vary dramatically, there are no standard procedures to follow. Most logistical tasks are included in the trip planning process. The following guidelines can be used as a generic guide for most adventure activities. During the orientation, the leader should:

a) Have participants complete all necessary paperwork, such as permission slips, waiver forms, medical forms, etc.

b) Complete a "hands-on check" of individual gear: It is not enough to read over a list in front of the group as a way of checking gear before entering the field. A leader must physically look at each individual's gear. Participants may not have the proper gear for various reasons. Maybe they simply forgot an item. Maybe they didn't know the proper gear to bring. Maybe they misunderstood the initial equipment list. Maybe they are so ingrained in old ways that they haven't taken the time to adhere to the suggested equipment list for your trip. Maybe they didn't know the environment and made incorrect choices.

c) Establish responsibility for equipment: The leader or participants should not assume how damaged or lost gear will be handled. The leader should facilitate a discussion on equipment responsibility and replacement. The discussion should include who is responsible for issued gear. Issued gear—i.e., stove, kitchen utensils, tarps, maps, tents, etc.—is the equipment that everyone in the group uses, and it is typically issued by the sponsoring organization. The discussion should also include who is responsible for personal gear that is used by the group. For example, if an individual brings a tent, stove, water filter, compass, etc., that is used by the whole group, who is responsible for the gear if it is damaged?

d) Establish how personal medication is to be handled. The leader should establish ground rules for the use of medication.
   (1) Who carries medication?
   (2) Where is extra medication packed?
   (3) If medication is taken, should the leader be informed? (For example, a participant may be accustomed to taking medication at home for a headache. In the wilderness, this habit could be dangerous if the leader is not informed. The aspirin may simply be masking more serious problems that the leader should know about; e.g., altitude sickness, dehydration, etc.)
   (4) Who has access to medications?

e) Ground rules (part of static norms): At some point during the initial orientation, ground rules must be established. Actual ground rules will vary from situation to situation and from leader to leader. One rule of thumb that should be kept in mind is to minimize ground rules and "boil" them down to the critical rules that must be observed. The leader must make ground rules clear without creating an environment that stifles individual freedom and enthusiasm. This can negatively affect learning and enjoyment. Basic rules may cover such issues as:
   (1) Using drugs and alcohol
   (2) Using lifejackets
   (3) Using correct camp skills (e.g., not placing self in situations without the group's or leader's knowledge of your location, correct stove use, correct sanitation procedures, etc.)

(4) Protecting the environment using practices that conform with outdoor ethics

(5) Forming or establishing exclusive relationships

(6) Using inappropriate language

B. The monitoring process. Once the trip is under way, it is the leader's responsibility to monitor the group at all times. A leader must focus his/her observations on key issues that will be presented in this section. (See fig. 24.2 for a summary of the monitoring process.)

1. The first issue to discuss is the concept of observation and what key items should be observed: "The purpose of observation is to clarify and improve the way in which the group is presently functioning through an objective assessment of the interactions among participants. Information about the group process is collected and then openly discussed so that modifications in group procedures and participants' behaviors can be made in order to improve group effectiveness" (Johnson and Johnson 2000, p. 64).

   a) A leader must observe a number of things:

      (1) The group process: How are participants communicating; e.g., how well does the group make decisions?

      (2) Task function: How does the group accomplish tasks; e.g., canoeing from point A to B, effectively/efficiently breaking camp in the morning, negotiating an off-trail hike.

      (3) Attention to safety: Does group keep safety at the forefront of decision making?

      (4) Attention to the environment: Does the group always take the environment into consideration?

      (5) Performance: How effective is the group in meeting the stated trip goals?

   b) A leader is constantly on duty as an observer. Observation of the five categories listed above is done on a daily basis. Observation is a skill that must be learned and practiced. Many times, involvement in the group as a participant negatively affects a leader's ability to observe with an objective eye. To observe objectively, the leader must be able to take a backseat. It would be the same as exercising a third eye that is like a video camera. The leader records individual behaviors and group actions based on the five categories. Observations will be played back (shared) to the group during meetings/debriefs.

   c) Steps for observation:

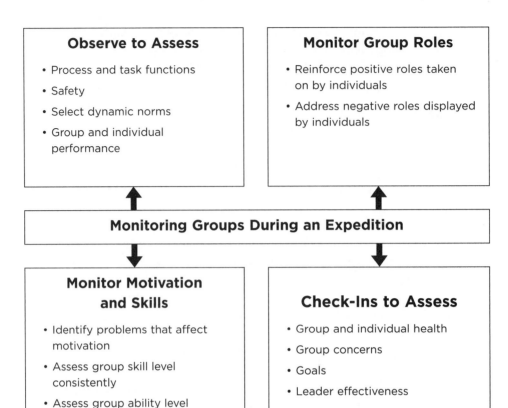

Observe to Assess

- Process and task functions
- Safety
- Select dynamic norms
- Group and individual performance

Monitor Group Roles

- Reinforce positive roles taken on by individuals
- Address negative roles displayed by individuals

Monitoring Groups During an Expedition

Monitor Motivation and Skills

- Identify problems that affect motivation
- Assess group skill level consistently
- Assess group ability level consistently

Check-Ins to Assess

- Group and individual health
- Group concerns
- Goals
- Leader effectiveness

FIGURE 24.2. Monitoring groups

(1) Observe participant behaviors without evaluative judgment initially. For example, you may observe that two participants tend to dominate most group conversations during group decision making, but do not make a value judgment that these two are being selfish and hogging the spotlight. Simply take note of the behavior. It is a good idea to make notes in a journal.

(2) Look for patterns. For example, are the same behaviors exhibited each time the group meets to make a decision? Pay close attention to how others react; e.g., become frustrated, quiet, or follow blindly.

(3) Once patterns are determined, use the data collected to give the group feedback. Follow rules for giving and receiving feedback—share information based on specific examples of behavior as

opposed to judgmental statements. Let the group formulate and articulate the positive and negative ramifications of the observed behavior.

(4) It should be the leader's goal to act as a sounding board for the group. The leader's observations are simply to raise group self-awareness. Raised self-awareness is critical if the group is to self-regulate and become more functional as a team in reaching its desired goals.

2. Monitoring your group by observing group member roles: Observing group roles will also help a leader monitor group process effectiveness, task accomplishment, safety, and protection of the environment. During the group process, a leader can monitor relationships and task productivity through awareness and recognition of group roles. A leader can reinforce positive group roles and confront negative group roles. Group roles should be monitored to help the group reach its goals. (See chapter 23, Group Development, for a list and description of positive and negative group roles.)

3. Monitoring your group by paying attention to levels of motivation and skill competence: "Two factors which you must constantly assess, and which will affect your leadership behavior, are the motivation of the crew and the competence of the crew" (North Carolina Outward Bound School 1993, p. 12).

a) Motivation waxes and wanes throughout an expedition. The leaders should monitor for the following to identify possible motivation problems:

(1) Participants are physically exhausted, hungry, and tired.

(2) "The relationship the student sees between the activity and something the student wants" (North Carolina Outward Bound School 1993, p. 13): e.g., the student practices knots so that he can participate in a multipitch climbing experience.

(3) "The relationship the student sees between the activity and something the crewmember wants to avoid" (North Carolina Outward Bound School 1993, p. 13): e.g., group member learns to construct a tarp in order not to get wet.

(4) "The expectance of success" (North Carolina Outward Bound School 1993, p. 13): e.g., the student does not want to climb because he does not think he can make it.

(5) "The degree to which the student was involved in the goal-setting process" (North Carolina Outward Bound School 1993, p. 13).

b) Competence involves effective communication, skill level, and abilities:

(1) Communication: Some participants may have great ideas to get the job done, but their ideas are not heard or are disregarded due to power struggles within the group.

(2) Skill level: If the group is having a difficult time accomplishing tasks, pay attention to skill level. Not being able to paddle at an appropriate level of competency is dangerous and may breed frustration or fear. This takes away from enjoyment.

(3) Ability level: Based on the maturity of individuals, they may deal with situations and conflict inappropriately; e.g., if you are witnessing a lot of conflict, teach conflict-resolution skills rather than always stepping in and dictating a solution. This empowers a group to solve its own problems in a mature way.

4. Monitoring your group by "checking in" on a regular basis: An important part of the monitoring process is to conduct periodic check-ins with the group. Check-ins are conducted for the following purposes:

a) To assess the physical health of individuals and the group: Many times participants will come to the leader to report physical ailments and to ask for help, but other times participants will not share physical problems with the leader. It is paramount that the leader closely monitors the physical health of participants. A simple headache, hot spot on the foot, or stomachache could turn into something very serious. A leader needs to continually check with individual participants throughout the trip and inquire about health. It is also a good idea to check in with the whole group during debriefs. Conduct a "sweep" (with the group seated in a circle, one person volunteers to begin, and everyone takes a turn sharing until you get back to the person who shared first) at the end of the day or first thing in the morning to actually hear everyone verbalize how he or she is feeling.

(1) Two important physical issues to monitor while on the trail:

(a) The importance of water consumption during a wilderness experience cannot be stressed enough. Dehydration is the precursor to many problems. Dehydration affects the morale and safety of the group. A leader should constantly remind the group to drink water. One of the best ways to monitor appropriate water intake is through the quality and quantity of urination. Urination should be clear and copious. Strong smelling, dark yellow urine is a sure sign of dehydration. It is the leader's responsibility to relay this information to the group and monitor this issue by directly asking participants about the quantity and quality of urination. While this may be uncomfortable for some, the leader needs to remember that he or she plays many roles as leader. The health-monitor role is paramount. For example, make a ritual out of drinking water. It is called the "toasting game." Start this ritual at the beginning of the trip during orientation. Tell participants that a toast can be made anytime during the experience. Whenever someone proposes a toast, the entire group pulls out water bottles and drinks to the occasion. It is a great way to celebrate accomplishments, gratitude, or the beauty of nature. It also forces participants to keep water handy.

(b) The other key issue to monitor that affects group morale and safety is food intake. Low blood sugar from lack of food affects our attitude and ability to think clearly. Statistics show that most accidents occur during activities in the middle of the day and in the late afternoon. One of the primary reasons for this is low blood sugar because participants are tired and hungry. The leader must insist on snacking throughout the day. Sitting down and consuming a large meal three times a day in the field is not the best way to treat our bodies. Because the level of physical activity is rigorous and constant during a wilderness experience, our bodies burn calories at a much higher rate. We must constantly replace calories by eating to keep blood sugar and energy levels up.

b) To assess group dynamics: During a morning or evening debrief, have individuals share issues and concerns. An open forum of this nature is very effective in defusing situations that may grow and result in a major conflict.

c) To assess goal accomplishment: As discussed in the goals section, check-ins can be used to assess goal accomplishment throughout the trip.

d) To assess leadership effectiveness: If the leader has established a positive, supportive environment, the leader can use the check-in to assess his or her effectiveness. Participants should be given the opportunity to provide the leader feedback. This is a tough thing for many leaders to do, but a leader who is open to feedback and acts on that feedback is role modeling healthy communication skills. This role modeling allows participants to engage more freely in similar behavior. The leader is also able to make adjustments in style, communication patterns, and in other areas to improve the quality of the trip. Leaders should also monitor each other with timely feedback.

III. Instructional Strategies

A. Timing. Teaching the skills required to orient and monitor a group is a challenging task. One of the most effective ways to accomplish the task is through a Leader of the Day (LOD) experience. The information can also be presented in a lecture designed to prepare students for the LOD experience. This content should also be discussed whenever the topic of expedition leadership is discussed. It is also important to role model orienting and monitoring tasks so that future leaders experience the process.

B. Activities

1. LOD exercise: Assign participants as LODs throughout a trip. LODs can practice setting tone and daily goal setting each day they serve as LODs. They can also practice monitoring skills as part of their duties. LODs can then reflect on their experiences in a journal and should receive feedback from the instructor and other participants at the end of the LOD experience.
2. Group discussion: Later during the trip, ask the group to reflect back on the beginning of their trip. Discuss how the orienting aspect of leadership was conducted.
3. Journal exercise: Have participants reflect through their journals on the orienting process and monitoring process by posing related questions (e.g., how was the tone for our group set; what group norms were established and how; identify specific group roles and explain how these roles affect the group process).
4. Full Value Contract: Create a Full Value Contract on some item that can be carried throughout the trip. A bandanna, the back of a map, a group journal, or a T-shirt can be used. Have individuals express their commitment by making their mark (e.g., signature, drawing, trail name, etc.).

C. Materials

1. Journals
2. Written criteria outlining duties of the LOD

CHAPTER TWENTY-FIVE

Group Processing and Debriefing

I. Outcomes

A. Outdoor leaders provide evidence of their *knowledge* and *understanding* by:

1. Describing the purpose of debriefing
2. Describing the major considerations in organizing daily briefing and debriefing sessions
3. Describing the major components of successful briefing and debriefing sessions
4. Explaining the purpose of the "processing" component of the debriefing

B. Outdoor leaders provide evidence of their *skill* by:

1. Conducting successful briefings and debriefings in the field
2. Planning and organizing briefing, debriefing, and processing sessions, taking into consideration their major components

C. Outdoor leaders provide evidence of their *dispositions* by:

1. Modeling willingness to process experience
2. Modeling willingness to learn from their own successes/mistakes and the successes/mistakes of others
3. Modeling competence in planning and conducting briefing, debriefing, and processing sessions

II. Content

A. Why we debrief. Processing our experiences is a critical component of becoming an outdoor leader as it is one of the most important activities in developing judgment.

1. Through debriefs participants get to analyze and evaluate experiences and learn from each other's successes and failures.
2. Debriefs are one of the most effective processes to help us improve as outdoor leaders. By looking back at what has happened we can explore what went well, what we want to remember to do again next time, what didn't work, and what we want to make sure we don't do next time.

B. Organizing the session. Many of the basic considerations for organizing a briefing or debriefing are identical to those involved in setting up a formal class presentation. (See chapter 1, Teaching and Learning, for more detail.)

1. Timing of the session
   a) The session is best conducted at a regular time each day so that it becomes a ritual—an established, integral part of the daily camp routine.
   b) Early-morning debriefs tend to be more objective because time has allowed emotions to subside and tempers to cool. Evening debriefs can be more emotionally charged as people are frequently tired, things are fresher in people's minds, and emotions may still be high if the day was stressful in any way. As leader you can use this knowledge to help decide whether to debrief late in the day or early the next day.
   c) Early morning is often a good time, since participants should be alert and the previous day's activities will still be relatively fresh in their memories.
   d) Should early-morning travel be necessary, the session can be held along the trail during an extended break. This is often preferable to skipping the daily session entirely or trying to hold it after a long day of travel when participants are tired.
2. Location of the session
   a) The session site should be an area sheltered from the elements and away from any distractions.
   b) The meeting should be located away from areas of high traffic use within the campsite (e.g., cooking and kitchen areas) to minimize human impact on any given area.
   c) The meeting site should be large enough to accommodate all participants comfortably and so all group members can have eye contact.

3. Preparation for the session
   a) All participants should know the time and location of the day's briefing/debriefing site well in advance.
   b) All participants should be informed of the routine and reminded to always bring:
      (1) Appropriate clothing
      (2) Notebook and pencil
      (3) Sitting pad or camp chair
   c) Participants should be reminded of any special materials they will need to bring to the session, such as:
      (1) Maps and a compass
      (2) Resource books
      (3) Special reports (e.g., logger's notes, etc.)
      (4) Journals
   d) All participants who may have to make presentations or reports during the session should be reminded of their responsibilities so they can be organized and ready.
   e) Participants should be discouraged from bringing food or drinks to the session as they are distracting. In addition, participants who worked hard to get their meals completed before the meeting often resent the inefficiency of others.
   f) Punctuality for all group activities is an issue that must be addressed early in the trip. Efficiency should be balanced with enjoyment and a nonstressful atmosphere.

C. Planning the session

1. The Leader of the Day (LOD) (see chapter 24, Group Orienting and Monitoring) should have a clear idea of the general components of the session, as well as a specific set of objectives to be met during the session.
2. In general, all sessions are comprised of three broad components, each with its own essential function. Although the order in which these components are addressed may differ, they all should appear in virtually every meeting.
   a) Informational component: Each session should include the information participants will need to prepare and plan adequately for the day's activities and for any future events that may require preplanning.
      (1) A specific itinerary for the day might be announced. This might include times, location of specific classes, moving of camp, etc.
      (2) Assignments for the day: The LOD might make and announce all special assignments/tasks for the day (e.g., sweep, logger, scout,

etc.) so participants can be prepared for their tasks.

    (3) Classes for the day: Participants responsible for making special presentations during the day can be reminded of their assignments.

b) Logistical component: Depending on the trip objectives and the leader's leadership style, briefing sessions might include an opportunity for group participation in the detailed planning of day trips, moving camp, travel routes, etc.

    (1) Participants can discuss and select the best routes, identify significant topographic features, estimate bearings, and write out Time Control Plans (see chapter 43, Travel Technique: An Introduction to Travel).

    (2) Participants can discuss individual and group gear to be taken on a trip and determine who will carry them.

    (3) If the group is splitting up for the day's travel, participants can discuss the objectives of the trip and the route, apportion group gear, determine group membership, and submit written emergency evacuation plans.

c) Educational component: One of the most important functions of a debriefing session is the opportunity for group members to share and process their experiences.

    (1) All sessions should include a quick "check-in" that surveys the mental and physical status of each participant. (See the SPEC Teacher's Tool Bucket in chapter 1 for a more complete description of a "check-in.")

        (a) All expedition members should know how others are feeling mentally and physically so that group plans and activities may take this into account.

        (b) Participants should recognize the session as an appropriate arena for airing personal views and settling interpersonal differences. An atmosphere of objective openness, tolerance, and compassion must be maintained at all sessions so that group members feel comfortable expressing their thoughts and feelings.

    (2) Sessions should include an analysis and evaluation of the various decision-making opportunities of the previous day. This particular aspect of the session is absolutely crucial to the development of effective decision-making skills. This "processing" phase of the session requires a high degree of skill and therefore requires discipline in preparing and guiding the discussion. (See "Conducting the session," below, for more detail on processing.)

D. Conducting the session

1. General guidelines and suggestions

   a) Proper technical and mental preparation are essential for a successful session. Refer to chapter 1, Teaching and Learning, to review aspects of communication that may prove helpful in conducting an effective session.

   b) A small notepad with brief reminders of important information or topics is very useful for reference during the session.

   c) Writing out specific objectives beforehand helps to focus the leader's attention on what must be done and will help clarify what is or is not relevant discussion during the meeting.

   d) Keep the session moving by insisting that participants focus on the issues at hand and refrain from clearly unnecessary banter or inappropriate comments. Don't be timid about diplomatically curtailing a rambling discussion. If necessary, designate a "taskmaster" to keep the discussion focused.

   e) To maintain group attention, try to keep sessions as short as possible (approximately thirty minutes), allowing time for stretching or bathroom breaks if necessary.

   f) Above all else, be professional in presentation and demeanor. A good-humored but essentially businesslike approach to the session will set an appropriate educational tone.

2. The "processing" component: Considerations for leading the analysis/evaluation phase of the session

   a) Fundamental to the development of decision-making skills is the ability to "process" experience (i.e., an ability to reflect on, describe, analyze, and communicate in some way that which was recently experienced). The analysis/evaluation phase of each debriefing is an opportunity for each participant to process the previous day's experience and share in the evaluative judgments that come out of the discussion (Quinsland and Van Ginkel 1984).

   b) If all participants are to process their own experiences successfully, they all must take part in the discussion concerning the previous day's experience. The individual who leads the discussion should be aware of the skills and techniques necessary for leading an effective group discussion. The "sweep" is an effective tool for inviting participation by all group members. (For more detailed suggestions on leading a discussion, see chapter 1, Teaching and Learning.)

   c) "Processing" should begin with a brief chronological recounting of the previous day's activities. This helps refresh memories for journal writing, allows the group to develop a common interpretation of the shared experience that may bind the group together, and identifies those moments of decision making, crisis, or conflict that need to be explored.

d) Once the previous day's events have been established, the process of analyzing those events may proceed.

    (1) Participants should be encouraged to specifically identify those moments when significant decision-making situations arose. As these moments are identified, the discussion leader should ask questions that focus on why each decision was made:

        (a) What factors influenced the decision?

        (b) What personal considerations had to be taken into account?

        (c) What possible options were open to the decision makers?

        (d) Who made the decision?

    (2) At this stage of the discussion, hasty conclusions about whether a decision was "good" or "bad" should be discouraged.

e) At some stage during the discussion, the decision makers (frequently the LOD) should be invited to critique their own performance and explain the rationale for their actions. Decision makers should be given an opportunity to fully explore and communicate their own interpretations of events before the group moves on to the evaluation stage.

f) Once the group understands the various factors that entered into the making of a specific decision and the decision makers have had an opportunity to explore and explain the rationale for their actions, then the discussion leader should invite comments that are evaluative:

    (1) Was the decision a good one?

    (2) In what other ways may the situation have been successfully handled?

    (3) What did you learn from this situation?

g) Throughout the processing experience, it is important that the discussion leader try to keep the tone as constructive and positive as possible without sacrificing a truthful assessment of the decision maker's strengths and weaknesses. Conflict and injured pride resulting from group criticism are inevitable and, though unpleasant, an essential aspect of the educational process that leads to the development of quality decision-making abilities.

h) Good listening skills are essential to ensure that opinions are being heard and understood. Active and silent listening activities may be used if listening problems are encountered.

i) At the conclusion of the processing discussion, it may be helpful for the discussion leader to use some brief statements to summarize the conclusions made by the group. This highlights the main points of the discussion and also helps to depersonalize some of the criticism that may have been directed at one individual, turning the focus toward understandings that can benefit any leader.

III. Instructional Strategies

A. Timing. Since briefing and debriefing sessions begin at the outset of the expedition, instruction in briefing and debriefing technique can begin immediately through an example set by instructors. Student LODs may be expected to conduct all but the "processing" aspects of a debriefing by the third or fourth day of the expedition.

B. Considerations

1. Teaching briefing and debriefing through daily example seems to be one of the most effective means of helping participants learn this technique. As each discussion leader helps the group examine the briefing or debriefing style of the previous day's leader, instructors should emphasize positive suggestions and ideas that are brought out.
2. It is generally a good idea for instructors to conduct sessions for the first few days of the expedition. This not only sets a good example for participants to follow, but it also sets a tone of objective openness and candor when instructors lead the self-critical aspects and evaluation of their own performance. Participants will see that the ability to evaluate one's own strengths and weaknesses candidly is an essential element of quality leadership.

CHAPTER TWENTY-SIX

History of Outdoor Leadership

I. Outcomes

A. Outdoor leaders provide evidence of their *knowledge* and *understanding* by:

1. Describing the definitions of fundamental terms used by outdoor leaders
2. Describing the evolution of outdoor leadership before and after the Outward Bound movement
3. Describing the role Paul Petzoldt played in the development of outdoor leadership
4. Describing current organizations and services that promote leadership development
5. Explaining the meaning of key terms: experiential education, outdoor education, adventure education, and environmental education
6. Explaining the historical linkage between outdoor education and outdoor leadership
7. Describing the relationship between Outward Bound, the National Outdoor Leadership School, and the Wilderness Education Association and the purpose of each
8. Explaining the purpose and programs of outdoor leadership development services

B. Outdoor leaders provide evidence of their *skill* by:

1. Sharing an understanding of outdoor leadership history with participants

C. Outdoor leaders provide evidence of their *dispositions* by:

1. Sharing an understanding of and enthusiasm for the heritage of outdoor leadership
2. Celebrating the contributions of key individuals and organizations in the evolution of outdoor education

II. Content

A. Outdoor leadership. Terms that have influenced its development:

1. Experiential education: "Emphasizes direct experience as a resource that can increase the quality of learning through combining direct experience that is meaningful to the learner with guided reflection and analysis" (Raiola and O'Keefe 1999, p. 47).

   a) Outdoor education: "Outdoor education means learning in and for the outdoors. It is a means of curriculum extension and enrichment through outdoor experience" (Smith et al. 1972, p. 20).

      (1) Outdoor recreation: Participants engage in socially acceptable outdoor activities during their leisure time.

      (2) Environmental education: "A process that creates awareness and understanding of the relationships between humans and their many environments—natural, man-made, cultural, and technological. Environmental Education is concerned with knowledge, values, and attitudes and has as its aim responsible environmental behavior" (Environmental Protection Agency 1988, p. 3).

      (3) Adventure Education: No consensus has been reached concerning the exact definition of adventure education. Professional adventure educators agree that it does contain elements of excitement, uncertainty, real or perceived risk, effort, and interaction with the natural environment (Raiola and O'Keefe 1999).

         (a) Adventure education includes the development of two distinct relationships:

           i) Interpersonal relationships: How two or more people interact in a group. Group dynamics such as conflict, cooperation, communication, decision making, and leadership influence serve as content for the learner.

           ii) Intrapersonal relationships: Individual developmental attributes such as self-confidence, self-esteem, self-efficacy, spirituality, or leadership style (Priest 1999).

         (b) Outdoor adventure education has been articulated this way: "One of the most important themes in outdoor adventure education is that the participants should be provided with the necessary skills, both mental and physical, to enable them to experience success in using and preserving the outdoors . . . Some of the generally accepted goals are personal growth, skill development, excitement and stimulation, challenge, group participation and cooperation, and understanding one's relationship to the environment" (Cinnamon and Raiola 1991, p. 130).

B. Historical overview. A brief historical overview of outdoor education is needed to appreciate the roots of outdoor leadership. The following represents only a few key individuals among a whole host of educators who have shaped outdoor leadership development.

1. 1800s: The organized camping movement begins in the United States. Frederick Gunn and his wife found the Gunnery School in Connecticut and integrate camping as part of their school programming.
2. 1910: The Boy Scouts of America is incorporated. Ernest Seton is appointed the first Scout Chief. A naturalist and author, he creates a youth organization called Woodcraft Indians that emphasizes outdoor skill development.
3. 1920s and '30s: L. B. Sharpe integrates education into organized camping. The first director of Life Camps for underprivileged youth, "he began using the term outdoor education synonymously with public school camping" (Raiola and O'Keefe 1999, p. 49).
4. 1930s: John Dewey, an educator who emphasizes the importance of experience-based learning inside and outside the classroom, becomes a leader in the progressive education movement in the United States.

C. Overview of outdoor leadership organizations

1. Outward Bound (OB) (www.outwardbound.com)
   a) History
      (1) Kurt Hahn, born in Germany of Jewish descent, developed a reputation as a progressive educator. He spoke out against Hitler during World War II and was imprisoned for a short time, and then released with the help of influential friends. He was exiled from his native home and moved to England. He founded the Gordonstoun School in Scotland and later moved to Wales. Hahn integrated adventure into his curriculum (such as seamanship and mountain sports) as a way to help his young men develop morally and physically. Hahn felt strongly that service to the community should also be part of the educational process (North Carolina Outward Bound 1993).
      (2) Hahn and others created the first Outward Bound school as a way to properly prepare young British seamen for war. "Outward Bound grew out of the need to instill a spiritual tenacity and the

Table 26.1. COMPARISON OF OUTWARD BOUND, NATIONAL OUTDOOR LEADERSHIP SCHOOL, AND WILDERNESS EDUCATION ASSOCIATION

Organization	Date and Place Founded	Founder(s) and Other Key Players	Mission Statement	General Philosophy	Number of Branches/ Affiliates	Number of Students Per Year
Outward Bound International	1941 Aberdovy, Wales	Kurt Hahn	"... to help people discover and develop their potential to care for themselves, others and the world around them through challenging experiences in unfamiliar settings" (www.outward-bound.org/about_sub1_mission.htm).	"To foster the core values of courage, trust, integrity, compassion, and cooperation" (www.outward-bound.org/about_sub1_mission.htm).	Forty-one Outward Bound schools worldwide (www.outward-bound.org/about_annual.htm)	173,000 (www.outward-bound.org/about_annual.htm)
Outward Bound USA	1962 Marble, Colorado	Josh Miner Early key players: Paul Petzoldt Tap Tapley	"... to enhance individual character, promote self-discovery, and challenge students to cultivate self-reliance, leadership, fitness, compassion, and service through exceptional wilderness education"(www.lynnseldon.com/article119.html).	"To broaden enthusiasm for and understanding of self, others, and the environment. To enhance interpersonal communications and cooperation" (North Carolina Outward Bound 1993, p. 8).	Seven U.S. schools and centers	65,000 (www.outward-bound.com/pdf/2000-2001_Annual_Report.pdf)
National Outdoor Leadership School (NOLS)	1965 Lander, Wyoming	Paul Petzoldt Early key player: Tap Tapley	"... to be the leading source and teacher of wilderness skills and leadership that serve people and the environment" (www.nols.edu/about/values.shtml).	"The NOLS community—its staff, students, trustees, and alumni—shares a commitment to wilderness, education, leadership, safety, community, and excellence. These values define and direct who we are, what we do, and how we do it" (www.nols.edu/about/values.shtml).	Eleven branches worldwide	3,000 (www.nols.edu/about/history).
Wilderness Education Association (WEA)	1977 Lander, Wyoming	Paul Petzoldt Bob Christie Frank Lupton Chuck Gregory Early key players: Dr. W. Forgey Jack Drury	"... promoting the professionalism of outdoor leadership and to thereby improve the safety of outdoor trips and to enhance the conservation of the wild outdoors ..."(www.weainfo.org/welcome.html).	Through the processing and assessment of leadership experiences, the WEA prepares individuals to lead safe, enjoyable, and environmentally sound backcountry outings. The WEA provides leadership training through a decentralized network of colleges, universities, and outdoor programs.	Forty-four affiliate colleges, universities, and outdoor programs	200

will to survive in young British seamen being torpedoed by German U-boats during World War II. What began as a training exercise for apprentice British seamen and youth in Wales has since evolved into a modern-day program for self-discovery and personal development" (North Carolina Outward Bound 1993, p. 4).

    (3) Josh Miner brought Outward Bound to North America in 1962 and hired Paul Petzoldt as chief instructor for the Colorado Outward Bound school.

  b) Mission and philosophy

    (1) Outward Bound's mission is " . . . to enhance individual character, promote self-discovery, and challenge students to cultivate self-reliance, leadership, fitness, compassion, and service through exceptional wilderness education" (www.lynnseldon.com/article119.html).

    (2) Outward Bound's general philosophy is "to broaden enthusiasm for and understanding of self, others, and the environment. To enhance interpersonal communications and cooperation" (North Carolina Outward Bound 1993, p. 8).

  c) Branches/affiliates: Outward Bound has four wilderness schools (Outward Bound West, Hurricane Island, Voyageur, and North Carolina); two independent urban centers (New York City Outward Bound Center and Thompson Island Outward Bound Education Center); and the school-reform program, Expeditionary Learning Outward Bound, in the United States. There are approximately forty-one schools around the world today.

2. National Outdoor Leadership School (NOLS) (www.nols.edu)

  a) History

    (1) Frustrated by the lack of qualified instructors in the profession and responding to the growing public interest in backcountry travel, Paul Petzoldt founded the National Outdoor Leadership School in 1965.

    (2) In 1966 NOLS allowed women to be students on courses, a radical departure from current practices of that time period.

    (3) The 1970s were marked by rapid growth and expanded course offerings in Mexico, Alaska, the northern Cascades, and Idaho.

    (4) In addition to offering wilderness leadership courses, NOLS offers other services, such as publishing educational resources, conducting research, sponsoring the Wilderness Risk Manager's Conference, and partnering and supporting Leave No Trace.

b) Mission and philosophy
   (1) NOLS's mission is " . . . to be the leading source and teacher of wilderness skills and leadership that serve people and the environment" (www.nols.edu/about/values.shtml).
   (2) NOLS's philosophy is to share " . . . a commitment to wilderness, education, leadership, safety, community, and excellence" (www.nols.edu/about/values.shtml).
c) Branches/affiliates: NOLS currently operates from established bases located around the world (e.g., Patagonia, Kenya, Yukon, and the Pacific Northwest). NOLS headquarters is located in Lander, Wyoming.
3. Wilderness Education Association (WEA) (www.weainfo.org)
   a) History
      (1) In 1976 a group of Western Illinois University students led by Paul Petzoldt and Dr. Frank Lupton traveled through the Targhee National Forest of Wyoming and the Wind River Range on an experimental course that would later become the model for the WEA National Standard Program.
      (2) In 1977 Paul Petzoldt and a group of college professors discussed the need for college-level professional training programs for the development of wilderness leaders and educators. On October 9, 1977, the Wilderness Use Education Association (WUEA) was created.
      (3) In 1978 WUEA was incorporated as a nonprofit organization in the state of Wyoming. In 1980 it was officially renamed WEA, and Paul Petzoldt was appointed executive director.
      (4) WEA courses typically consist of students who are seeking professional outdoor leadership development. WEA Outdoor Leadership certification is awarded to students who successfully meet certification criteria.
   b) Mission and philosophy
      (1) WEA's mission is " . . . promoting the professionalism of outdoor leadership and to thereby improve the safety of outdoor trips and to enhance the conservation of the wild outdoors."
      (2) WEA's philosophy: Through the processing and assessment of leadership experiences, the WEA prepares individuals to lead safe, enjoyable, and environmentally sound backcountry outings. The WEA provides leadership training through a decentralized network of colleges, universities, and outdoor programs.
   c) Branches/affiliates: Forty-four organizations are accredited to offer WEA courses.

D. Paul Petzoldt

1. Paul Petzoldt played a major role in pioneering formal training and gaining recognition for professional outdoor leadership. Petzoldt saw a need for a new breed of outdoor leaders based on the growing use of the wild outdoors and progressive education programs instigated by Outward Bound.

2. Highlights of Petzoldt's life and accomplishments:

    a) An internationally recognized pioneer in the field of wilderness education, Petzoldt's early exploits as a mountaineer and wilderness guide provided the experience and background that became the foundation of his later teachings.

    b) He directed the Petzoldt-Exum School of American Mountaineering in the Teton Range during the 1920s.

    c) He was a member of the first American expedition to K2 in the Himalayas in 1938.

    d) He taught mountain evacuation and cold-weather dress to U.S. ski troops during World War II.

    e) He testified before the U.S. Congress to help bring about the 1964 Wilderness Act.

    f) He is the author of *The New Wilderness Handbook.*

    g) He and NOLS instructors developed some of the first Leave No Trace techniques to be practiced by wilderness leaders. He and his instructors were concerned about the ekistic relationship of users in a wilderness environment.

    h) He cofounded the Wilderness Education Association (WEA) in order to integrate outdoor leadership as a discipline in higher education.

    i) He founded the PPLS (Paul Petzoldt's Leadership School for Youth) outdoor program in Maine in 1996.

3. Paul Petzoldt was one of the first public voices to raise society's awareness of the need for qualified outdoor leaders. Petzoldt never ceased his effort to educate outdoor leaders to be safe, environmentally sound users of the wild outdoors until his death in 1999. In his lifetime, Petzoldt saw outdoor leadership rise to a respected level of professionalism. Now, a myriad of related organizations, enterprises, and services have evolved to support the outdoor leadership profession. The following represent only a few examples.

E. Other key professional organizations

1. Wilderness medicine certification providers

    a) Levels of certification: Basic Wilderness First Aid, Wilderness First Responder, Wilderness EMT

b) Examples of providers:
   (1) Stonehearth Outdoor Learning Opportunities (SOLO): www.soloschools.com/
   (2) Wilderness Medical Associates (WMA): www.wildmed.com/
   (3) Wilderness Medicine Institute (WMI)/NOLS: www.nols.edu/wmi/
2. Rock climbing and mountaineering certification and program accreditation
   a) American Mountain Guides Association (AMGA): www.amga.com/. This nonprofit organization seeks to represent the interests of American mountain guides by providing support, education, and standards.
   b) American Alpine Institute (www.mtnguide.com/): This organization is dedicated to helping climbers raise their skills, protect the environments in which they climb, develop good judgment, and safely gain access to the great mountains of the world.
   c) American Alpine Club (www.americanalpineclub.org/): This nonprofit organization is dedicated to promoting climbing knowledge, conserving mountain environments, and serving the American climbing community.
   d) National Outdoor Leadership School (NOLS): www.nols.edu. This organization offers specialized courses in rock climbing, mountaineering, caving, and boating.
3. White-water canoeing, kayaking, sea kayaking, and rafting certification: The American Canoe Association (ACA): www.acanet.org/
4. Accreditation services for outdoor education programs
   a) Association for Experiential Education (AEE): www.aee.org/
   b) American Camping Association (ACA): www.acacamps.org/
5. College and university preparation programs for outdoor leaders
   a) Wilderness Education Association Affiliates: www.weainfo.org. These affiliates of the WEA offer outdoor leadership certification for college credit.
   b) There are educational institutions that have created majors and minors specifically designed to train outdoor leaders.

III. Instructional Strategies

A. Timing. This topic is usually taught as time permits. It is particularly suitable for a rainy day or a rest day.

B. Activities

1. Lecture: This approach is most appropriate when participants have little or no knowledge of the topic. (See chapter 1, Teaching and Learning, for different teaching strategies.)

2. "The Minute in History": Using a chronology of events, students are asked to volunteer to prepare a short presentation (one to three minutes) based on a small portion of history. Other resources should be available to help the students expand on the rudimentary information, such as Petzoldt's biography, *On Belay,* or a copy of an Outward Bound instructor's manual. Each day a presentation can be given at the daily debriefing or at some other appropriate time.

3. Student-led presentations: Students are asked to take a portion of the lesson content and present it to the group. Students should be encouraged to use their creativity to make the presentations as interesting as possible (i.e., impersonations, skits, etc.).

4. Storytelling: If a staff or group member has personal knowledge of the evolution of outdoor or wilderness education, his or her personal experiences could be used as a basis for a storytelling/discussion approach to the topic. A campfire or other teachable moment may provide a good opportunity for this approach.

5. Organizational comparison activity: The instructor can provide participants with an example of a common outdoor activity that reflects the different philosophy of each organization. It should be pointed out that the differences are sometimes subtle, and an observer may find the distinctions among the programs blurred depending on the instructor, location, and/or situation. The following map and compass activity is an example.

   a) Outward Bound: The group is asked to travel from point A to point B. Participants are given minimal instruction in map and compass use. The focus of the exercise is to build group unity and individual confidence as group members work together to reach the objective. Participants debrief the experience in terms of their personal growth and group dynamics.

   b) National Outdoor Leadership School: The group is asked to travel from point A to point B. Participants are given extensive formal instruction in map and compass use, including the rationale behind the techniques used. The focus of the exercise is to teach specific map and compass skills. Debriefing and journaling of the activity may or may not occur.

   c) Wilderness Education Association: The group is asked to travel from point A to point B. Participants are given extensive formal instruction in map and compass use, including the rationale behind the techniques used. The focus of the exercise is to provide decision-making opportunities and teach specific map and compass skills. Participants debrief the experience in terms of the leadership and decision-making skills related to the activity as well as what they learned about navigation. Students are required to reflect on their experience through journaling.

6. See the Close Encounters: Wilderness Education in the United States challenge at the end of the chapter.

C. Materials

1. *On Belay* by Paul Petzoldt
2. An Outward Bound instructor's manual

Challenge

Knowledge Outcome	Title	Skill/Disposition Outcome
What do you want them to know?		**What skill/disposition do you want them to develop?**
The participants can describe the important philosophical perspectives of the Wilderness Education Association (WEA), Outward Bound (OB), and the National Outdoor Leadership School (NOLS) and trace their historic relationship through the life of Paul Petzoldt.	Close Encounters: Wilderness Education in the United States	Leadership: creatively seeks alternative, original, and imaginative ideas/solutions

Essential Question or Key Issue:

What are the perspectives of OB, NOLS, and WEA that distinguish each from the other as wilderness education organizations? How are all three linked by the historic influence of Paul Petzoldt?

Description of Challenge/Task/Performance:

This challenge involves a three-part process. The first step involves developing a base of knowledge regarding important topics related to the state of wilderness education in the United States today. The second step involves sharing the knowledge with others. The third step involves processing the shared knowledge and presenting it in a creative way.

Step 1. Creating a base of knowledge: Divide the group into three different teams. Each of these teams will become an "expert" on a different one of the following topics: organizational philosophy of OB, organizational philosophy of NOLS, and organizational philosophy of WEA. Every team is responsible for researching the role that Paul Petzoldt played within its organization. While researching their topic, each team should focus *only* on that information that is "most essential" to know as it relates to the essential question cited above. At the conclusion of the time allotted for research, all members of each expert team must agree on the "most essential" points of understanding for their topic.

Step 2. Sharing the "most essential" information of the experts: Take one expert from each of the expert teams and combine them into a new "sharing team." The new sharing teams now have somebody possessing the "most essential" information from each of the expert teams. Allot time for all members of the sharing team to share their expertise with the others in their group. At the conclusion of this sharing, all members of the various sharing teams should have a general level of understanding of all the information that was researched.

Step 3. Process the shared information and present it in a creative way: Return everyone back to his/her original "expert" team (the team that did the original research). Your task: Create a role play in which your team builds a campfire in such a way that it reveals the unique philosophy of the organization you researched (OB, NOLS, WEA). At the conclusion of the role plays, conduct a large-group discussion in which you trace Petzoldt's influence among the organizations and clarify any remaining questions about each of the organizations.

Criteria for Assessment and Feedback:

Form criteria:
- The role play has a point to make. The plot communicates the organizational philosophy in overt (perhaps exaggerated) terms.
- The actors portray their roles convincingly.
- The actors stay in character throughout the role play.

Content criteria:
- The role play accurately characterizes the philosophy of the organization being represented.

Knowledge:
- The participants recognize and can discuss the philosophical perspective of each of the organizations.
- The audience and group members can participate in the discussion about organizational philosophy and the influence of Paul Petzoldt.
- The audience and group members ask well-informed questions that reveal understanding of the topic.

Skill: Leadership: creatively seeks alternative, original, and imaginative ideas/solutions
- During preparation for the role play, each group member offers at least one idea for the role play that is different from the others.

Product Quality Checklist

Date: _____   Class Period: _____

Product Author(s):	Product Title/Name: Close Encounters: Wilderness Education in the United States	Evaluator Name(s):

Observed	Standard/Criteria	Possible Points	Rating
	The role play has a point to make. The plot communicates the organizational philosophy in overt (perhaps exaggerated) terms.		
	The actors portray their roles convincingly.		
	The actors stay in character throughout the role play.		
	The role play accurately characterizes the philosophy of the organization being represented.		
	Total		

Observations:

Elements of Questionable Quality:

Elements of Exceptional Quality:

CHAPTER TWENTY-SEVEN

Interpretation of the Natural and Cultural Environments

I. Outcomes

A. Outdoor leaders provide evidence of their *knowledge* and *understanding* by:

1. Describing the importance of interpreting the natural and cultural environments
2. Describing the components of an interpretative plan
3. Describing natural and cultural attributes ideally suited for interpretation
4. Describing specific communication and leadership skills necessary for effective interpretation

B. Outdoor leaders provide evidence of their *skill* by:

1. Effectively interpreting the natural and cultural environment
2. Developing a natural and cultural interpretation plan for an outdoor trip
3. Developing effective evaluation tools to determine the success of an interpretation plan
4. Exhibiting basic leadership skills that enhance the interpretative process

C. Outdoor leaders provide evidence of their *dispositions* by:

1. Exhibiting enthusiasm for interpretation of the natural and cultural environments
2. Modeling and communicating an appreciation for the natural and cultural environments
3. Modeling effective leadership skills and communication when acting as an interpreter

II. Content

A. The importance of natural and cultural interpretation

1. An outdoor leader has an ethical responsibility to interpret the natural and cultural environment during an outdoor trip. Interpretation of the natural and cultural environments brings about key benefits described by G. W. Sharpe (1976):

    a) To assist wilderness users in developing a keener awareness and understanding of, and appreciation for, their surroundings and the complexities of coexisting with that environment

    b) To make the outdoor experience rich and enjoyable

    c) To assist land managers in accomplishing management goals

    d) To broaden the participant's perspective beyond the immediate setting to encompass the larger natural resource environment

    e) To motivate the participants to protect the natural environment

    f) To instill an appreciation of a region's culture and heritage

2. Knudson, Cable, and Beck (1995) explain the importance of natural and cultural interpretation this way: "The heritage of any nation lies in its natural resources, its special historic sites, and its cultural collections. The vigor and strength of its future arise from its people's healthy attachment to their roots" (p. 14). The outdoor leader has the unique opportunity when leading participants into the wilderness to interpret cultural and natural resources in a unique and intimate way. This provides a realistic means of instilling genuine respect and care for our natural and cultural environments.

3. Examples of natural and cultural attributes that an outdoor leader could interpret during a wilderness trip:

    a) Natural attributes

       (1) Flora and fauna: Identification and understanding of flora (wildflowers, trees, shrubs, grasses, algae, fungus) and fauna (mammals, birds, amphibians, reptiles, fish, insects) found in particular environments or ecosystems

           (a) Learn common names to deepen appreciation for the interconnectedness of all living things

           (b) Learn about a plant's or animal's function in the ecosystem and about the habits of particular animals

           (c) Discover benefits of specific flora and fauna

           (d) Explore how the flora and fauna have been affected by humans

(e) Discover unique characteristics to enhance appreciation and knowledge of the organism and, in some cases, alleviate irrational fears and stereotypes (e.g., snakes, spiders, leeches)

(f) Explore how the flora and fauna have affected human development and activity in a particular region (e.g., logging, fishing, hunting, trapping, industry, etc.)

(2) Geology: Explore the geological formations that characterize the region, such as mountains, valleys, canyons, lakes, streams, rock formations, caves, etc.

(a) Explore the age and formation process of geological features

(b) Discover how the geology of an area influences the ecosystem

(c) Explore how the geology has affected human development and activity in that region

(3) Ecosystems: Explore the unique aspects of particular environments, such as deciduous forests, marine environments, alpine systems, tundra environments, desert environments, etc.

(a) Study forest succession, the role of fire, the role of disease, and other factors related to the life and health of a forest

(b) Study estuaries, tides, waves, beaches, coastal erosion, etc.

(c) Study alpine or tundra plant and animal life as a system, or discuss why alpine and tundra environments are so fragile

(d) Discover unique characteristics of a desert environment and how plants and animals adapt, etc.

(e) Explore how nonnative/exotic species influence the ecosystem

(4) The sky and beyond

(a) Discuss unique weather patterns and phenomena (see chapter 48, Weather)

(b) Take advantage of natural occurrences or events, such as eclipses, sunspots, or meteor showers

(c) Explore and learn constellations

(d) Discuss the moon's cycle and its effects

(e) Discuss various cultural interpretations (e.g., myths, lore) of weather and astronomical features

b) Cultural attributes
   (1) Indigenous people: Explore the history and culture of the indigenous people of the region. Explore customs, beliefs, cultural connection to the environment, uses of natural materials, or human influence on the land.
   (2) Local population: Explore the beliefs and customs of the area's current inhabitants. Discuss the culture of the local population, intercultural differences and impacts, or cultural effects on the natural resources.
   (3) Historic events: Explore historic events that shaped the character of the region.
      (a) Visit archaeological sites, such as ruins, petroglyphs, pictographs, or old villages
      (b) Discuss how historic events affected the local culture and the natural environment

B. The interpretative plan. An outdoor leader must plan and conduct background research to adequately incorporate interpretation of the natural and cultural environments into a wilderness experience.

1. Components of an effective plan:
   a) First phase: Create learning objectives. The outdoor leader should develop clear, specific, and feasible objectives to enhance learning. This includes making decisions on what aspects of the cultural and natural environment will be interpreted and prevents the leader from haphazardly interpreting the environment while on a trip. Without predetermined objectives, the effectiveness of interpretation is compromised.
   b) Second phase: Research the trip area. The outdoor leader should research and become familiar with the specific natural and cultural attributes of the proposed trip area.
   c) Third phase: Create a plan. The leader should determine how to actually impart natural and cultural information to trip participants. It is during the planning phase that the leader should determine the educational methods to be used during the trip. The following are examples of methods that might be implemented:
      (1) Bring books chronicling the cultural history of an area to be read as a group during an evening program or during down time
      (2) Provide flora and fauna identification books, and other appropriate books, for group members to use
      (3) Schedule time during the trip for interpretative walks to identify and discuss the natural environment

    (4) Develop games and activities that enhance interpretative education

    (5) Schedule an outside speaker (local authority) to meet the group for a lecture, a story, or an interactive activity

    (6) Plan the itinerary and route with adequate time and opportunity to visit significant natural or cultural sites

    (7) Develop plant and animal checklists

d) Fourth phase: Implement the plan. The leader must obtain the supporting resources (e.g., books, star charts) to effectively implement the plan. It is up to the leader to properly sequence activities and lectures so that the educational process is effective. The leader should also be sensitive to teachable moments by taking advantage of opportunities for interpretation as they present themselves.

e) Fifth phase: Evaluation and revision. The leader should consider using one or more evaluation tools to determine the success of his or her interpretative efforts. The following serve as suggestions for possible evaluation techniques:

    (1) Student journaling: Ask participants to reflect on the natural and cultural environment

    (2) Identification checklist: Use checklists to track participant progress

    (3) Assessment activities: Design fun, interactive games that test participant knowledge of the surrounding environment

    (4) Participant debriefing: Encourage participants to debrief thoughts and feelings that surface during a trip about issues related to the cultural and natural environments

    (5) Observation of participants: Observe each participant's behavior as a trip progresses to determine if the initiative to learn is self-motivated and independent from the leader

    (6) Revision of the plan: After determining the effectiveness of the plan, revisions can be made to improve the interpretative aspect of future trips

C. Leadership and communication skills necessary for effective interpretation of the natural and cultural environments

1. An outdoor leader's job is to communicate information regarding the natural and cultural environment in order to impart knowledge and influence the attitudes and behaviors of the participants. (See chapters 1 and 29 for suggestions on how to communicate effectively.) The following leadership considerations are specific to interpretation, according to G. W. Sharpe (1976):

a) It is critical that the leader role model interest and enthusiasm in the exploration process in order to ensure participant participation.

b) The leader should create a plan and activities that will capture the attention of each participant.

c) The leader should create an atmosphere of ease. For example, do not force someone to interact with plants or animals in an uncomfortable way.

d) The leader should cater to diverse interests and not assume everyone will be interested.

e) The leader should create messages that are meaningful and that touch people's lives.

f) The leader should realize that in an unfamiliar setting most people tend to reject new ideas.

g) The leader should not assume that he or she will reach everyone.

2. For outdoor leaders interested in further developing their natural interpretation skills and strategies, a text entitled *The Interpreters Guidebook* is recommended as a resource (Regnier, Gross, and Zimmerman 1992).

III. Instructional Strategies

A. Timing

1. Pretrip consideration: Participants can be given information or reading assignments before the trip. Books, magazine articles, and Web sites that document the natural and cultural aspects of an area provide valuable background information to prepare for a trip.

2. Pretrip consideration: Places of historical, cultural, and environmental interest should be incorporated into the trip itinerary. Arrangements should also be made to schedule meetings with potential speakers during the trip.

3. Formal lessons: Schedule times during the day to have formal flora and fauna interpretative lessons. Also, schedule time to read from books and other literature about the region during formal group meetings. Pack applicable plant and animal identification books and other guidebooks as part of the trip library.

4. Teachable moments (opportunity teaching): Take advantage of natural events and historical features during the trip. Stop to identify and discuss plants and wildlife along the route.

B. Considerations

1. Assessment strategies
   a) Use journaling for participants to reflect on natural and cultural issues. Participants should be encouraged to document fauna and flora that is identified.
   b) Create interactive quizzes to assess the ability of participants to identify local fauna and flora. For example, common games such as Jeopardy, I Spy, or 20 Questions can be adapted.
   c) Assign an identification checklist to be completed by the end of the trip.
   d) Facilitate evening discussions on the cultural and environmental issues of the area.

C. Activities

1. Evening readings: Have participants take turns reading excerpts out of books that describe the history and culture of the region. It is a powerful way to share actual stories of people and events that characterize or shaped the region.
2. Plant of the day: Introduce the group to a new tree or flower each day. Learn to identify the plant and discuss its unique characteristics. It is necessary to carry plant and animal identification materials to give participants a chance to make the introductions.
3. Flora and fauna checklist: Develop a checklist of common plants and animals of the region. Create a competition or simply challenge the participants to complete the checklist by identifying all items.
4. Guest speakers: Local authorities, land managers, storytellers, and local residents can be met along the route. Land managers or local residents can bring deeper appreciation for a region through stories.
5. Stargazing: Take advantage of a clear night and sleep as a group in an open area. Identify stars, planets, and constellations and share associated stories or facts, or have participants make up their own constellation characters.
6. Night walks: Schedule a hike at night in an appropriate area. Hiking at night allows students to experience the "nightlife" of the natural environment. Discussions of nocturnal wildlife and related issues can be facilitated.
7. Poetry and creative writing: Have participants create stories and poetry related to the natural and cultural environment. These works can be written in a journal and shared during evening meetings.

CHAPTER TWENTY-EIGHT

Knots: An Introduction

I. Outcomes

A. Outdoor leaders provide evidence of their *knowledge* and *understanding* by:

1. Describing the fundamental knots used in a camp setting
2. Describing the strengths and weaknesses for basic camp knots
3. Describing the appropriate application for basic camp knots
4. Describing appropriate terminology to teach the art of knot tying
5. Describing the four categories of knots
6. Describing the three basic concepts for creating effective, efficient knots
7. Comparing the fundamental use and functions for each knot
8. Comparing advantages and disadvantages of basic camp knots
9. Critiquing a knot's level of efficiency and effectiveness after it is tied
10. Critiquing any context or application where a camp knot is needed

B. Outdoor leaders provide evidence of their *skill* by:

1. Competently tying basic camp knots in a variety of settings
2. Applying the appropriate knot in the correct situation
3. Identifying the appropriate category for each knot tied
4. Teaching the art of knot tying using standard terminology

C. Outdoor leaders provide evidence of their *dispositions* by:

1. Correctly tying knots
2. Using the correct knot in the appropriate situation

II. Content

A. Rope materials

1. Natural fibers: Rope has been made of plant fibers since its inception more than 10,000 years ago. Fibers commonly associated with natural fiber ropes include flax, jute, sisal, cotton, and abaca (the Manila-hemp plant). Although not nearly as common as it once was, it is still not uncommon to see small-diameter cordage made of natural fibers. (See table 28.1 for a comparison to synthetic fibers.)

2. Synthetic fibers: Man-made fibers were initially developed in the 1930s with new ones still being created. Common synthetic fibers include nylon (polyamide), polyester (Dacron), and polypropylene.

B. Types of rope

1. Laid: Typically three stands are twisted together. Varying the tension of the twist will affect the flexibility and handling of the rope.

2. Braided: Typically ranging from eight to sixteen plaits (braids) that when braided together make for a rope that is more flexible and less likely to kink. Some braided ropes are hollow, and some have a separate core that can add a variety of positive characteristics, including strength and resistance to abrasion.

3. Sheath and core (kernmantel): Made with a kern (inner core) of twisted nylon threads covered by a mantel (jacket or sheath). The core absorbs energy and stretches under a sudden load, providing most of the rope's strength. The mantel protects the core and helps determine much of the rope's handling characteristics.

C. Rope care

1. Reduce exposure to sun whenever possible
2. Store in cool, dry, dark place
3. Keep away from chemicals (gas, bug spray, suntan lotion, etc.)
4. Try not to step on the rope
5. Coil appropriately
6. Wash with mild detergent when needed
7. Avoid sharp edges to avoid cutting/fraying the rope

D. Four categories of knots

1. Knots: Configurations on rope that do not move (e.g., figure eight or bowline)
2. Bends: Connect two rope ends together (e.g., square knot)

Table 28.1. ROPE COMPARISON CHART

	Natural Fibers			Synthetic Fibers		
	Sisal	Cotton	Hemp	Nylon	Dacron	Polypropylene
Shock loading	Poor	Poor	Fair	Excellent	Fair	Fair
Handling	Poor	Excellent	Fair	Excellent	Excellent	Fair
Durability	Poor	Excellent	Excellent	Excellent	Excellent	Fair
Rot and mildew resistance	Poor	Poor	Poor	Excellent	Excellent	Excellent
UV resistance	Excellent	Excellent	Excellent	Poor	Excellent	Poor
Acid resistance	Poor	Poor	Poor	Excellent	Excellent	Excellent
Alkali resistance	Poor	Poor	Poor	Excellent	Excellent	Excellent
Abrasion resistance	Poor	Poor	Fair	Excellent	Excellent	Fair
Melting point	N/A	N/A	N/A	482°F (250°C)	473°F (245°C)	302°F (150°C)

3. Hitches: Tie around something (e.g., taut-line hitch or clove hitch)
4. Decorative knots: Arts and crafts, like weaving a bracelet (e.g., macramé)

E. Three basic concepts to remember when tying camp knots

1. A good knot should be relatively easy to tie.
2. A good knot should serve the purpose for which it is designed and used.
3. A good knot should be relatively easy to untie.

F. Knot terminology. It is important to establish a common language when teaching knots. Using standard reference points will help simplify the complicated process of explaining knot construction. The following terms are recommended. See figure 28.1 for an example of each term.

1. Standing end: The part of the rope that you do not work with while tying a knot. The standing end could be several inches to a hundred feet in length.
2. Working end: The part of the rope that you work with, usually one end of the rope.
3. Loop: When the rope crosses under or over itself.
4. Bight: A bend in the rope where the rope does not cross itself to form a loop.

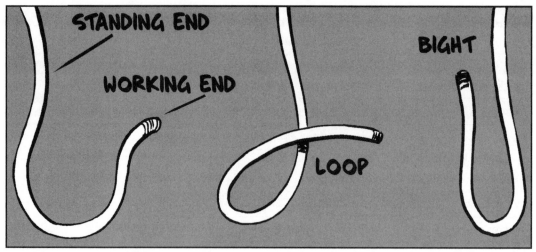

FIGURE 28.1. Knot terminology

5. Slippery: When you finish a knot with a bight that allows the knot to be untied by just pulling the end (e.g., bow, slippery taut-line hitch, and slippery trucker's hitch; see fig. 28.12).

G. Common knots used in an outdoor setting. While there are literally hundreds of different knots, if the average outdoorsperson can master ten to fifteen knots, he or she will undoubtedly have the right knot to handle nearly every situation. We have listed eleven knots. Some of them have limited uses (the overhand, half-hitch, and overhand loop), and we share them merely to help understand the basics, while others have very specific tasks for which they are ideally suited (such as the slippery taut-line hitch and the trucker's hitch).

1. Overhand
   a) Description: This is the most elementary of knots and is demonstrated primarily to help develop a basic understanding of knots. It is said that the Native Americans described this knot as "the knot that ties itself" because it is what happens naturally to garden hoses, electrical cords, etc. (see fig. 28.2).
   b) Uses: Securing a thread to a needle, tying the corner of a bandanna, stopper knot to keep a knot from sliding through a hole.
   c) Strengths: It is easy to tie.
   d) Limitations: It has limited uses and is difficult to untie when put under tension.
2. Half-hitch
   a) Description: Another basic knot that is really nothing more than an overhand knot tied around or through an object (see fig. 28.3).

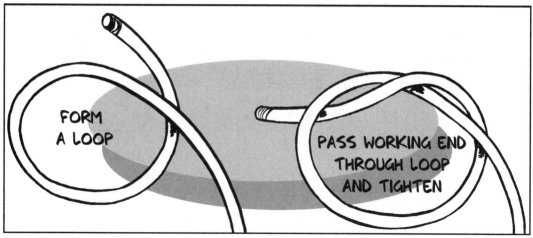

FIGURE 28.2. Overhand knot

    b) Uses: Although this knot has limited or trivial uses, it has many uses when combined with a second (or double) half-hitch (see below).

    c) Strengths: It is easy to tie and usually easy to untie.

    d) Limitations: It has limited uses.

3. Double half-hitch

    a) Description: The double half-hitch is the tried and trusted means to secure a rope to nearly anything (see fig. 28.3).

    b) Uses: Tying a rope to a post, ring, tree, or nearly anything (e.g., putting up a clothes line).

    c) Strengths: It is easy to tie, works well for numerous purposes, and is usually easy to untie.

    d) Limitations: It is not designed to hold heavy weights or for use where safety is a concern.

4. Square knot

    a) Description: Another basic camp knot that has a variety of uses around camp. This knot works best with ropes of equal size (see fig. 28.4).

    b) Uses: A good knot for securing wound bandages, bundles, and packages, or for tying the ends of a bandanna together.

    c) Strengths: It is relatively easy to tie ("right over left, then left over right") and untie.

    d) Limitations: It can come undone too easily, so it must not be used where safety is an issue.

5. Bowline

    a) Description: The bowline is arguably the most useful knot available when you want a loop that will not slip under force and will remain easy

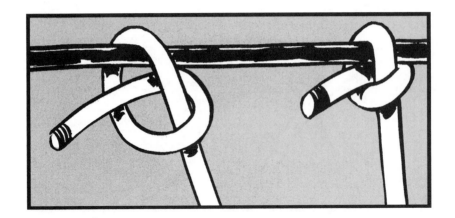

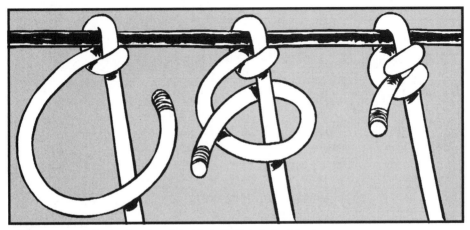

FIGURE 28.3. Half-hitch (above) and double half-hitch (below) knots

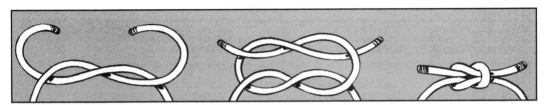

FIGURE 28.4. Square knot

to untie under virtually all conditions. Learning to tie this knot any-where at anytime will go a long way in making a true outdoorsperson (see fig. 28.5).

b) Uses: It serves as an excellent knot to anchor the rope to almost any object (e.g., tying a line through a grommet, tying a rope around a tree).

c) Strengths: It is extremely versatile as it will not slip or jam.

d) Limitations: The working end can sometimes loosen up, so it should be tied off with an overhand knot in some circumstances.

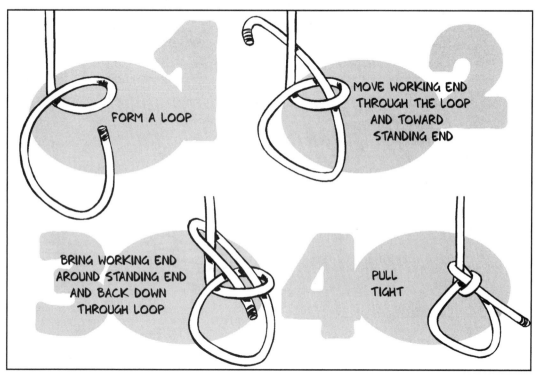

FIGURE 28.5. The bowline

6. Overhand loop

a) Description: A basic knot that has a multitude of uses but can be very difficult to untie once it has been under tension (see fig. 28.6).

b) Uses: Anytime you need a simple loop, this knot can be used.

c) Strengths: This is an extremely easy knot to tie and is very functional.

d) Limitations: With smaller-diameter line or when put under tension, this can be a very difficult knot to untie.

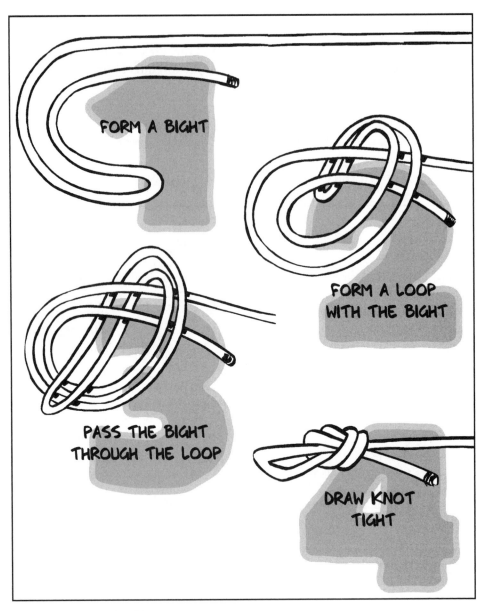

FORM A BIGHT

FORM A LOOP
WITH THE BIGHT

PASS THE BIGHT
THROUGH THE LOOP

DRAW KNOT
TIGHT

FIGURE 28.6. The overhand loop

7. Figure 8 on a bight
   a) Description: Like the bowline and overhand loop, this knot is used to
   form a loop. It is a very strong knot, but it is more difficult to untie
   than the bowline once the knot is weighted. It can be tied very simply,
   but for rock climbing purposes it must be learned to be tied as a "follow-through" knot. (See fig. 28.7 and fig. 28.8)

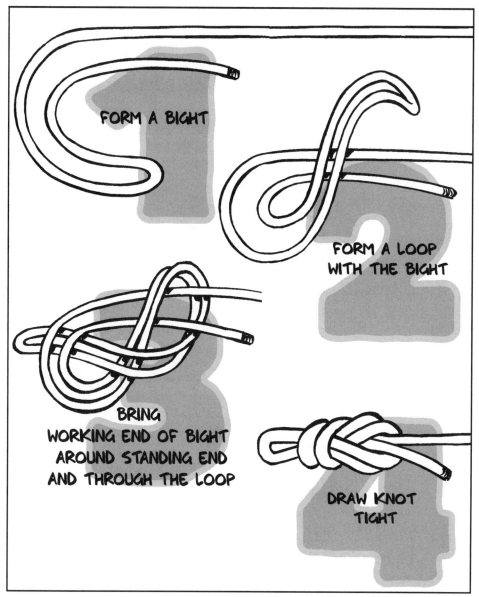

FORM A BIGHT

FORM A LOOP
WITH THE BIGHT

BRING
WORKING END OF BIGHT
AROUND STANDING END
AND THROUGH THE LOOP

DRAW KNOT
TIGHT

FIGURE 28.7. Figure 8 on a bight

b) Uses: When a simple loop is needed, this knot is nearly as easy to tie and easier to untie than the overhand loop. It is one of the most common knots used for rock climbing.

c) Strengths: It is easy to tie.

d) Limitations: When put under tension, it can be difficult to untie.

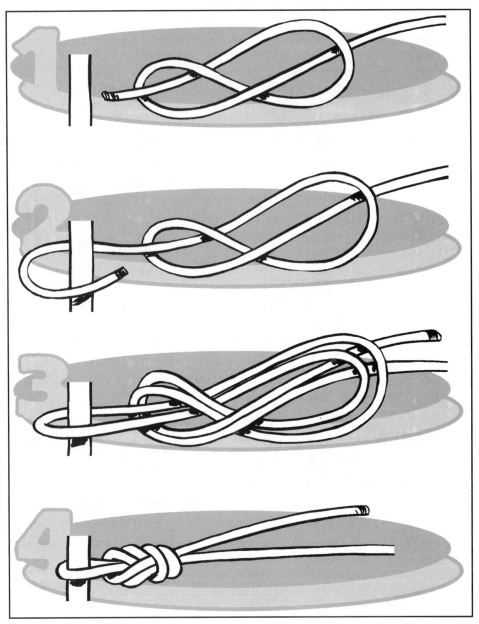

FIGURE 28.8. Figure 8 on a bight follow-through

8. Clove hitch

    a) Description: A knot that rivals the bowline in its usefulness and versatility, a clove hitch tightens as force is applied. There are two basic ways to tie a clove hitch: When tying a clove hitch around a post or pole, you can slide it over the top (see fig. 28.9); however, another method must be used when the rope can't be slipped over an object and must be tied around it (e.g., a large tree) (see fig. 28.10).

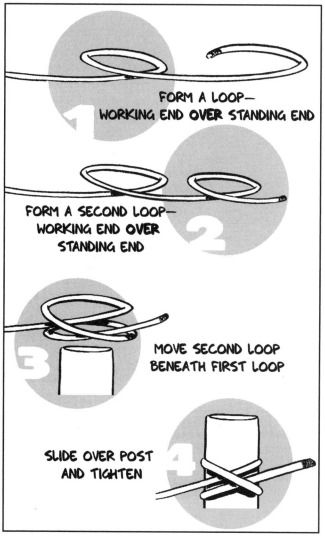

FORM A LOOP—
WORKING END OVER STANDING END

FORM A SECOND LOOP—
WORKING END OVER
STANDING END

MOVE SECOND LOOP
BENEATH FIRST LOOP

SLIDE OVER POST
AND TIGHTEN

FIGURE 28.9. Clove hitch over a post

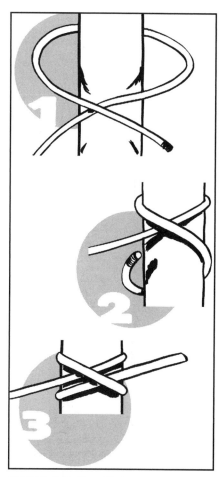

FIGURE 28.10. Clove hitch around a post

b) Uses: It is an excellent knot to place over a tent stake, around a tree or pole, or around the top of a nylon food bag to hang in a tree.

c) Strengths: It is relatively easy to tie and has numerous uses.

d) Limitations: Like most hitches, it can loosen if the tension is not consistent.

9. Taut-line hitch

a) Description: This knot is a handy camp knot because it is easily adjustable. You can tighten or loosen a line by simply sliding the knot up or down the standing end of the rope. The taut-line works by applying friction when it is under tension (see fig. 28.11). We like to use the slippery version of this knot (see fig. 28.12).

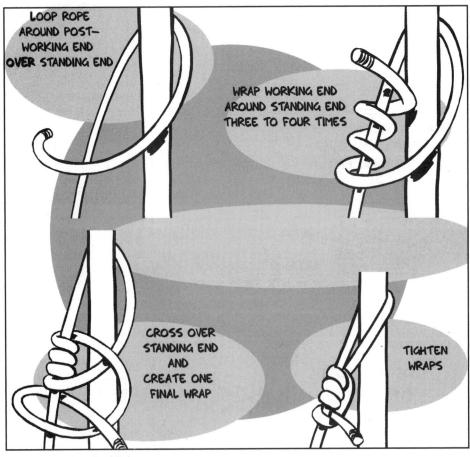

LOOP ROPE AROUND POST— WORKING END OVER STANDING END

WRAP WORKING END AROUND STANDING END THREE TO FOUR TIMES

CROSS OVER STANDING END AND CREATE ONE FINAL WRAP

TIGHTEN WRAPS

FIGURE 28.11. Taut-line hitch

The Backcountry Classroom

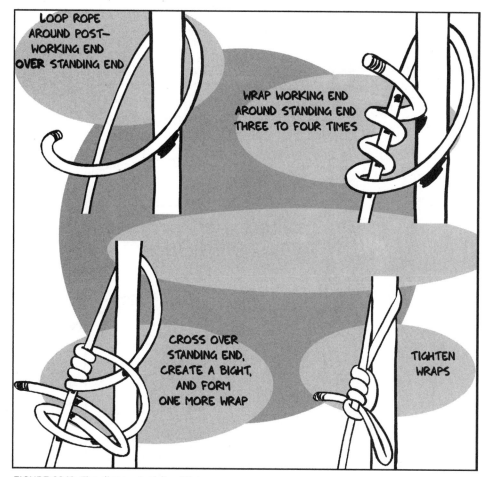

FIGURE 28.12. The slippery taut-line hitch

b) Uses: Excellent for erecting rain tarps and securing tents.

c) Strengths: Its adjustability and ease of tying and untying make this a useful knot.

d) Limitations: It can loosen up in some cases and may need to be readjusted.

10. Trucker's hitch

a) Description: The trucker's hitch is an excellent knot when a lot of tension is needed in the rope. This knot is easily adjustable and can be untied very quickly. Like the taut-line hitch, we like to make the trucker's hitch slippery (see fig. 28.13).

b) Uses: It can be used to safely secure items, such as a canoe or kayak, onto a car or truck (thus its name). It can also be used in setting up a rain tarp or for a tight clothesline.

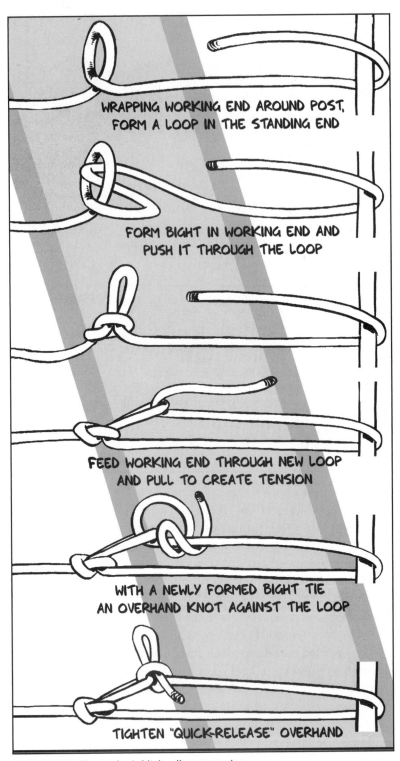

WRAPPING WORKING END AROUND POST, FORM A LOOP IN THE STANDING END

FORM BIGHT IN WORKING END AND PUSH IT THROUGH THE LOOP

FEED WORKING END THROUGH NEW LOOP AND PULL TO CREATE TENSION

WITH A NEWLY FORMED BIGHT TIE AN OVERHAND KNOT AGAINST THE LOOP

TIGHTEN "QUICK-RELEASE" OVERHAND

FIGURE 28.13. The trucker's hitch—slippery version

c) Strengths: If tied properly, it is very secure and easy to untie.

d) Limitations: If the loop created to cinch the item down is not created properly, it can be very difficult to untie the knot.

III. Instructional Strategies

A. Timing

1. This lesson should be broken down into smaller parts. Participants will be overwhelmed if too many knots are taught at once.

2. Teach knots as they are needed. For example, when establishing your first campsite, demonstrate two to three knots while demonstrating shelter construction.

B. Considerations: Assessment strategies

1. Knot tying is an excellent skill to include in a skills checklist assessment.

2. Assess each participant's knots as part of shelter construction, trailer loading, or during any activity that requires knot tying.

C. Activities

1. This is an excellent skill for the participants to teach. Divide the knots among the participants and work with them individually to develop a lesson around a specific knot.

2. Create a knot relay race by dividing the group into smaller teams. Design a competition relay race to test their knot skills.

3. Place participants in pairs and have them teach one another the knots as the instructor provides the initial demonstration.

4. Create a ritual where a new knot is taught or a previously taught knot is reviewed every morning at the end of the daily brief or debrief.

5. Have students tie knots while blindfolded or behind their backs to test their skills.

D. Materials. Issue a 3- or 4-foot length "knot rope" to each participant that is to be used exclusively for learning and practicing knots. Expect group members to have their "knot rope" with them at all times.

CHAPTER TWENTY-NINE

Leadership

An older student struggling to balance the challenge of getting the task done (task behavior) and keeping people happy (relationship behavior) once said, "You know, this leadership is complex stuff. When I was foreman of a construction crew and someone wasn't getting the job done, I'd just hit them alongside of the head with a two by four. I see now that leadership is a lot more complex than that." We believe that leadership is indeed complex stuff, but that it is a skill that can be learned, developed, and nurtured. The research bears this out. The dispositions of leadership are essential. Good leaders must be disposed to value the characteristics of leadership listed in this chapter. We believe that these dispositions must be modeled if learners are to value them and incorporate them into their actions. The components of leadership have to be recognized, practiced, and observed. Feedback needs to be largely self-reflective, but feedback from all the people involved is essential as well. This chapter provides a foundation of knowledge about leadership and some tools and ideas for learning and developing leadership skills.

I. Outcomes

A. Outdoor leaders provide evidence of their *knowledge* and *understanding* by:

1. Describing and comparing definitions of leadership
2. Describing and comparing leadership styles
3. Describing and critiquing leadership traits
4. Explaining the Situational Leadership model
5. Describing their own strengths and limitations as a leader
6. Describing the role of followership
7. Describing communication and explaining the role it plays in leadership
8. Describing the basic decision-making process

9. Describing decision-making styles and explaining the role they play in leadership
10. Explaining the value of having a designated leader
11. Explaining how different leadership situations require different leadership styles

B. Outdoor leaders provide evidence of their *skill* by:

1. Exercising good judgment
2. Making and implementing good decisions
3. Demonstrating confidence and trust in group members
4. Maintaining credibility
5. Providing a safe forum for group members to express themselves
6. Identifying outcomes and prioritizing tasks
7. Distinguishing between fact, opinion, and assumption
8. Organizing information, time, space, materials, people, and tasks effectively
9. Delegating tasks efficiently and equitably
10. Setting and meeting deadlines
11. Combining and blending theory and experience to create new knowledge, action, or values (synthesis)
12. Recognizing and identifying leadership and decision-making styles in themselves and others
13. Communicating effectively
14. Balancing organizational tasks with individual needs and interpersonal relations
15. Proactively confronting and dealing with potential conflict, and managing conflict effectively when it occurs
16. Implementing various leadership styles and adapting them to various situations

C. Outdoor leaders provide evidence of their *dispositions* by:

1. Regularly self-assessing
2. Seeking alternative, original, and imaginative ideas
3. Setting and modeling high standards
4. Putting the group's needs above one's own interests
5. Being flexible
6. Challenging conventional thinking
7. Confronting difficult issues
8. Seeing humor and fun as part of learning

9. Implementing low-impact camping practices
10. Celebrating diversity
11. Modeling the behaviors they want in their followers
12. Being trustworthy individuals with integrity and ethical character
13. Having and sharing a vision
14. Valuing people
15. Taking appropriate risks
16. Empowering others

II. Content

Part 1. What Is Leadership, and What Does It Take to Be a Leader?

A. Defining *leadership*

1. "Leadership is a process which assists an individual or a group to identify goals and objectives and to achieve them. The leadership process is further defined by the need for some specific action, decision, or initiative by one or more persons acting in the leadership role. Outdoor Leadership means that the setting and program focus are directly related to the natural or cultural environment" (Buell 1983, p. 6).
2. "Any action that focuses resources toward a beneficial end" (Rosenbach and Taylor 1984, p. xv).
3. " . . . the ability to plan and conduct safe, enjoyable expeditions while conserving the environment" (Petzoldt 1984, p. 42).

Each of the cornerstones of leadership, described in the following section, requires leaders to demonstrate competency by providing evidence of their knowledge, skills, and dispositions. While the importance of knowledge and skills is obvious, dispositions are probably of greater importance. They are an indication of what an individual values, values which are then reflected in an individual's utilization of their abilities. It is the recognition that learning requires leaders to demonstrate competence in each of these three areas that has inspired us to create the knowledge, skill, and disposition outcomes used at the beginning of each chapter in this edition of the book.

B. The cornerstones of leadership

1. Definition and characteristics

   a) The cornerstones of leadership—critical thinking, personality, knowledge, and psychomotor skills—are what we have found to be the critical components that determine and influence an individual's ability to lead.

   b) These cornerstones do not stand alone. They are connected by and work in harmony with leadership qualities and traits that together form a solid and balanced foundation for further leadership development.

   c) As with all characteristics of leadership, no single person has perfected all these characteristics. The challenge is to understand our strengths and weaknesses, work on improving areas of weakness, and surround ourselves with people whose strengths complement our weaknesses.

   d) Weakness in one area does not necessarily mean our leadership is unsound. Just as a coach recognizes strengths and weaknesses and discovers how to win by maximizing one and minimizing the other, so too must leaders acknowledge their own strengths and weaknesses.

2. The four cornerstones

   a) Critical thinking: Good outdoor leaders are good critical thinkers.

   (1) When a group of international experts was asked to reach consensus on the meaning of critical thinking, the following definition evolved: Critical thinking is understood to be "purposeful, self-regulatory judgment which results in interpretation, analysis, evaluation, and inference, as well as explanation of the . . . considerations upon which that judgment is based" (Facione 2004). The ideal critical thinker is:

   (a) Habitually inquisitive

   (b) Well informed

   (c) Trustful of reason

   (d) Open minded

   (e) Flexible

   (f) Fair minded in evaluation

   (g) Honest in facing personal biases

   (h) Prudent in making judgments

   (i) Willing to reconsider

   (j) Clear about issues

   (k) Orderly in complex matters

   (l) Diligent in seeking relevant information

   (m) Focused in inquiry

   (n) Persistent in seeking results which are as precise as circumstances permit

(2) Key attributes (i.e., indicators that will tell you that critical thinking is taking place) (Mobilia 1999). Critical thinkers:
    (a) Analyze information and events objectively and develop verification procedures
    (b) Discern cause and effect
    (c) Distinguish fact from opinion
    (d) Synthesize information and ideas
    (e) Seek to be well informed
    (f) Seek reasons
    (g) Judge the credibility of a source, use credible sources, and accurately credit resources
    (h) Are open minded
    (i) Ask questions for clarification
    (j) Deduce and induce
    (k) Make and evaluate value judgments
    (l) Identify assumptions

b) Personality: Good outdoor leaders consistently display certain desirable personality traits.
    (1) Personality can be defined as the distinctive emotional, behavioral, and temperamental traits that make up an individual. (See "personal qualities," below, for examples.)
    (2) These qualities and traits are considered part of an individual's personality. While they can be developed and modified, they are a part of the individual's makeup regardless of whether or not the person is in a leadership position.
    (3) A dedicated leader recognizes his or her personality strengths and weaknesses and works on developing the positive personal qualities necessary to be an effective leader. (For example, an individual has little patience but, realizing this, works on improving that characteristic in order to be a more effective leader.)

c) Knowledge: Good outdoor leaders have a broad base of knowledge, both theoretical and experiential.
    (1) Theoretical knowledge:
        (a) Knowledge that is learned by reading, observation, and listening.
        (b) One of the limitations of theoretical knowledge is that, without experience, it provides too small a base for decision making, thus forcing the leader to be extremely conservative if objectives of safety and environmental protection are to be met.

(2) Experiential knowledge:
   (a) Knowledge that is gained/accumulated through doing.
   (b) If used appropriately, this is an excellent means of rein-
       forcing knowledge and refining the decision-making
       process.
   (c) This is limited by the fact that, unless experience is
       processed, it is worthless. In other words, we don't learn
       from our mistakes unless we make a conscious effort to
       do so.
d) Psychomotor skills: Good outdoor leaders have the physical abilities
   necessary to conduct the specific outdoor activities of the trip.
   (1) Psychomotor skills encompass the physical ability to do things,
       often among the most enjoyable parts of outdoor ventures.
   (2) Although not necessarily the most critical component of outdoor
       leadership, psychomotor skills are important to:
       (a) Provide for the safety of the group
       (b) Pass on knowledge
       (c) Provide a positive role model

C. Leadership qualities and traits

1. There is largely unanimity of opinion about the inclusion of many ideal
   qualities and traits.
2. We have broken these traits down into the following: essential leadership
   qualities, leadership traits, and personal qualities.
   a) Essential leadership qualities: These qualities are critical to effective
      leadership. (See fig. 29.1.)
      (1) Quality decision-making ability
          (a) Probably the most critical factor in leadership is the abil-
              ity to make quality decisions and facilitate the decision-
              making process. (See chapter 10, Decision Making, for a
              detailed discussion of the decision-making process.)
          (b) Leaders with good decision-making abilities and knowl-
              edge of their own limitations will be more likely to lead
              safe, enjoyable adventures.
      (2) Knowledge of one's strengths and limitations, sometimes defined
          as metacognition (thinking about thinking)
          (a) This ability is sometimes called self-regulation because it
              requires that leaders constantly self-assess themselves in
              order to evaluate their own strengths and weaknesses.

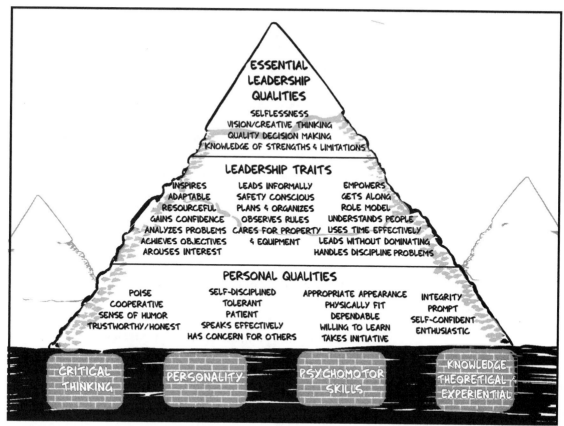

FIGURE 29.1. Essential leadership qualities

Unless leaders can stay within their own limitations, they will not be truly safe leaders.

(b) "Know what you know and know what you don't know" is a phrase frequently used by Paul Petzoldt in describing this characteristic to potential outdoor leaders.

(c) Leaders must be realists and not bluff either themselves or their followers. Famous humorist Will Rogers said it well when he stated, "It isn't what we don't know that gives us trouble, it's what we know that ain't so" (Canadian Conservative Forum n.d.).

(3) Selflessness: To be effective in achieving group objectives, it is essential that leaders have the ability to put group needs above their own interests.

(4) Vision/creative thinking: The ability to anticipate or to "see what might be" is invaluable in helping to come up with unique ways to solve problems. Leaders with vision see where the group needs to go and find original ways to get them there.

   (a) Vision can be defined as having unusual foresight. Creative thinking can be defined as the ability to generate new, diverse, and elaborate ideas (Infinite Innovations Ltd. 1999–2003).

   (b) Key attributes (i.e., indicators that will tell you that creative thinking is taking place) (Mobilia 1999):

   i) Seeking alternatives to "in the box" thinking (i.e., thinking in new and nontraditional ways)

   ii) Expanding on existing ideas

   iii) Seeking the original

   iv) Synthesizing old ideas into new or unique approaches

   v) Integrating seemingly unrelated ideas

   vi) Using intuition, metaphor, and extrapolation to broaden the scope of one's thinking

   vii) Taking risks

b) Leadership traits: These qualities are generally recognized as desirable in a leader. An effective leader:

   (1) Achieves objectives

   (2) Understands people's needs

   (3) Gets along with people

   (4) Is resourceful

   (5) Gains the confidence of others

   (6) Has the ability to analyze problems

   (7) Is adaptable to situations

   (8) Has the ability to arouse and develop interest

   (9) Leads without dominating

   (10) Has the ability to handle disciplinary problems

   (11) Has the ability to inspire others

   (12) Has the ability to lead informally

   (13) Empowers/encourages leadership in others

   (14) Has the ability to plan and organize

   (15) Observes rules and regulations

   (16) Takes proper care of equipment and property

   (17) Uses time effectively

(18) Is safety conscious but permits freedom of adventure

(19) Has the ability to serve as a role model

c) Personal qualities: The distinctive traits that make up the individual (Buell 1983). An effective leader:

    (1) Has a sense of humor

    (2) Is trustworthy/honest

    (3) Has poise

    (4) Has a cooperative attitude

    (5) Has self-discipline

    (6) Is tolerant

    (7) Is patient

    (8) Has concern for others

    (9) Models appearance appropriate for the task

    (10) Is physically fit

    (11) Is dependable

    (12) Has a willingness to learn

    (13) Has an ability to speak effectively

    (14) Has integrity

    (15) Is prompt

    (16) Has self-confidence

    (17) Is enthusiastic

    (18) Takes initiative

D. The Leadership Challenge. The research-based book *The Leadership Challenge*, by James Kouzes and Barry Posner (San Francisco: Jossey-Bass Publishers, 1995), reinforces our own leadership experience. There is extraordinary consistency between the work of these authors in the world of business leadership and our wilderness leadership experience.

1. Kouzes and Posner speak of surveying several thousand business and government executives about the values they found most important in good leadership. Their research consistently shows four characteristics at the top. Leaders need to be:

    a) Honest

    b) Forward looking

    c) Inspiring

    d) Competent

2. From this research, they also found "five fundamental practices that enable leaders to get extraordinary things done" (pp. 8–9):

    a) Challenge the process: Good leaders find ways to do things better. They learn from failures and successes alike.

b) Inspire a shared vision: Good leaders see what can be, enthusiastically share the vision with others, and inspire them to reach for it.

c) Enable others to act (empower): "Leaders enable others to act, not by hoarding the power they have but by giving it away" (p. 12). Good leaders build relationships based on trust and confidence.

d) Model the way: Good leaders are good examples. Their actions speak louder than words.

e) Encourage the heart: Good leaders "breathe life into the hopes and dreams of others . . . Leaders communicate their passion through vivid language and an expressive style" (p. 11).

Part 2. Leadership Styles and Leadership Implementation

A. Leadership styles. One of the keys to effective leadership is mastering various leadership styles and developing the ability to adapt them to various situations. While it is important to recognize one's dominant leadership style, it is even more important to recognize that different leadership situations require different leadership styles. Effective leaders are able to adapt their leadership style to the situation.

1. Examples:
   a) A moderately experienced (autocratic leaning) leader is leading a group of peers; i.e., a group of similar age with similar skill and experience levels. When the leader arrives at the first night's campsite, instead of telling everyone where to camp, how to dispose of waste, and whether or not they can use campfires, she asks a series of questions to take advantage of the group members' expertise. Recognizing the situation, she doesn't tell them what to do but rather hears what they recommend and builds consensus that is consistent with outdoor-ethics camping practices. (Note that even though the leader is most comfortable with an autocratic leadership style, she recognized that this situation called for consensus or democratic-oriented leadership style. In this case, she would have stepped in only if the group's recommendations were inconsistent with outdoor-ethics camping practices.)
   b) A group of outdoor leadership students has arrived late at a reration point in a moderate rain due to a series of problems, including getting lost and having to take a trail that was much more difficult than anticipated. The leader (who tends to always want to reach consensus) assigns tasks fairly and efficiently without input. He moves around the various

groups, letting them know exactly what they have to do and when he hopes they will be done. He shares with them his desire to get the tasks done correctly and as soon as possible so they can quickly move to their campsite, get out of the rain, and relax for the balance of the day. (In this case, knowing that the group was tired and not in a mood to sit down and reach consensus on who was going to fill peanut butter containers and who was going to refill spice containers, the leader used a more autocratic style in assigning tasks and timelines. The followers could recognize and appreciate that by listening to the leader and following his "orders," they had a better chance of getting into camp early, where they would then be able to get a good hot meal and relax.)

2. The leadership continuum

   Leadership styles fit on a continuum (see fig. 29.2). At one end of the continuum, the leader makes the decision and tells the group what to do. At the other end, the group makes the decision and takes total responsibility for it.

3. Primary leadership styles: Historically, this continuum has been broken down into the following three primary leadership styles:

   a) Autocratic

      (1) The decision-making function resides primarily with the assigned leader (Buell 1983).

      (2) Characteristics:

         (a) Fast process

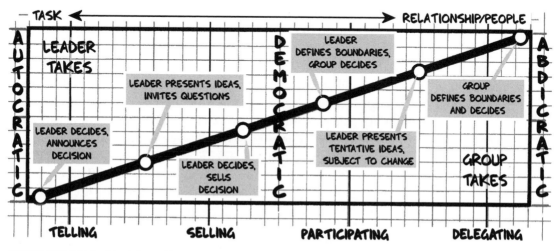

FIGURE 29.2. Leadership style continuum

(b) Discourages a group commitment

(c) Does not promote spontaneity or creativity within the group

(3) This is an effective method when the assigned leader has the most knowledge and experience. It is also effective in a dangerous situation when quick, decisive action must be taken. It is probably the most efficient style in terms of time and communication.

(4) Example: An outdoor leader is working with a young and inexperienced group of campers (ten to twelve years old). The leader sets down very specific rules and clear consequences. The leader makes it clear that while he wants the group to have fun, safety must come first. The leader has determined where they are going to go and the schedule, and he has given the campers some choice of games and activities and some dinner options from which to choose. (Note that the leader has primarily used an autocratic style by making the big decisions for the group [itinerary and schedule]. On the other hand, he recognizes that, in order to encourage the group's commitment and participation, he may want to give them some choice. In this case, he has given the group some choices regarding meals and the games they might play.)

b) Democratic

(1) The decision-making function resides with the group (Buell 1983).

(2) Characteristics:

(a) Slow process

(b) Encourages a group commitment to the outcome

(c) Produces greater initiative

(d) May produce a disenchanted minority

(3) This style may be appropriate when the objective is to build group cohesiveness or when time is available. The democratic style is an important one to use when it is desirable to have a shared commitment or have the group accept responsibility for decisions.

(4) While a democratic style may imply a group "vote," consensus can often be used more effectively and is the ultimate expression of democracy. Consensus implies unanimity—that the whole group has agreed with the decision. Although it is often difficult and time consuming to reach, consensus eliminates the disenfranchised minority of a democracy and maximizes group commitment.

(5) Example: The group has to decide how to get to the final pickup

destination. Looking at the map, it is clear that there are a number of possible routes and that some are much more challenging than others. The leader, understanding the need for the group to commit to the selected route, reminds people of the course objectives, and then carefully facilitates a democratic group decision-making process on what route to take. The options are carefully explored so that the group understands the pros and cons of each one. The group finally uses the "thumb tool" (see chapter 1, Teaching and Learning, for a description of the thumb tool and its use) to ratify the decision and selects one of the more difficult routes. (Note that the leader, who has more knowledge and experience and could have easily selected the route, understood the importance of getting a commitment to the route and therefore encouraged a group decision. Although it took a long time to make the decision, there was no complaining once they started the arduous trip because they all had ownership of the decision. It should be pointed out that the leader had to keep in mind that if the participants selected a route that was unsafe or too challenging, then she would have had to step in and perhaps be more autocratic.)

c) Abdicratic or laissez-faire (Lunenburg and Ornstein 1991)

    (1) The decision-making function has been relinquished and resides with the individual.

    (2) This style should not be confused with consensus decision making. Consensus assumes unanimity, while laissez-faire permits each individual to go his or her own way independent of others within the group.

    (3) Characteristics:

        (a) Inhibits a sense of common group purpose

        (b) Inhibits the development of group cohesion

        (c) Allows for maximum individual freedom

    (4) In wilderness education, an adaptation of this style may be used by instructors to empower a member of the group or the group as a whole with the decision-making prerogative.

    (5) Example: A wilderness leadership instructor is struggling to get students to use an effective decision-making process. As a result, when the students come to a trail intersection and want to take a trail that takes them in the opposite direction of their destination, she nonchalantly shrugs her shoulders and says, "Okay, if you're sure that's the way to go." After walking about fifteen minutes in the

wrong direction the instructor says she needs to stop to put some moleskin on a potential blister. While she is tending to her foot, a couple of students look at their maps and figure out they are going in the wrong direction. After a short discussion, they turn back in the correct direction toward their destination. That evening they debrief the decision-making process. (Note that the instructor temporarily appeared to abdicate her decision-making responsibility, by design, in order to get the students to become aware of the decisions they make and how they are making them. Rather than wait until the group had gone miles out of their way, the instructor found a subtle way to get the students to look at their maps and figure out that they were going in the wrong direction.)

B. Situational Leadership® (Hersey and Blanchard 1982; see fig. 29.3)

1. A leadership model based on three things:
   a) The amount of direction (task behavior): The degree of specific guidance and instruction the leader must give the group to get a specific task accomplished. Regarding task behavior, the leader might ask, "What do I have to do to make sure the task gets done efficiently and correctly?"
   b) The amount of socioemotional support (relationship or people behavior): The degree of encouragement and instruction required to help the group work together effectively to accomplish its task. Here the leader might ask, "What do I have to do to keep the group happy so they can do a good job?"
   c) The level of "readiness" of the group members: The ability and readiness of individuals or a group to take responsibility for directing their own behavior. This time the leader might ask, "How involved in this task do I have to be? Can the group handle it with minimum support from me, or do I need to take a very hands-on approach in this particular case?"
2. This model allows the leader to assess the group's readiness to accept responsibility for directing its own behavior, as well as monitor its progress through the stages of group development.
3. Situational Leadership reinforces the fact that there is no "best" style of leadership and provides four styles:
   a) Telling: Leader-centered. The leader "tells" the group what to do.
   b) Selling: Problem-oriented versus people-oriented leadership. The leader proposes solutions to problems.
   c) Participating: Shared decision making. The leader actively involves the group in identifying and solving problems.

Situational Leadership®
LEADER BEHAVIORS

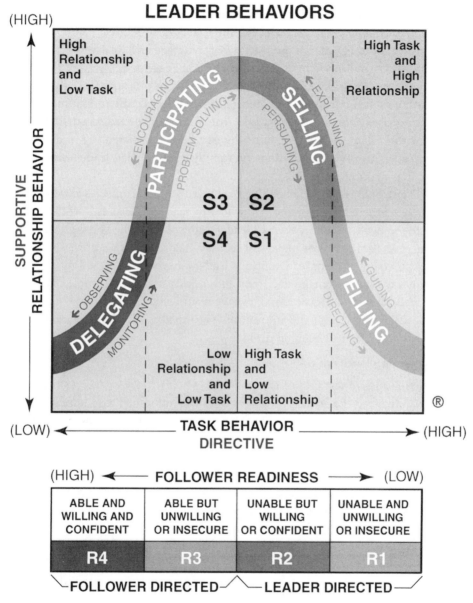

d) Delegating: The leader delegates decision making and assumes a supportive role.

4. The Situational Leadership styles parallel Jones's group development theory. (See chapter 23, Group Development, for more details.)

5. The Situational Leadership model is very practical and relatively easy to understand and implement. The principles are easy to apply across a variety of settings. Many like its emphasis on the concept of leader flexibility and treating each subordinate uniquely based on the task at hand. Some feel that the use of the model must take into account the need to push followers with a relatively low level of readiness to use a participating or delegating leadership style so that they can rapidly increase their leadership and decision-making abilities.

a) Example: Based on Hersey and Blanchard's model, on the second day of a wilderness leadership course students' readiness level is low; therefore, theoretically, a telling style of leadership would be the appropriate style to use. An instructor may want to use a delegating style, however, thus immersing student leaders in the leadership role and providing opportunity for them to make decisions and quickly grasp the complex nature of leadership and decision making. We would encourage the use of a delegating style so that the amount of learning about leadership and decision making will be maximized.

C. Implementing leadership

1. The role and importance of the leader

a) Quite often the leader is thought of as the individual who handles emergencies. While this ability is of the utmost importance, it is the exceptional responsibility. The definitions of leadership imply a much broader role.

b) The leader is not the person at the front of the line, but rather the person floating among the group and checking that everything is all right.

c) The leader is an organizer who anticipates and tries to make things go smoothly, becoming a problem solver as the need arises.

d) Individual versus team leadership:

(1) In many instances, team or consensus-based leadership may work, but one person needs to be in charge and take responsibility when a crisis develops.

(2) Without one individual taking overall responsibility for the group, the potential for problems greatly increases. As President Harry Truman said, "The buck stops here," referring to the fact that as

president he was ultimately responsible for what happened in the federal government.

e) There are some trips that operate on a leaderless philosophy. We do not endorse this philosophy and strongly feel that someone has to take responsibility for the overall leadership of a group. Saying that your group has no leader is a recipe for creating a trip that will have more negative memories than positive.

2. Communication

a) A leader will rarely get into trouble by effectively overcommunicating but may often get into trouble by undercommunicating.

b) There is a tendency to overestimate the group's understanding of situations. If in doubt, explain it again a different way. Find ways to determine how well you are understood. Ask them to paraphrase what you have just said in their own words. When complex tasks are given to individuals or groups, one of the first things to do is ask them to "chunk" the task; i.e., to explain what the different components (chunks) of the task are. It is a way to determine how well the task is understood.

c) Leaders should take the time to explain as much as possible in every given situation. For example, if the group is taking a break, the leader should let everyone know how long it will be and why the group is taking it here and now. Or, if unforeseen circumstances change the objectives of the trip, the leader should communicate those changes.

d) Communicating minimizes misunderstanding and lessens individual and group frustration.

e) Keep in mind that only 7 percent of a message is provided by the words you speak. Tone of voice provides 38 percent of the message, and facial expression provides 55 percent (Mehrabian 1971). Understand/be aware of the nonverbal messages you are/may be sending.

f) Half the job of communicating is listening. Frequently, people in a position of authority are too busy sharing what they consider to be the important information to listen well. Leaders who paraphrase what they think they heard back to the person talking to them demonstrate and model the ability to listen (e.g., "This is what I understand you to be saying . . . ").

g) Remember: It takes as much or more energy to listen as it does to speak.

3. The leader as a role model

a) A leader does not have the choice whether or not to be an example. The choice is whether to be a good or bad example (Resource Ministries International 1999).

b) A leader must serve as a role model and must not follow the creed, "Do as I say, not as I do."

c) Double standards must be minimized. If they must exist at all, the reason should be communicated and explained to the group.

   (1) Example: Perhaps an instructor may leave the expedition at a reration point in order to attend his daughter's birthday party. Students may be upset that the instructor gets to leave the course for personal reasons and they can't. If the instructor is able to effectively explain to the students that he has taught these courses for ten years while it is a one-time-only experience for them, and also that being able to attend his daughter's birthday is an important family event, perhaps the participants will be more understanding and less resentful.

d) The leader who serves as a good role model will develop a group of excellent followers.

e) An adaptation of what author Robert Fulghum says in *All I Really Need to Know I Learned in Kindergarten* says it all: "Don't worry that your followers don't listen to you; worry that they are watching everything you do" (Fulghum 1990).

4. Followership

   a) Definition: "The American Camping Association defines followership as the ability to serve in a democratic group situation under leadership of a member of that group but still retain the capacity to suggest, criticize, and evaluate, as well as serve in the project" (Buell 1983, p. 8). Buell also lists additional qualities for being a follower:

      (1) Stress the importance of the individual
      (2) Accept a lesser role so the group can reach its goals
      (3) Keep communication open with leaders and other followers

   b) Good followership is as important as good leadership. Individuals should be committed to followership because:

      (1) Without followers, goals will not be met.
      (2) Being a good follower allows a leader to develop empathy for followership.
      (3) Most people go through life primarily as followers. Unfortunately, just as leaders are frequently not formally trained, neither are followers.

5. Leading versus instructing: Does a good leader have to be a good teacher? Does a good teacher have to be a good leader? It is generally recognized that a good teacher does not have to be a good leader, but a good leader must be

a good teacher. Many feel good leaders are even better teachers.

6. Recognizing and identifying leadership styles: An important means of developing positive leadership abilities is to recognize and identify the leadership styles of others. This can be done through observation and documented through debriefings and journaling.

7. Credibility and leadership

   a) To be credible is to be believable or trustworthy. Leaders do things that either increase their credibility, becoming more believable and trustworthy, or decrease their credibility. Think of it as a savings account. When you lead by acting and speaking in believable ways to your followers, you make deposits into your credibility savings account and gain credibility. When you act or speak in unbelievable ways, you make withdrawals from your credibility savings account. The problem is that it only takes a few withdrawals to outweigh all your deposits. It takes many believable and honest actions and a long period of time to make up for one or two unbelievable or dishonest actions. This is why it is important to be as believable and honest with your followers as possible.

   b) There is a very simple, yet often difficult, thing a leader can do to gain credibility: Do what you say you are going to do. In other words, if you don't think you can get something done, don't offer to do it. It means saying "no" sometimes, but most people would prefer that to hearing someone say they are going to do something and then not have it get done.

8. Identifying outcomes and prioritizing tasks

   a) Leadership, by definition, is about helping people determine outcomes and achieve them. Sometimes the outcomes are predetermined (e.g., a college course), and sometimes they need to be determined (e.g., a family trip). In either case, the job of the leader is to communicate or facilitate what it is the group hopes to accomplish.

   b) Once the outcomes are determined, the challenge is then to prioritize the tasks that will help accomplish the outcomes.

   c) Tasks will need to be reprioritized through a process of constant assessment. This is an incredibly important and necessary step in accomplishing outcomes.

9. Delegation and leadership

   a) Some leaders struggle to delegate and want to have their hand in every activity related to the task. Others delegate readily but struggle to monitor what their followers are doing. The challenge is to find a balance that allows the leader to delegate many of the tasks while monitoring and supporting ongoing activities.

b) Avoiding micromanagement
  (1) Micromanagers try to oversee every detail of every activity. They think that this is their job, but what they really do is discourage the followers' sense of their ability to make a contribution and possibly strip them of an identity with the task. The followers get frustrated because of their lack of sense of purpose. They develop a sense of, "why bother, because he'll redo it anyway."
  (2) Frequently, the reasons leaders micromanage are:
      (a) There is no clear understanding of who is supposed to do what. Job or task descriptions are helpful in preventing micromanagement.
      (b) Many leaders fall victim to the belief that if they don't do it, no one else will, or no one will do it as well. Leaders need to recognize that there is more than one way to do something. The leader is better off making sure the task is clear and that standards for quality are clear, then getting out of the followers' way.
  (3) One way to cut down on micromanaging is to allow followers to regularly give anonymous feedback to the leaders. In this way, they will become aware that they are doing it.
  (4) President Theodore Roosevelt said it well: "The most effective executive is one who hires good people and then has the good sense to stand back and watch them do their work" (Daniels 2002).
10. Setting quality criteria: What do we mean by quality criteria? The simplest way to determine quality criteria is to ask the simple question, "What things will we see or hear that will tell us we have done a good job?" Taking the time to have that discussion will increase the chances of the group having a safe, environmentally sound, and enjoyable experience.
  a) Example: Suppose the task was to find a route to the next food drop. Quality criteria might be:
      (1) We arrive with energy to spare and don't get too exhausted.
      (2) The route is safe.
      (3) We get to see new and unique countryside.
      (4) We get to see some culturally and historically interesting sites.
      (5) We camp in environmentally sound campsites.
Having quality criteria allows us to debrief the experience and accurately measure our success.
11. Appropriate risk taking: Competent leaders use good judgment to balance many factors while still allowing for acceptable risk taking.

III. Instructional Strategies

A. Timing. Although the teaching of leadership starts on day one of a course and is reinforced daily with the activities listed below, the content of this chapter is usually taught once all the students have had an opportunity to be Leader of the Day (LOD) at least once. The activities below can be used in the classroom before the course or within the first half of a trip.

B. Considerations

1. Teaching leadership: In teaching leadership there are two important components:
   a) Instructors need to make sure that students understand leadership theory.
   b) Instructors must provide opportunities for students to lead and have students reflect on their leadership experiences and of those around them.
2. Typical activities that need to take place on a wilderness course for students to be able to learn about leadership include:

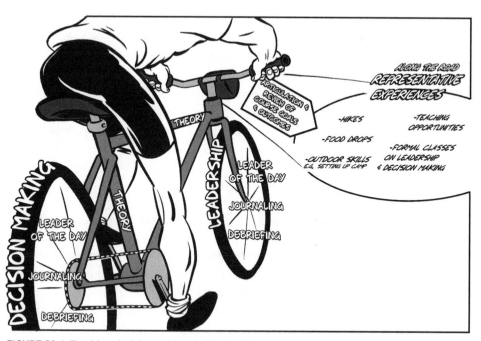

FIGURE 29.4. Teaching decision making and leadership

a) Articulation of course outcomes: Participants need to understand the role and importance of leadership in relation to the course outcomes. Is it clearly communicated that leadership is an important learning outcome within the course? Our experience dictates that this needs to be done at the beginning of a wilderness course and at least once more during the course.

b) Review of the assessment process: Participants also need to understand the role and importance of the assessment process as it relates to the assessment of leadership. How will they receive feedback, when will they receive feedback, and what role will their leadership ability play in grading, certification, or other forms of evaluation?

c) Journals: Writing in journals encourages participants to formally identify and analyze their own leadership of others. The journals provide instructors with an opportunity to see into the student's mind and observe whether he or she sees the decisions that are being made and whether he or she is beginning to grasp how decisions are being made.

d) Leader of the Day (LOD): This provides opportunities for each student to take on the leadership role. For participants to develop their leadership abilities to the greatest extent possible, it is important to:

   (1) Let the LODs take as active a role as possible.
   (2) Let them take charge with as little interference as possible.
   (3) Let them make mistakes, and then help them constructively and positively learn from them.
   (4) Have the LOD and the group evaluate leadership roles in terms of successes and failures. Also, have the LOD and the group describe the leadership styles, cornerstones, traits, and personal qualities exhibited.
   (5) Encourage future LODs to build on the previous leaders' strengths and weaknesses.
   (6) Give participants time to grow.
   (7) Communicate to the participants what they can do to improve.
   (8) Be objective: Avoid letting personal likes and dislikes interfere with evaluating someone's leadership.
   (9) Be cautious and understand that, in group discussions, the instructor's words carry more weight than the words of students.

e) Debriefings: Daily group debriefings give participants the opportunity to share and reflect on their analysis of leadership observed during the day. (See chapter 25, Group Processing and Debriefing, for more information on debriefing.)

f) Leadership theory lesson: This lesson usually takes place after students have been the LOD at least once. This lesson allows the students to begin to understand the theoretical aspects of leadership and to view leadership both theoretically and practically through the lens of their own experience. This lesson can be taught with a traditional or SPEC approach. (See chapter 1, Teaching and Learning, for more information on teaching strategies.)

g) Opportunities for students to lead: These are the daily activities that take place naturally or are designed by the instructor that provide the grist of leadership for the mill of reflection. We have provided a sample list of activities that typically occur on a course that provide such opportunities:

    (1) Student-led hikes: Trail and off-trail hikes, with and without instructor supervision, provide a multitude of opportunities for students to take on leadership roles.

    (2) Reration/food drops: The numerous tasks associated with this activity provide numerous opportunities for leadership.

    (3) Use of daily "camping skills": Finding a tent site, preparing meals, packing the pack, and most of the other camp skills also provide opportunities for taking on leadership roles.

    (4) Designing lessons: As students design teaching lessons for a variety of learners, they also engage in the leadership process.

3. Assessment: Observation and feedback

a) The above activities take place within a framework of instructor observation and feedback. Instructor observations provide participants with feedback concerning their progress in mastering the role of leader.

b) Peer feedback affords participants additional input from the group concerning their role as leader.

C. Activities

1. The Outdoor Leaders R' Us challenge (see the end of the chapter)
    a) Purpose:
        (1) To develop an understanding of leadership styles and traits
        (2) To explore alternative, original, and imaginative ideas
2. The Ideal Outdoor Leader challenge (see the end of the chapter)
    a) Purpose:
        (1) To develop an understanding of leadership characteristics
        (2) To practice the synthesis of ideas and information

Challenge

Knowledge Outcome	Title	Skill/Disposition Outcome
What do you want them to know? Participants will have a deeper understanding of leadership styles and traits and the link between theory and practice.	Outdoor Leaders R' Us	**What skill/disposition do you want them to develop?** Decision making: considers the pros and cons of options

Essential Question or Key Issue:

What is the link between leadership styles and traits and good outdoor leadership?

Description of Challenge/Task/Performance:

Outdoor Leaders R' Us, the world's premier outdoor leadership training organization, has asked your advertising agency to create a recruitment brochure/booklet to attract the best outdoor leaders from this year's graduating class of college outdoor leadership programs in the United States. Outdoor Leaders R' Us takes great pride in hiring trainers that embody the essential qualities and characteristics of leadership as defined in *The Backcountry Classroom*. They are especially interested in attracting people who have both a deep understanding of leadership theory and styles, and the capacity to make this knowledge come to life in the field through skillful practice.

Outdoor Leaders R' Us wants you to produce a brochure/booklet that communicates their image of an ideal outdoor leader and attracts candidates who have those same attributes. In its finished form, the brochure should be no larger than a four-fold 8" by 14" brochure or an eight-page 5" by 8" booklet (two pieces of 8" by 11" paper). You may make a larger mock-up for presentation purposes out of easel paper. It is crucial that the content of the brochure addresses all the leadership issues mentioned above.

Since they want to start recruiting as soon as possible, Outdoor Leaders R' Us would like you to present a mock-up of your brochure/booklet to their marketing team on _____.

Criteria for Assessment and Feedback:

Form criteria:
- The product is either a four-fold brochure made of paper no larger than 8" by 14" or an eight-page booklet not larger than 5" by 8". (A mock-up for presentation purposes may be made out of easel paper.)
- The product is colorful and dramatic—it attracts attention.
- The product message is clear, easy to understand, appropriate to its audience, and free of grammatical and spelling errors.

Content criteria:
- It contains language that will attract potential staff.
- It makes the connection between the four cornerstones of leadership and the jobs at Outdoor Leaders R' Us.
- It makes connections between essential and desirable leadership qualities and traits and the jobs at Outdoor Leaders R' Us.
- It makes connections between the various theories of leadership styles and the jobs at Outdoor Leaders R' Us.
- It makes clear links between theory and practice.

Knowledge:
- The participants will have a deeper understanding of leadership styles and traits and the link between theory and practice.
- The brochure/booklet will accurately reflect the four cornerstones of leadership, leadership qualities and traits, and leadership styles.
- The brochure/booklet will accurately show a link between outdoor leadership theory and practice.

Skill: Decision making: considers the pros and cons of options
- Every group member will be able to describe the pros and cons that were considered regarding at least one decision made in the preparation of the brochure/booklet.

Product Quality Checklist

Date: _____   Class Period: _____

Product Author(s):	Product Title/Name: Outdoor Leaders R' Us	Evaluator Name(s):

Observed	Standard/Criteria	Possible Points	Rating
	The product is either a four-fold brochure made of paper no larger than 8" by 14" or an eight-page booklet not larger than 5" by 8". (A mock-up for presentation purposes may be made out of easel paper.)		
	The product is colorful and dramatic—it attracts attention.		
	The product message is clear, easy to understand, and appropriate to its audience.		
	It contains language that will attract potential staff.		
	It makes connections between the four cornerstones of leadership and the jobs at Outdoor Leaders R' Us.		
	It makes connections between essential and desirable leadership qualities and traits and the jobs at Outdoor Leaders R' Us.		
	It makes connections between the various theories of leadership styles and the jobs at Outdoor Leaders R' Us.		
	It makes clear links between theory and practice.		
	Total		

Observations:

Elements of Questionable Quality:	Elements of Exceptional Quality:

Challenge

Knowledge Outcome	Title	Skill/Disposition Outcome
What do you want them to know? The participants can describe and critique a variety of leadership traits.	The Ideal Outdoor Leader	**What skill/disposition do you want them to develop?** Leadership: seeks alternative, original, and imaginative ideas

Essential Question or Key Issue:

What are the characteristics of the ideal outdoor leader?

Description of Challenge/Task/Performance:

With the assistance of your teacher/instructor, form small groups. In your team/group, discuss what you think are some of the most desirable qualities of an "ideal" outdoor leader. On one piece of poster paper, make a creative caricature of an "ideal" outdoor leader that highlights the traits the team has discussed. Be as specific as possible. As an expression of your originality, make sure each team poster is different from all the others.

Each team member should be prepared to interpret his/her team poster for the entire group and explain why the highlighted traits were chosen and not others.

Criteria for Assessment and Feedback:

Form criteria:
- The poster is made of only one piece of paper.
- The poster's message is clear.
- The poster is unique—no other in the group is like it.

Content criteria:
- The poster contains creative imagery representing the "ideal" outdoor leader.
- The traits of outdoor leadership are readily identifiable.

Knowledge:
- The participants can describe and critique a variety of leadership traits.
- The poster depicts traits commonly associated with effective outdoor leadership.
- Team members can explain why they chose to depict selected leadership traits rather than others.

Skill: Leadership: seeks alternative, original, and imaginative ideas
- The representation of the "ideal" outdoor leader is unique and different from all the other groups.

Developed by Leading EDGE, LLC for The Backcountry Classroom. *For more information log on to* www.realworldlearning.info.

Product Quality Checklist

Date: _____   Class Period: _____

| Product Author(s): | Product Title/Name:

The Ideal Outdoor Leader | Evaluator Name(s): |

Observed	Standard/Criteria	Possible Points	Rating
	The poster is made of only one piece of paper.		
	The poster's message is clear.		
	The poster is unique—no other in the group is like it.		
	The poster contains creative imagery representing the "ideal" outdoor leader.		
	The traits of outdoor leadership are readily identifiable.		
	Total		

Observations:

Elements of Questionable Quality: | **Elements of Exceptional Quality:**

CHAPTER THIRTY

Navigation: Map Folding

I. Outcomes

A. Outdoor leaders provide evidence of their *knowledge* and *understanding* by:

1. Explaining the rationale for using a particular map-folding technique
2. Describing techniques and explaining reasons for protecting maps

B. Outdoor leaders provide evidence of their *skill* by:

1. Demonstrating an appropriate map-folding technique
2. Demonstrating proper care and storage of a map

C. Outdoor leaders provide evidence of their *dispositions* by:

1. Modeling proper care, use, and folding of maps

II. Content

A. Demonstration of map folding

1. Fold the map in half lengthwise so that the printed side of the map faces in. (See fig. 30.1, step 1.)
2. Fold back half of one length so that the map's side margin is parallel with the first fold. (See fig. 30.1, step 2.) The printed side should face up, and the quadrangle name should show at the bottom. Turn the map over and do the same with the other side of the map.
3. The map should now be folded lengthwise in quarters with the printed side facing out. Fold the map in half so that the quadrangle names face each other and the top and bottom map margins meet. (See fig. 30.1, step 3.)

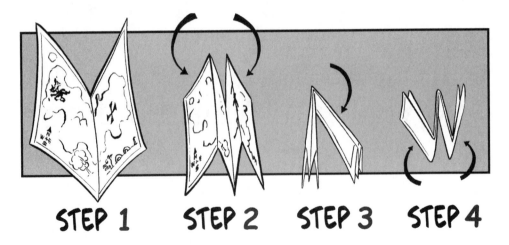

FIGURE 30.1. The fine art of map folding

4. Fold back one half of each folded half of the map so that the quadrangle names are facing out. (See fig. 30.1, step 4.) Turn the map over and do the same on the other side. The quadrangle name should now face out.

B. Why the map is folded this way

1. It allows easy identification of the map.
2. The original creases can be used to refold the map and see any one section of the map at a time.
3. Most maps that are folded this way will fit into a shirt pocket.

C. Map storage

1. Although some maps are available in waterproof materials, most maps are still printed on paper. In order to keep the map dry and usable, it is wise to use a simple plastic bag with an overhand knot or a zippered plastic bag as an effective and inexpensive method of storing and protecting the map.
2. Reinforce the need to keep the map stored in the bag nearly all the time, even when it is not raining. Perspiration, as well as any other type of moisture, will rapidly shorten the life of the map.
3. Maps may also be protected from moisture by sealing them with a commercial waterproofing agent such as Aquaseal, Map Seal, or Thompson's Water Seal. While they all work reasonably well, they do have limitations.
   a) Never allow coated maps to be pressed hard together for prolonged periods of time. This could result in the maps getting permanently stuck together.

b) Thompson's Water Seal makes maps water-repellent, not truly water-proof.

III. Instructional Strategies

A. Timing. This is an excellent lesson for a teachable moment. When maps are issued to participants, it is an excellent time to teach them how to fold them. It is also appropriate for student instruction as it is a relatively simple lesson but requires good communication skills and the ability to give a demonstration.

B. Strategies

1. Walk through each step with the participants (i.e., make one fold, and then have them make the fold). Make sure they are following each step—don't get ahead.
2. To avoid a mix-up of maps, ask participants to write their names above or below the name of the map.
3. Ask participants why they think the map is folded this way.

C. Materials

1. An unfolded map
2. Plastic bags
3. Map seal, if available

CHAPTER THIRTY-ONE

Navigation: Map Interpretation

I. Outcomes

A. Outdoor leaders provide evidence of their *knowledge* and *understanding* by:

1. Describing the uses for a topographic map
2. Identifying and correctly locating features on a topographic map
3. Identifying and correctly describing elevation symbols
4. Identifying key information provided on the margins of a map

B. Outdoor leaders provide evidence of their *skill* by:

1. Using map interpretation skills to safely navigate in the backcountry

C. Outdoor leaders provide evidence of their *dispositions* by:

1. Modeling effective map interpretation for safe backcountry travel

II. Content

A. General background

1. A map is "a reduced representation of a portion of the surface of the earth" (Kjellstrom 1976, p. 8).
2. A topographic map is a map that shows the three-dimensional features of the land's surface in two dimensions. "Topos" = place; "graphein" = to write or draw (Kjellstrom 1976).

3. Where to acquire maps: While the best known recreational maps in the United States are the USGS topographic "quadrangle" maps, there are many maps produced regionally that are excellent for backcountry travel. We like to provide a variety of different maps on our trips so participants gain confidence in reading different types and scales of maps.

    a) USGS Earth Science Information Centers (ESIC) (http://geography.usgs .gov/esic_index.html), which are located in the following cities:

        (1) Anchorage, Alaska

        (2) Denver, Colorado

        (3) Menlo Park, California

        (4) Reston, Virginia

        (5) Rolla, Missouri

        (6) Sioux Falls, South Dakota

    b) Local outdoor/sporting goods stores

    c) Online: The USGS Store, http://store.usgs.gov/; http://topomaps.usgs .gov/ordering_maps.html

    d) Mapping software: Numerous mapping programs are available that allow the customization and printing of specific maps for the region you are traveling; waterproof paper is available for printing the maps

B. Map margin information. Participants should be able to identify each of the following:

1. Name of the map

2. Names of adjacent maps

3. Location of the map on the earth's surface

    a) Longitude, note meridians

    b) Latitude, note parallels

4. Date of the map: Note possible changes that may have occurred since the map was drawn and field tested

5. Map scale/series: Note how the scale is drawn

    a) Scale ratio: Inches/cm on map = inches/cm in the field

        (1) 1:24,000: A good map for detailed study of a small area

           1 inch = 2,000 feet in field

           Approximately 2½ inches = 1 mile

           1 cm = 240 m; 4 cm =1 km

        (2) 1:25,000: Used in metric series and similar to 1:24,000 scale

           1 cm = 250 m

        (3) 1:62,500: Good general-purpose map, although not as common as it once was

Approximately 1 inch =1 mile in field

1 cm = 625 m; 1½ cm = 1 km

b) Map series

(1) 15″ (minute) series: Covers a section of the earth's surface 15″ of longitude × 15″ of latitude (note longitude and latitude marks on map to confirm size)

(2) 7½″ series: Note that it takes four 7½″ maps to equal a 15″ map

(3) 7½″ × 15″ series: Metric series, currently only available for a few areas of the United States

6. Map datum: The map datum describes the model that was used to match the location of features on the ground to coordinates and locations on the map. For recreational purposes it is only important to know what map datum your map is based on when using GPS (Global Positioning System) receivers.

C. General map details. Identify the location of each detail on a sample map:

1. Map symbols

a) Cultural symbols: Symbols of human-made objects, represented by the color black:

(1) Roads

(2) Railroads

(3) Churches

(4) Trails

(5) Buildings

(6) Cemeteries

(7) Bridges

(8) Schools

(9) Quarries/mines

b) Water symbols: Represented by the color blue:

(1) Lakes

(2) Streams

(a) On 7½″ maps, for a stream width of more than 40 feet (12 meters), both shores are shown.

(b) On 15″ maps, for a stream width of more than 80 feet (24 meters), both shores are shown.

(3) Springs

(4) Marshes/swamps

c) Map directions

(1) True north: This is the north that is shown on a map.

(2) Magnetic north: This is the north that attracts the compass needle. Subsequent navigation lessons (see chapters 32 and 33) discuss true north, magnetic north, and declination in more detail.

(3) Place name designations: Note the different styles of lettering used for area names, elevation figures, political boundaries, etc.

2. Elevation markings: Represented by the color brown:

a) Contour lines: "An imaginary line on the ground along which every point is at the same height above sea level" (Kjellstrom 1976, p. 23). Note the altitude numbers located along some contour lines.

(1) Index contour: Heavier brown contour lines, usually spaced at 100-foot elevation intervals (50 meters on metric maps).

(2) Intermediate contours: The contour lines between index contours.

(3) Contour interval: "The distance in height between one contour line and the one next to it" (Kjellstrom 1976, p. 23). Intervals vary from map to map.

b) Contour shapes (see fig. 31.1)

(1) Hills and mountains

(2) Passes

(3) Steep areas

(4) Flat areas

c) Depression contours are contours showing the edges and slope in an area that lies at a lower elevation than all of the surrounding terrain. Short ticks are drawn at right angles to the contour lines. The ticks point downslope toward the bottom of the depression.

d) Interpreting elevation change

(1) Contours forming Vs generally point uphill. Contours forming Us are usually ridges and point downhill

(2) Streams that come together forming Vs generally point downhill.

e) Benchmarks: "BM" represents the location of a marker in the field where altitude or distance has been verified. The number next to "BM" indicates the elevation.

(1) Horizontal: There are several names for horizontal control points: triangulation stations, traverse stations, trilateration stations, and intersection stations, depending on which kind of horizontal control system was used in establishing them and the amount of precision they represent. This type of control point can be a small brass or aluminum disk, concrete post, iron pin, or bolt, but also a radio tower, water tower, church spire, mountain top, or any other type of object that can be identified from a distance.

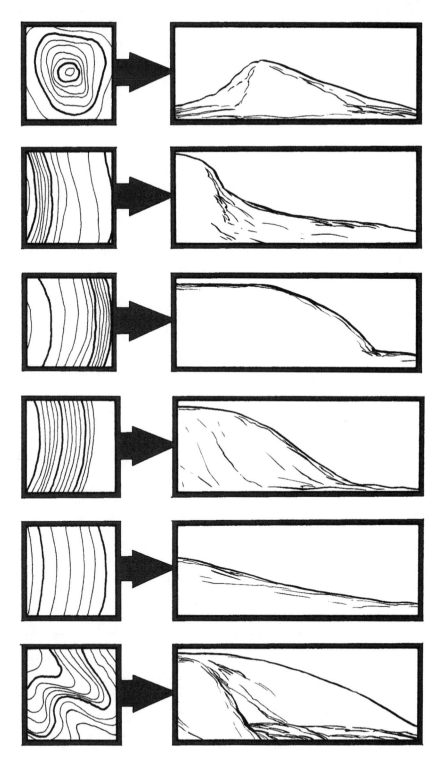

FIGURE 31.1. Contour shapes

U.S.G.S. Common Topo Map Symbols

BOUNDARIES

National	
State or territorial	
County or equivalent	
Civil township or equivalent	
Incorporated city or equivalent	
Federally administered park, reservation, or monument (external)	
Federally administered park, reservation, or monument (internal)	
State forest, park, reservation, or monument and large county park	
Forest Service administrative area	
Forest Service ranger district	
National Forest System land status, Forest Service lands	
National Forest System land status, non-Forest Service lands	
Small park (county or city)	

BUILDINGS AND RELATED FEATURES

Building	
School; house of worship	
Built-up area	
Ranger district office	
Guard station or work center	
Racetrack or raceway	
Airport, paved landing strip, runway, taxiway, or apron	
Paved/Unpaved landing strip	
Well (other than water), windmill or wind generator	
Tanks	
Covered reservoir	
Gaging station	
Located or landmark object (feature as labeled)	
Boat ramp or boat access	
Roadside park or rest area	
Picnic area	
Campground	
Winter recreation area	
Cemetery	Cem

CONTROL DATA AND MONUMENTS

Principal point	3-20
U.S. mineral or location monument	USMM 438
River mileage marker	Mile 69

Boundary monument

Third-order or better elevation, with tablet	BM 9134 BM 277
Third-order or better elevation, recoverable mark, no tablet	5628
With number and elevation	67 4567

Horizontal control

Third-order or better, permanent mark	Neace Neace
With third-order or better elevation	BM 52 Pike BM393
With checked spot elevation	1001
Coincident with found section corner	Cactus Cactus
Unmonumented	

Vertical control

Third-order or better elevation, with tablet	BM 5280
Third-order or better elevation, recoverable mark, no tablet	528
Bench mark coincident with found section corner	BM 5280
Spot elevation	7523

CONTOURS

Topographic

Index	6000
Approximate or indefinite	
Intermediate	
Approximate or indefinite	
Supplementary	
Depression	
Cut	
Fill	

RIVERS, LAKES, AND CANALS

Perennial stream	
Perennial river	
Intermittent stream	
Intermittent river	
Disappearing stream	
Falls, small	
Falls, large	
Rapids, small	
Rapids, large	
Masonry dam	
Dam with lock	
Dam carrying road	
Perennial lake/pond	
Intermittent lake/pond	
Dry lake/pond	
Narrow wash	
Wide wash	Wash
Canal, flume, or aqueduct with lock	
Elevated aqueduct, flume, or conduit	
Aqueduct tunnel	
Water well, geyser, fumarole, or mud pot	
Spring or seep	

SUBMERGED AREAS AND BOGS

Marsh or swamp	
Submerged marsh or swamp	
Wooded marsh or swamp	
Submerged wooded marsh or swamp	
Land subject to inundation	Max Pool 431

SURFACE FEATURES

Levee	Levee
Sand or mud	Sand
Disturbed surface	
Gravel beach or glacial moraine	Gravel
Tailings pond	Tailings Pond

ROADS AND RELATED FEATURES

Primary highway	
Secondary highway	
Light duty road	
Light duty road, paved	
Light duty road, gravel	
Light duty road, dirt	
Light duty road, unspecified	
Unimproved road	
Unimproved road	
4WD road	
4WD road	
Trail	
Highway or road with median strip	
Highway or road under construction	Under Const
Highway or road underpass; overpass	
Highway or road bridge; drawbridge	
Highway or road tunnel	
Road block, berm, or barrier	
Gate on road	
Trailhead	

RAILROADS AND RELATED FEATURES

Standard gauge railroad, single track	
Standard gauge railroad, multiple track	
Narrow gauge railroad, single track	
Narrow gauge railroad, multiple track	
Railroad siding	
Railroad in highway	
Railroad in road	
Railroad in light duty road	
Railroad underpass; overpass	
Railroad bridge; drawbridge	
Railroad tunnel	
Railroad yard	
Railroad turntable; roundhouse	

TRANSMISSION LINES AND PIPELINES

Power transmission line; pole; tower	
Telephone line	Telephone
Aboveground pipeline	
Underground pipeline	Pipeline

VEGETATION

Woodland	
Shrubland	
Orchard	
Vineyard	
Mangrove	Mangrove

MINES AND CAVES

Quarry or open pit mine	
Gravel, sand, clay, or borrow pit	
Mine tunnel or cave entrance	
Mine shaft	
Prospect	
Tailings	Tailing
Mine dump	

GLACIERS AND PERMANENT SNOWFIELDS

Contours and limits	
Formlines	
Glacial advance	
Glacial retreat	

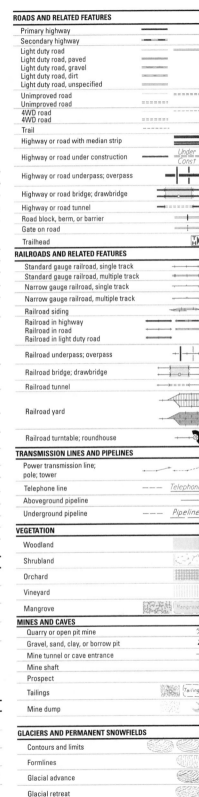

FIGURE 31.2. USGS map symbols

(2) Vertical: The vertical control point is for precisely establishing the elevation at a given location. This type of control point is usually, but not always, a small brass or aluminum disk, concrete post, iron pin, or bolt that is permanently attached to a boulder or bedrock.

III. Instructional Strategies

A. Timing. Map interpretation skills may be introduced to participants almost immediately while traveling during the first few days of the course. A more formal class is usually taught in conjunction with a trailless hike or mountain climb when skills can be applied immediately.

B. Considerations

1. Early map skills can be developed along the trail and during breaks. Calling attention to prominent topographic features and then locating them on the map arouses interest, introduces map terminology, and encourages participants to become more aware of their natural surroundings. Asking participants to predict upcoming terrain features encourages them to continue map use on the trail. Asking participants to measure distance traveled encourages awareness of map scale and builds a base of experience for later Time Control Plan (see chapter 34) development.

2. Formalized map classes may be a combination of lecture and discussion depending upon the extent of participant knowledge. The class should focus on a general overview of all map features and their identification on sample maps. Instructors may ask participants to conduct a theoretical journey across the map and describe the identifiable map features, obstacles, or land forms that they will encounter along the way.

3. More advanced map skills are best developed in practice on a trailless hike where participants must concentrate on observing terrain features in order to follow progress on their maps. Treeless mountaintops make excellent classroom sites for understanding contouring, distance, and how terrain may have changed over time. Ask participants to orient their maps without the use of their compasses, thereby using the opportunity to identify prominent land features.

4. Use the knuckles to describe contours. Draw lines on knuckles with the hand in a fist, and then open the hand to show how the lines look on a topographic map.

5. Use a sand pile to describe contours.

C. Materials

1. A map for at least every two participants. All maps should be of the same area, at least initially. Once participants gain expertise reading one map, then it is a good idea to show them different types of maps of the same area.

2. Blank paper and pen. In lieu of a blackboard, this can come in handy to help describe map symbols and features.

CHAPTER THIRTY-TWO

Navigation: An Introduction to the Compass

I. Outcomes

A. Outdoor leaders provide evidence of their *knowledge* and *understanding* by:

1. Describing the function of a compass in finding direction in the field
2. Identifying and properly describing the function of the parts of a compass
3. Explaining how to take a field bearing

B. Outdoor leaders provide evidence of their *skill* by:

1. Using a compass to safely navigate in the backcountry
2. Properly demonstrating how to take a field bearing
3. Properly demonstrating how to set and follow a field bearing

C. Outdoor leaders provide evidence of their *dispositions* by:

1. Modeling the use of a compass to navigate safely in the backcountry

A. Concept of "direction"

1. Direction is defined as the line of travel or sight from point A (present location) to point B (destination).
2. Direction is expressed in terms of the 360 degrees of a circle.
   a) Present location is assumed to be the center of the circle. (See fig. 32.1.)
   b) Any direction can be expressed in terms of the degrees of an angle measured clockwise from a point at the top of the circle to the point on the circumference representing the direction.
   c) For two or more people to describe a direction to each other accurately, they must establish a common "top of the circle" from which degrees will be measured. True north has been universally identified as the top of the circle.

Give examples of directions N, S, E, and W in degrees.

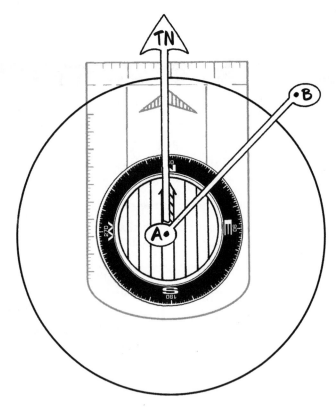

FIGURE 32.1. The concept of direction. "A" represents location; "B," destination; and "TN," true north.

B. Parts of the compass (based on the Silva Polaris Type 7 and similar compasses). (See fig. 32.2.)

1. Base plate
   a) The rectangular, transparent piece of plastic upon which all compass parts rest.
   b) This plate typically has millimeter and inch markings along the edge for measuring.
   c) The edges of the base plate are parallel to the "direction of travel" arrow, which is imprinted on it.
2. "Direction of travel" arrow
   a) Imprinted arrow on the base plate that runs from the edge of the compass housing to one end of the base plate.
   b) Compass bearings or degree readings are taken from the point where the base of the "direction of travel" arrow touches the numbers on the edge of the compass housing.
   c) Whether using the compass in the field or on a map, the "direction of travel" arrow must always point toward the intended destination.

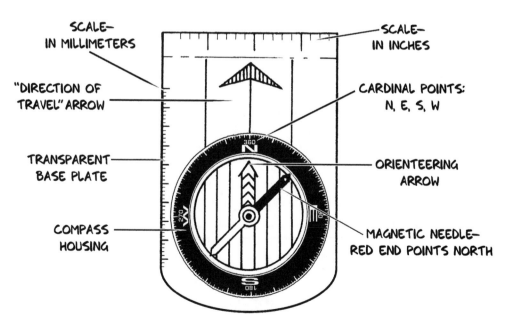

FIGURE 32.2. Parts of the compass

3. Compass housing
   a) Circular, rotating rim found in the middle of the base plate.
   b) The compass housing has the initials of the four cardinal points—N, S, E, and W—on the upper rim and degree lines on the outer rim.
   c) Most compasses have lines representing increments of two degrees of angle with every twentieth degree numbered. Some smaller compasses have only five-degree increments.
4. Magnetic needle
   a) The magnetic needle is suspended on a bearing in the middle of the liquid-filled, plastic-cased housing.
   b) This needle points to magnetic north when the compass is held steady and level.
5. Orienting arrow and orienting/meridian lines
   a) Usually in blue or white, these are represented by the outline of an arrow. They are also the parallel lines engraved in the plastic bottom of the housing.
   b) The arrow points directly to the 360°/0° mark on the compass housing.
   c) The compass is said to be "oriented" or "boxed" when the compass housing is turned so that the magnetic needle lies directly over the orienting arrow and both the arrow and the needle simultaneously point to the letter *N* on the compass housing rim.
   d) The orienting lines run parallel to the orienting arrow and are used in establishing map bearings.

C. Function of the compass

1. The magnetic needle of the compass always points to magnetic north. This provides a constant and common reference point (360°/0°) from which all directional degree designations may be measured.
2. By facing true north, then pointing to an intended destination (B in fig. 32.1), an imaginary angle is formed by the line pointing to true north and the line pointing to the destination. The meeting point of these two legs of the angle is the observer's present location (A in fig. 32.1).
3. The primary function of the compass is to assist the backcountry traveler in establishing the direction of north and thereby measuring the angle or "bearing" of the intended line of travel to the destination.

D. Using a "field bearing"

1. A "field bearing" is the angle of the line of travel established when the compass alone is used to sight a destination in the field.

2. Taking a field bearing
   a) Squarely face the distant point that is the intended destination.
   b) Hold the compass level in the palm of one hand and at midchest height with the direction of travel arrow pointed directly at the destination.
   c) Orient or "box" the compass by turning the compass housing until the magnetic needle rests squarely over the orienting arrow.
      (1) Both the magnetic needle and the orienting arrow should point to N.
      (2) Make sure to turn only the compass housing—do not move the base plate or turn your body away from the direction of travel to your intended destination.
   d) Once the compass is oriented and the magnetic needle comes to rest, read the degree marking on the rim of the compass housing where it intersects the tail of the direction of travel arrow and where it usually says READ BEARING HERE. This degree reading is the "field bearing" that should be written down for reference and followed during travel to the destination.
   e) When taking bearings, be sure the compass is not exposed to metal objects, iron deposits, or magnetic fields that may cause the magnetic needle to function improperly.

E. Following a field bearing

1. Once a field bearing is established, travel may proceed along the line of travel on a relatively straight course (depending upon the terrain) by following the "direction of travel" arrow.
2. Since the sight of the original destination point may be lost during travel, it is important to start the trek by spotting a clearly visible landmark that is nearby and is on the same bearing as the destination.
   a) By moving toward a nearby landmark, checking the bearing, and then moving on to the next sighted landmark, the traveler can proceed along the line of travel without constantly following the exact path indicated by the compass.
   b) This "leapfrog" method of travel allows the traveler to circumvent hazards or obstacles while still holding to the correct line of travel.
3. Once the destination is reached, a return route may be easily established by adding or subtracting 180 degrees to or from the original bearing. This "back bearing" just reverses the original line of travel and allows the traveler to proceed back along the original route to the starting point.

III. Instructional Strategies

A. Timing. This lesson is usually taught after participants have gained some experience with maps and their use.

B. Considerations

1. While on the trail, introduction to the compass can start with simple exercises that establish the location of north, the general direction of travel along the trail, etc. Compass terminology may also be introduced during breaks.
2. Early formal classes on the compass should combine lectures and demonstrations with an immediate opportunity for practice. Following instruction in the technique of establishing field and map bearings, participants should immediately apply this knowledge in the surrounding environment by taking bearings on easily visible landmarks and matching them on their maps.
3. Once participants have gained confidence in taking bearings, a short compass course or simple trailless hike will allow participants to practice following a bearing in the field. Special care should be taken to ensure that the compass course area is completely safe so that disoriented students cannot get lost. Students should be teamed up so that route determination is a group effort. This allows for mutual teaching, reinforcement, and confidence building.

C. Activity: Three-legged compass walk

1. Have participants work alone or in pairs.
2. In a fairly open area (field or open forest), have each participant or pair randomly select their own compass bearing under 120 degrees and set their compass at their selected bearing.
3. Have them follow their bearing for fifteen paces (the first leg).
4. From their current location they should add 120 degrees, set their compass to their new bearing, and walk another fifteen paces (the second leg).
5. From this location they should add another 120 degrees, set their compass to their new bearing, and walk another fifteen paces (the third leg). This should bring them back to where they started.
6. If they did not arrive back where they started, have them try to determine why. Sometimes we will ask participants to leave something on the ground (a coin or other small item) and see how closely they come back to it.

D. Materials

1. One compass per student
2. Paper and pen (in lieu of a blackboard, this can be very handy to describe parts and functions of the compass)
3. Cord
   a) This can be useful in describing the concept of bearings as angles.
   b) Ideally, a different color cord could represent a different radius of the angle of a bearing.

CHAPTER THIRTY-THREE

Navigation: Combining the Map and Compass

I. Outcomes

A. Outdoor leaders provide evidence of their *knowledge* and *understanding* by:

1. Explaining how to take a map bearing
2. Explaining how to orient a map with a compass
3. Explaining how to apply declination
4. Explaining how to convert map bearings to field bearings and vice versa

B. Outdoor leaders provide evidence of their *skill* by:

1. Combining knowledge of map and compass effectively for safe travel in the backcountry
2. Demonstrating how to take a map bearing
3. Demonstrating how to orient a map with a compass
4. Demonstrating how to convert map bearings to field bearings and vice versa

C. Outdoor leaders provide evidence of their *dispositions* by:

1. Modeling the use of the map and compass to navigate safely in the backcountry

II. Content

A. Philosophy. Once experience has been gained with maps and compasses separately, the two skills can be combined to maximize their potential. It is important to keep in mind that when used together, however, both should be relied upon and not one without the other.

1. Use the map to find easier routes that are close enough to the original bearing and the destination. Don't blindly follow a bearing that goes through swamps and up cliffs.
2. Don't take the easiest route if it contradicts the bearing.
3. Generally speaking, when in doubt, rely on the bearing. The terrain can be deceiving, while a correct bearing is generally not.

B. Using map and compass

1. Taking a map bearing
    a) The compass may be used as a protractor when attempting to establish a bearing for travel from one known place on a map to another.
    b) Place the compass on the map with one of the long edges of the base plate connecting the starting point of the trip with the destination. Be sure the "direction of travel" arrow is pointing in the direction of the destination. (See fig. 33.1.)
    c) Turn the compass housing until the orienting arrow and the meridian lines (or "map aid" lines) within the housing are parallel with the nearest north/south longitudinal line (meridian) on the map.
        (1) The only true north/south lines are those printed on the map margins (and the "ticks" that mark the "neat" lines). It is important for participants to understand that the grid lines on a map are not true north/south meridian lines. It is best to use the edge of the map or any line parallel to the edge for taking a map bearing.
        (2) Be sure the orienting arrow is pointing to true north at the top of the map.
    d) Read the map bearing from the rim of the housing where it intersects with the direction of travel arrow. This reading is called a "map bearing"; i.e., the angle measured in degrees formed by a line of travel on a map in relationship to true north (top of map).
    e) Some like to draw parallel north/south lines on the map in pencil to insure accuracy when taking bearings, although, as will be seen shortly, a better method may be employed.
2. Declination: Using a map bearing

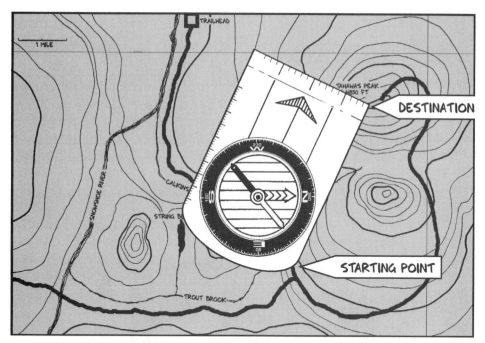

FIGURE 33.1. Taking a map bearing

a) Before understanding how a map bearing can be used in the field as a guide for travel, declination should be understood and must be taken into consideration.

b) Declination is the difference, expressed in degrees of an angle, between the location of true north (as found on a map) and that of magnetic north (as shown by a compass) measured from any given location on the globe.

    (1) The declination for any given area is recorded on the bottom of that area's map.

    (2) This measurement must be checked and accounted for before wilderness travel by map and compass is undertaken.

c) If, as is the case for much of the eastern United States, magnetic north is located some degrees west of the North Pole (true north), then:

    (1) Declination + map bearing = field bearing. For instance, in New York State, where the average declination is fourteen degrees, that fourteen degrees must be added to any map bearing before it can be used accurately in the field to find the way. (The reverse would be done west of zero-degree declination: declination – map bearing = field bearing.)

    (2) Field bearing – declination = map bearing. Again, in New York

State, with an average declination of fourteen degrees, fourteen degrees must be subtracted from any field bearing before that measurement may be accurately used to find a location on a topographic map. (The reverse would be done west of zero-degree declination: field bearing + declination = map bearing.) (See fig. 33.2.)

d) Drawing pencil lines parallel to magnetic north/south (i.e., parallel to the margins) across the map will eliminate the need to add or subtract

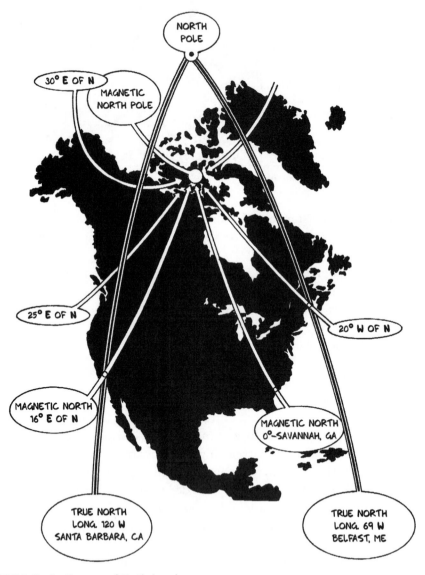

FIGURE 33.2. Declination map of North America

when taking map bearings. However, this method is discouraged until participants have a thorough understanding of why and when to add or subtract when taking map bearings and plotting field bearings.

3. Orienting a map with the compass

   a) When observing terrain features in the field, it is frequently helpful to line up the map so that it faces the same way as the observer. This lining up of the features of the map with those in the field is known as "orienting the map."

   b) Orienting the map can be easily accomplished with the compass.

      (1) Set the compass "direction of travel" arrow at the appropriate declination for the area.

      (2) Place one of the long side edges of the compass base plate along either of the north/south margins of the map. Make sure the "direction of travel" arrow is heading in a northerly direction.

      (3) Turn the map, with the compass on it, until the magnetic needle is "boxed" by the orienting arrow. Both the compass and the map are now oriented.

III. Instructional Strategies

A. Timing. This class is best taught after participants have a good understanding of both map and compass and are ready to combine the two.

B. Considerations

1. Teaching declination should inspire especially creative efforts from instructors. Since this concept is difficult for some to grasp, instructors should be prepared to use a number of approaches to illustrate the idea.

2. Visual aids (diagrams) and props (colored shoestrings representing true north, magnetic north, and line of travel) should be employed to help visualize the concept in different ways.

3. Mnemonic phrases may help participants remember how to convert map bearings to field bearings (e.g., FM Stereo = Field to Map, Subtract).

4. A skit can be used where participants play the following roles: true north, magnetic north, the East Coast, St. Louis, and California. Angles and declination can be demonstrated by using "St. Louis" as zero degrees.

C. Materials

1. Maps
2. Compasses
3. Visual aids as needed

CHAPTER THIRTY-FOUR

Navigation: Route Finding with Map and Compass

I. Outcomes

A. Outdoor leaders provide evidence of their *knowledge* and *understanding* by:

1. Explaining how to apply compass and map skills to the planning and proper execution of an off-trail hike
2. Describing how factors such as terrain, comfort of participants, and time requirements must be taken into consideration when planning an off-trail hike
3. Describing factors taken into consideration when developing a Time Control Plan and explaining why a Time Control Plan might be used

B. Outdoor leaders provide evidence of their *skill* by:

1. Planning a safe off-trail hike
2. Applying appropriate map and compass skills when hiking off trail
3. Applying appropriate route finding skills when hiking off trail
4. Preparing a Time Control Plan

C. Outdoor leaders provide evidence of their *dispositions* by:

1. Modeling appropriate map and compass skills when traveling off trail
2. Modeling appropriate route finding skills when hiking off trail
3. Modeling the use of a Time Control Plan when planning an off-trail hike

II. Content

A. Terrain considerations

1. The safety of the group must be of paramount concern during route planning. Obviously, dangerous obstacles such as cliffs, large rivers, and crevasses should be avoided.
2. Alternate routes should be anticipated if these areas or other questionable areas (such as swamps or bogs) are deemed unsafe to travel through.

B. Comfort. When planning, match the group's strengths and physical condition to the difficulty of the anticipated route.

1. How much altitude must be gained?
2. Is water available along the route?
3. How thick might the forests be?
4. Will the terrain be very wet or insect ridden?

C. Time and distance. It is important to accurately predict how much time will be required to travel the desired distance.

1. Terrain features: Features such as steep terrain, thick woods, and wet swamps all slow down travel time considerably.
2. Routes: Choose routes that ensure that the group has adequate time to accomplish the objective, even if a minor emergency occurs.
3. Establish guideposts: Select routes that allow the traveler to look for clearly identifiable landforms and features to use as guides, thus minimizing the opportunity for getting lost. (See fig. 34.1.)
   a) Handrails
      (1) Select land features that parallel the line of travel to the left or right.
      (2) If a traveler crosses over a handrail, it should indicate that he or she has drifted off to the left or right of the chosen path.
   b) Backstop
      (1) Select a landform to serve as a "dead end" or "gone too far" barrier.
      (2) Hitting this landform indicates that a turn was missed or the objective was passed.
   c) Checkpoints
      (1) Selected terrain landforms (i.e., checkpoints) along the line of travel can be used to confirm the traveler's exact location.
      (2) These checkpoints can be used frequently to evaluate progress and determine on a map whether or not travel is going as planned.

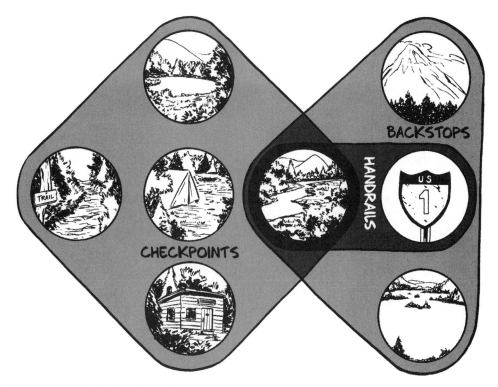

FIGURE 34.1. Checkpoints, handrails, and backstops

Travelers should use the map to keep constant track of their location.

4. Altitude gain or loss
   a) The gain or loss of altitude along a route must be properly estimated in order to make an accurate Time Control Plan and can be another clue about the accuracy of the route chosen.
   b) The group can count contour lines from the starting point to the destination to get an idea of the ruggedness of the terrain.
5. Distance
   a) The distance of the proposed route should be measured on the map using a string and the distance scale.
   b) Distance naturally figures into the Time Control Plan.
6. Time Control Plan: A detailed itinerary of the day's travel, known as a Time Control Plan (TCP), is extremely helpful in encouraging participants to closely examine the potential route and anticipate what the day is going to be like. It is also helpful to participants in developing their map interpretation skills, estimating travel times, and developing judgment and decision-making skills, as well as being a reference in case of emergency.

We encourage students individually (or in pairs) to create their own TCP, and then the instructor collects them. At the end of the day, the Leader of the Day (LOD) gives them back out and perhaps rewards the "winning" TCP; i.e., the one that is closest to predicting the actual time while still being comprehensive.

A thorough TCP might include:

a) The number of people in the group, the day's designated leader, and other assigned roles (e.g., scout, sweep, etc.).

b) A counting of the number of contour lines that will be crossed going uphill and the number crossed going downhill with a computation of the elevation gained, elevation lost, and the net elevation gain or loss. (This is a good activity to do as a large group so that everyone begins to understand how to determine whether a given contour line indicates uphill or downhill travel.)

c) Starting point, destination, and the computed distance to be traveled.

d) A brief description of unique characteristics of the day's travel route, including obstacles and hazards (e.g., forest types, swamps, river crossings, etc.).

e) A written estimate of the time it will take to reach the destination, broken down into estimated travel time, rest time, and meal breaks.

f) Contingency plan: What if you can't make your destination, get lost, or have an emergency? Where might you camp, find water, get help, etc.?

7. Travel time guidelines:

a) On a flat trail with a relatively heavy pack, most groups can travel at about 2 miles per hour.

b) When off-trail hiking, most groups can travel at about 1 mile per hour.

c) At altitudes up to 7,000 feet, add one hour of travel time for every 1,000 feet of elevation gained.

d) At altitudes between 7,000 feet and 11,000 feet, add one and a half hours of travel time for every 1,000 feet of elevation gained.

e) For every 1,000 feet of elevation lost, add thirty minutes of travel time.

III. Instructional Strategies

A. Timing

1. As their confidence builds, participants should be encouraged to plan and execute progressively more difficult off-trail hikes. Planning sessions for trips should include instruction and discussion of the following:

a) Terrain considerations in route planning

b) Identifying potential "handrails," "backstops," and "checkpoints"

c) Altitude loss or gain and counting contour lines

d) Estimating distances

e) Developing Time Control Plans

2. Participants should be encouraged to submit written estimates or predictions for each area of concern. During debriefings, these can be compared to the actual travel experience, which helps build a base of experiential knowledge.

B. Materials

1. Map

2. Compass

3. Notebook and pencil

CHAPTER THIRTY-FIVE

Navigation: Triangulation with Map and Compass

I. Outcomes

A. Outdoor leaders provide evidence of their *knowledge* and *understanding* by:

1. Explaining the reason for using triangulation with a map and compass
2. Describing how to triangulate using map and compass

B. Outdoor leaders provide evidence of their *skill* by:

1. Demonstrating how to determine their location by triangulation with a map and compass

C. Outdoor leaders provide evidence of their *dispositions* by:

1. Modeling the competent use of a map and compass to triangulate

II. Content

A. Definition of triangulation. The process of locating an unknown point by using intersecting bearings taken on three or more known points.

B. Steps

1. Using a topographic map of the area, positively identify two or three known landmarks that can be seen both in the field and on the map.
2. Take a field bearing of landmark number one. Write this bearing down and convert it to a map bearing. (Be sure to consider the area's declination.)
3. Set the compass for the map bearing of landmark number one.
   a) Place the edge of the compass base plate with the "direction of travel" arrow facing landmark number one on the map.
   b) Keeping the front tip of the base plate on landmark number one, rotate the compass base plate around the landmark until the orienting arrow and the orienting/meridian lines are pointing to true north/south on the map.
   c) Draw a pencil line on the map along the compass base plate edge that touches landmark number one. (This line may have to be extended.)
   d) The present location lies somewhere along this line.
4. Repeat the same procedure for landmarks number two and number three.
   a) Once all three bearings are recorded on the map, the lines should intersect or at least form a small triangle at some point on the map. This area is the approximate location from which the three bearings were taken (i.e., the present location).
   b) Participants should not be discouraged if the lines do not meet precisely at some given point. Given the level of sophistication of normal compasses and the participants' skill level, an approximate location should suffice to satisfy the need to know "where we are."

III. Instructional Strategies

A. Timing. This is an advanced map and compass technique and should be taught once participants have some degree of familiarity with both map and compass.

B. Considerations

1. Triangulation is best taught on treeless mountaintops or at least in areas of open visibility where clearly distinguishable landmarks can be seen.

2. For practice, participants can triangulate an already known location.

3. The instructor can provide bearings to identify a hypothetical "unknown" location on the map.

4. Participants should attempt to locate their approximate position at some convenient time on an off-trail hike using triangulation.

C. Materials

1. At least one map for every two participants

2. One compass for each participant

3. Pencil

CHAPTER THIRTY-SIX

Navigation: An Introduction to GPS

I. Outcomes

A. Outdoor leaders provide evidence of their *knowledge* and *understanding* by:

1. Describing what the Global Positioning System (GPS) is and how it originated
2. Describing the uses and limitations of the GPS
3. Describing how to use a GPS receiver

B. Outdoor leaders provide evidence of their *skill* by:

1. Setting up a GPS receiver for land or marine use, specifying the units of measure, and being ready to use a GPS receiver
2. Using the GPS receiver in conjunction with maps and compass to navigate

C. Outdoor leaders provide evidence of their *dispositions* by:

1. Recognizing and communicating both the value and limitations of GPS devices
2. Reinforcing the idea that the GPS is just another tool in the navigator's tool belt, that its limitations must be recognized, and that how to use a map and compass is essential

II. Content

A. An overview

1. GPS stands for "Global Positioning System."

2. GPS is a satellite navigation system that consists of twenty-four satellites that orbit the earth, transmitting information about precise time and position.

   a) GPS development originated in the 1970s with the U.S. Department of Defense, but it is now managed by the Interagency GPS Executive Board (IGEB; www.igeb.gov).

   b) It was developed to provide continuous worldwide positioning and navigation data to U.S. military forces. GPS also has a variety of nonmilitary uses of interest to the general public, such as hiking, fishing, boating, and auto travel.

   c) Originally the U.S. government built into the GPS what is called Selective Availability, which is the intentional degradation of the GPS signals. It prevented civilian users of the GPS from the highest levels of position accuracy, i.e., the ability to determine exactly where you are. In May 2000 the U.S. government turned off Selective Availability. The military reserves the right to turn on Selective Availability when it feels necessary. It can also change the datum, rendering the GPS completely useless in order to prevent people from using it to direct planes and missiles. In general, however, civilians can now utilize the same precise data that was formerly available only to the military, allowing for a level of accuracy with a GPS receiver that surpasses the resolution of USGS quad maps; i.e., approximately 50 feet (15 meters).

   d) Most of today's GPS receivers are designed to be accurate to 50 feet (15 meters), although WAAS-enabled units can provide position accuracy of 10 to 16 feet (3 to 5 meters) 95 percent of the time. WAAS stands for Wide Area Augmentation System, a system of satellites and ground stations that provide GPS signal corrections (called Differential GPS or DGPS) in order to improve position accuracy. WAAS was developed by the Federal Aviation Administration for aviation purposes. WAAS satellite coverage is currently only available in North America, although plans are under way in other parts of the world to develop similar systems.

3. Position and navigation information is inherently valuable for a broad range of activities, including hiking, hunting, camping, boating, surveying, aviation, national defense, and vehicle tracking.

4. Other systems, like map, compass, and altimeter, have traditionally been used to gather this information. Since GPS receivers are electronic and are vulnerable to damage, their use should never be depended on as the sole means for determining location or for navigation. They are best used as a backup or supplement to a map, compass, and altimeter.

a) Different models of GPS receivers also have different temperature limits and may not work in extreme heat and cold. A receiver may not work in consistently freezing weather (which also drains the battery life) or in desert climes. Check to make sure the GPS receiver you purchase meets your performance criteria needs.

b) Obstructions may also limit the use of a GPS receiver, so, for example, it may not work in areas that are densely forested, in areas where much of the sky is blocked by land formations, or inside buildings.

c) GPS receivers are designed to operate most effectively with a clear sky view. Anytime you compromise with less than a full sky view, you are compromising the operation of the GPS and the accuracy of your position fix. There is no GPS that can be trusted to perform well at all times in heavy tree cover or in steep and narrow valleys where GPS satellite signal masking can be present. GPS satellites move continuously and may one day be in an excellent position and the next in a poor reception situation. In general, with today's state-of-the-art receivers, there is little difference in "heavy tree cover" performance between the various models.

B. How the GPS works

1. The complete system consists of twenty-four satellites orbiting about 12,000 miles above the earth and five ground stations to monitor and manage the satellite constellation.

2. These satellites provide twenty-four-hour-a-day coverage for both two- and three-dimensional positioning anywhere on Earth.

a) Information received from three satellites yields a two-dimensional fix (latitude and longitude).

b) Information received from four satellites is required for three-dimensional positioning (latitude, longitude, and altitude).

3. Each GPS satellite sends coded signals regarding the exact time and its position. These signals are processed in your GPS receiver, enabling the receiver to compute position, velocity, and time.

4. A GPS receiver receives these signals from three or more satellites at once to determine the user's position on Earth (Dana 2000).

C. Features of the GPS receiver. Planes, automobiles, and large boats generally use GPS receivers that are built in and run off the engine battery. Backpackers, mountaineers, sea kayakers, and canoeists use portable receivers that run on batteries. Portable, handheld units can often fit in a pocket and are usually waterproof. (See fig. 36.1.) Recently, a wristwatch has been marketed that contains a GPS.

1. Common features of a state-of-the-art portable GPS unit available at press time:
    a) Water-resistant: Submersible to 1 meter for thirty minutes
    b) Weight: approximately 5.4 ounces with batteries
    c) Color/backlit display
    d) Built-in compass
    e) Built-in altimeter/barometer
    f) Operating temperature range: approximately 5°F to 158°F (-15°C to 70°C)
    g) Receiver: WAAS enabled, twelve parallel channels
    h) GPS accuracy: < 49 feet (15 meters), 95 percent
    i) DGPS accuracy: 10 to 16 feet (3 to 5 meters), 95 percent
    j) Map storage: 56 MB
    k) Battery life: Up to twenty hours of typical use
    l) Hunting/fishing calendar and sunrise/sunset times
    m) Geocaching navigation mode
    n) Geolocation games
    o) Multiplatform navigation; i.e., can be used on foot, in a boat, or in a car
    p) Accepts data from other map sources
    q) Fifty reversible routes, 10,000 track points, and 1,000 waypoints
    r) Elevation computer provides current elevation, ascent/descent rate, minimum and maximum elevation, total ascent and descent, average and maximum ascent and descent rates
    s) Trip computer provides odometer, stopped time, moving average, overall average, total time, max speed, and more

D. Understanding the GPS receiver

1. GPS receivers allow the user to set up navigational units of measurement in terms of statute, metric, or nautical units. This allows for land use (statute miles per hour [mph] or kilometers per hour [kph]) or for marine use (nautical miles per hour [knots]). Users must also set up bearings for either true or magnetic north.
2. GPS receivers have different map datums (Grubbs 1998).
    a) The map datum describes the model that was used to match the location of features on the ground to coordinates and locations on the map.

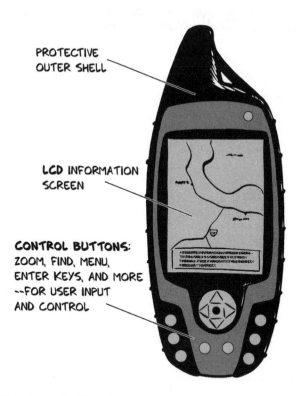

FIGURE 36.1. Features of a GPS unit

b) Most USGS topographic maps are based on an earlier datum called the North American Datum of 1927, or NAD 27.

c) While the world is converting to a common datum, WGS 84 (World Geodetic Standard 1984), this process will take some time to complete.

d) Since the difference between WGS 84 and NAD 27 can be up to 200 meters, you should always make sure your GPS unit's datum is matched to the datum of the map you are using.

3. The GPS receiver reads a variety of coordinate systems. (See section E for more information on coordinate systems.)

a) In North America there are two common systems:

(1) Latitude/longitude (lat/long)

(2) Universal Transverse Mercator (UTM)

b) Like the map datum, you must also set your GPS receiver to the coordinate system that corresponds to your maps.

4. While portable GPS receivers vary in size and in the number of functions they can perform, there are a number of commonalities. Table 36.1 lists many of the common functions found on a GPS receiver, as well as the terms and abbreviations for land and marine use.

Table 36.1. COMMON GPS FUNCTIONS AND ABBREVIATIONS		
Function	**Marine**	**Land**
Speed	SPD (speed)	SOG (speed over ground)
Bearing	BRG	BRG
Distance	DST	DST
Heading	HDG	COG (course over ground)
Velocity Made Good	VMG	VMG
Course to Steer	CTS	CTS
Estimated Time of Arrival	ETA	ETA
Recorded Position	LANDMARK	WAYPOINT

5. The receiver screen depicts the data for different functions. The user can often specify an array of data to display. The typical GPS unit has a number of displays, including a compass display, travel display, and map display.

E. Coordinate systems

1. Latitude/longitude: The traditional, and still most widely used, map coordinate system is latitude/longitude.

   a) Latitude is measured in degrees from the equator (0) to each of the poles—90 degrees north for the North Pole and 90 degrees south for the South Pole. Lines of latitude are parallel as they circle the earth; i.e., they never intersect.

   b) Longitude is measured east or west of the prime meridian (0), which runs through Greenwich, England. Longitude is expressed in degrees from 0 to 180 east or west. Lines of longitude all intersect at the North and South Poles.

   c) Latitude and longitude are expressed in terms of degrees (⅟₃₆₀ of the circumference of the earth), minutes (⅟₆₀ of a degree), and seconds (⅟₆₀ of a second). For example, the coordinates for Beavercreek, Ohio, are 39° 44' 25" N, 084° 04' 26" W.

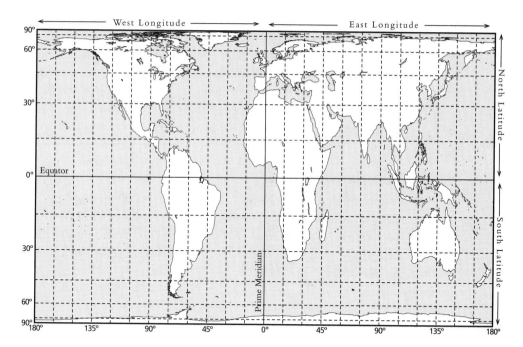

FIGURE 36.2. Longitude/latitude map

    d) Each degree of latitude is 60 nautical miles; each minute is 1 nautical mile. This is true uniformly from the equator to each pole. Degrees, minutes, and seconds of longitude, however, are wider at the equator and narrower as you approach the poles, making use of this system somewhat difficult.

2. Universal Transverse Mercator/UTM: The UTM system divides the earth into sixty zones, each zone being 60 degrees wide, to equal 360 degrees to describe the circumference of a circle.

    a) Each zone contains a Central Meridian running down the center of the zone. The Central Meridian of each zone is set at 500,000 meters east so that all coordinates have a positive value.

    b) UTM maps have basic grid lines, both horizontal and vertical, drawn 100,000 meters (100 km, or about 62 miles) apart. Depending on the scale and purpose of the map, there may also be 10,000-, 1,000-, or even 100-meter lines.

    c) All vertical grid lines run parallel to the central meridian; all horizontal lines run parallel to the equator. While the latitudinal lines on a UTM map are all parallel, the longitudinal lines are not due to distortion in projecting a round globe onto a flat map surface.

d) It is easy to identify locations on UTM maps since coordinates are specified in terms of zone and grid lines. Vertical lines (latitude) are specified in numbers from 0 to 1,000,000 within a specific zone. Horizontal lines (longitude) are specified in terms of meters from the equator.

 (1) For example, the coordinates for Beavercreek, Ohio, would be written 16 0750882 4402816, where 16 is the zone, 0750882 is the easting (the east-west coordinate), and 4402816 is the northing (the north-south coordinate).

 (2) To specify location to the nearest kilometer (1,000 meters, 0.62 mile), all you have to do is drop the last three digits. Thus, Beavercreek would be specified as 16 0750 4402. The first number is the zone, the second set of numbers is the easting, and the third set is the northing.

e) UTM does not cover the poles. UTM maps stop at 84° North and 80° South.

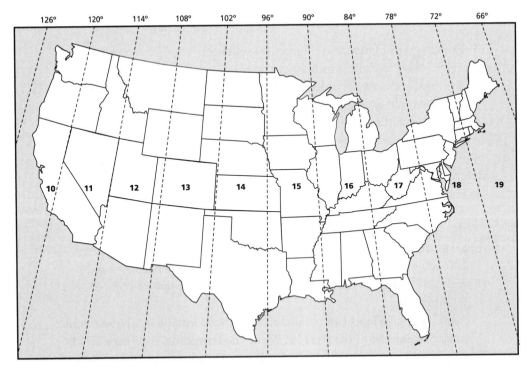

FIGURE 36.3. UTM zones of the United States

F. Coordinating GPS use with map and compass

1. It is best to use GPS along with map and compass to create a redundant set of information. This provides a backup, as well as a validity check, of your computations.

2. In some situations, like when you cannot see landmarks (e.g., fog, desert, or other settings with few distinguishing features), the GPS provides valuable information hard to determine otherwise.

3. In other situations, use of map and compass provides a faster and easier means to determine or confirm your location. Consider, for example, hiking on a trail that is going downhill, with a stream at the bottom, using a map that has both the trail and the stream located on it.

4. There are also times when the two systems complement each other. For example, speed of travel can be estimated using a map and compass when the features are indistinct or when crossing a large lake in a canoe on a windy day, but when more precise information is needed, a GPS receiver can give accurate information about SOG (speed over ground). COG (course over ground), and even time or distance to destination (if your GPS receiver has these options and you have programmed in the coordinates of your destination).

5. Using the GPS receiver takes time and practice. As with any equipment, don't rely on it until you have familiarized yourself with its use prior to a trip—and, even then, use judgment.

III. Instructional Strategies

A. Timing. GPS is an optional topic and should only be taught well after participants are competent with both maps and compass. Participants are usually curious about GPS, and exposure to it can be a valuable learning experience.

B. Considerations

1. This lesson can be taught in many small pieces. Using this strategy, the instructor might introduce the concept of GPS as the concluding part of a map and compass class. This might be followed up in another class with the basic functions of GPS, with a look at a GPS receiver, and with a small demonstration. A third component of this skill-development sequence could be to have students use the GPS to locate their present location (e.g., base camp) and record this waypoint in the GPS memory, assuming that the GPS has this function.

On the trail, the navigator of the day can use the GPS as a second method for determining distance traveled, speed of travel, or location. As a more advanced lesson, the navigator can input waypoints and order them to create a route for the day, following the GPS indications and using the map and compass as a backup.

2. To give a demonstration of how a UTM map is constructed, a demonstration involves cutting an orange. Imagine that the orange is the earth. Cut a small circle from the top and bottom of the orange (representing the poles). Now, make a series of vertical cuts in the orange. To simulate the UTM system, you'd need a big orange and sixty sections of orange.

Each section should look like figure 36.4. Next, flatten out each piece and you'll have a representation of zone. Take the marker and draw a line down the center of this section—that is the central meridian for this zone. Draw a horizontal line to represent the equator and mark the top 84° North and the bottom 80° South. Note that each of the sixty sections (hypothetically, in this case, since you probably won't be able to get sixty sections from your orange) is six degrees in width.

Next, overlay a grid. This can be done by drawing lines on a piece of clear plastic wrap, using a piece of window screening (which you may also be using to screen cooking leftovers during washing), or even by making a grid of twigs. You can even bring pieces of overhead transparency sheets for this or make sure course manuals have clear plastic covers that can double as transparency sheets (a china marker works well for writing on this surface). The result will conceptually look like figure 36.5, which simulates the UTM map.

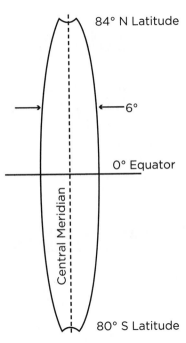

FIGURE 36.4. A section of an "orange" meridian

3. Assessment strategies: We have found that the best way to assess students' skills with GPS is to assess the accuracy of students in completing the tasks outlined in the section on teaching strategies above. For example, each stu-

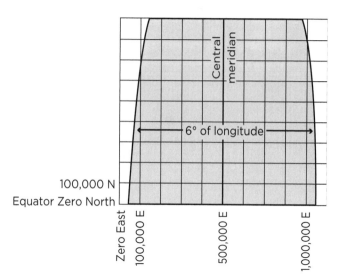

FIGURE 36.5. A simulation of the UTM system

dent could independently find the position of base camp and record the coordinates. Students could then compare the coordinates that they recorded. In this case, the instructor will see which students have recorded the correct coordinates.

Throughout this assessment process, when students have incorrect data it is often instructive to have them explain how they arrived at their answers. Often, problems with logic or computations will become apparent and can be easily corrected.

As the navigator for the next day plans and reviews the route and inputs waypoints into the GPS, the instructors can check the coordinates for each waypoint. As part of the end-of-day debriefing, the navigator of the day can review his/her computations using map and compass as well as GPS. Any inconsistencies between the numbers generated by each system can be discussed.

C. Materials

1. GPS receiver
2. Map
3. Compass
4. A knife, an orange, a piece of clear plastic wrap or screen, a sheet of overhead transparency, and a marking pen for the UTM demonstration

CHAPTER THIRTY-SEVEN

Personal Hygiene

Many illnesses and injuries can be avoided with the practice of proper personal hygiene. Illnesses all too often get spread throughout camping groups due to improper hygiene. A number of factors, including environmental factors and one's immunity, affect the amount of impact these illnesses have on individuals. This chapter is designed to help learners prevent/minimize illness and injury due to poor hygiene practices.

I. Outcomes

A. Outdoor leaders provide evidence of their *knowledge* and *understanding* by:

1. Describing the role that personal hygiene plays in the success of a backcountry trip
2. Describing techniques that prevent potential health problems or unwanted negative group dynamics

B. Outdoor leaders provide evidence of their *skill* by:

1. Practicing socially acceptable personal hygiene techniques in the backcountry

C. Outdoor leaders provide evidence of their *dispositions* by:

1. Modeling a concern for personal hygiene and its role in maintaining sound health and positive group dynamics

II. Content

A. Importance of personal hygiene

1. Practicing good personal hygiene:
   a) Helps prevent and/or minimize the chance of illness
   b) Contributes to positive expedition behavior
   c) Shows consideration for tent mates and other group members
   d) Helps to raise spirits and contributes to a feeling of overall well-being
   e) Contributes to the positive role-model image that leaders should maintain

B. The microbes that make us ill

1. Viruses
   a) Characteristics
      (1) Viruses are extremely tiny organisms; they account for more than 50 percent of all acute respiratory illnesses (e.g., the common cold).
      (2) They require living cells in order to reproduce and are usually species specific; i.e., they are only found in living animals and tend to be found only in one species.
      (3) In the wilderness, viruses are virtually always transmitted by hand to mouth. When someone has a "bug"-like viral illness and he or she handles water bottles, bug-repellent containers, and other containers, and also frequently shares bags of trail food, the organism could be transmitted. Others then touch these items or reach into the food bags, becoming ill by hand-to-mouth contact or eating the contaminated food. It is far more likely you will catch an infectious disease by this mechanism than from drinking untreated water—so wash your hands!
   b) Examples
      (1) Norwalk virus (the cause of most food- and water-transmitted viral illnesses)
      (2) Hepatitis (types A, B, and C)
      (3) Mumps
      (4) Influenza
      (5) HIV
   c) Prevention
      (1) All the viruses we need to worry about in North American wilderness areas are inactivated with sufficient heat, ultraviolet light, and some sanitizers.

      (2) Typical wilderness prevention includes boiling water and thoroughly washing hands, ideally with hot water and soap and/or the use of hand sanitizers.

      (3) To prevent the transmission of viruses, you should refrain from sharing water bottles and reaching in food bags to eat nuts, raisins, and similar foods. Provide individual supplies of things like trail mix and avoid sharing them.

      (4) Pour food into people's hands or personal cups and wash hands frequently.

  d) Treatment

      (1) Generally, antibiotics are not effective against viruses, and most, like influenza, the common cold, and gastrointestinal viruses, have no "cure."

      (2) Most viruses must run their course until the body's defenses can defeat them. Medicines relieve some of the symptoms.

2. Bacteria

  a) Characteristics: Bacteria are microscopic, single-cell plants that can grow and reproduce, unlike viruses, outside of any mammalian hosts.

  b) Examples of conditions caused by bacteria:

      (1) Wound infections

      (2) Boils and abscesses

      (3) Some intestinal infections (e.g., salmonella or shigella)

      (4) Some forms of pneumonia

  c) Prevention

      (1) Handling food properly

      (2) Keeping food at the proper temperature

      (3) Keeping both large and small wounds clean, and applying topical antibiotics

      (4) Using sanitizers, high temperatures, and ultraviolet light (most are killed this way)

  d) Treatment: Antibiotics are effective in treating most forms of bacterial infections.

3. Fungi and yeast

  a) Characteristics

      (1) They are primitive plants that are usually found in moist environments.

      (2) Fungi and yeast feed on living plants, decaying organic matter, and animal tissue.

      (3) They are frequently bothersome but rarely debilitating.

b) Examples
  (1) Athlete's foot
  (2) Ringworm
  (3) Yeast infections
c) Prevention: Keep susceptible areas of the body clean and dry.
d) Treatment: Fungicidal powders and ointments usually work well.
4. Protozoa
  a) Characteristics
    (1) A phylum of single-celled animals.
    (2) Most cases of protozoan illness are transmitted, like viral diseases, by hand to mouth.
  b) Examples
    (1) Giardia lamblia
    (2) Cryptosporidium
  c) Prevention
    (1) Since the evidence is becoming clearer that most cases of both giardia and cryptosporidiosis are transmitted by hand-to-mouth spread, the first line of defense should be a thorough washing of hands, ideally with hot water and soap, and/or using hand sanitizers. This is of particular importance in the case of giardia, as it is now known that many people can carry and spread this organism and have absolutely no symptoms (i.e., they are asymptomatic carriers).
    (2) To prevent the transmission of giardia or cryptosporidiosis, you should refrain from sharing water bottles and reaching in food bags to eat nuts, raisins, and similar foods. Provide individual supplies of things like trail mix and avoid sharing them.
    (3) Pour food into people's hands or personal cups and wash hands frequently.
    (4) Bringing water to a boil is an effective way to treat water suspected of having giardia and cryptosporidium in concentrations high enough to make someone ill.
    (5) Protozoa can be filtered out of the water with virtually all commercially available backpacking filters.
    (6) While halogens (chlorine and iodine-based treatments) are effective against virtually all bacterial and viral pathogens likely to be encountered in the backcountry of North America, protozoa are another issue. "Giardia lamblia in the adult active form is mostly sensitive to halogens; the quiescent oocyst form is moderately

resistant to halogens. The pathogen Cryptosporidium parvumin in its common oocyst form in surface waters, on the other hand, is very resistant to halogens even at high concentrations. Do not trust a halogen to rid your water of Cryptosporidium" (www.dcsar .org/featuredbooks.html). On the other hand, there is absolutely no evidence that cryptosporidium has ever been a problem for healthy users of North American backcountry water.

    d) Treatment

        (1) Giardia: The antibiotic metronidazole, sold under the brand name Flagyl, is the most common treatment.

        (2) Cryptosporidiosis: There is no specific treatment for cryptosporidiosis. However, some people may respond to certain antibiotics.

C. The number one priority in maintaining health in the outdoors (in case we haven't made it clear yet): WASH YOUR HANDS—WASH YOUR HANDS—WASH YOUR HANDS

1. Make sure to wash your hands before preparing meals and after defecating. Save a bandanna exclusively for drying your hands after a good washing, or carry a small absorbent towel. Towels that pack easily and absorb wonderfully are available in many outdoor specialty stores. Simply allowing hands to air dry is another option.

D. Preventing the spread of illness

1. Spare the group from exposure to your germs. Sneeze and cough into your elbow, not into your hand. Remember, your hand is the primary backcountry kitchen tool, so keeping it as clean as possible is even more critical when traveling with a group.

2. Do not share bandannas, toothbrushes, razors, water bottles, eating utensils, and the like.

3. Bringing water to a boil is the only treatment necessary for water suspected of contamination in the backcountry of North America.

4. Food preparation precautions

    a) Wash hands prior to food preparation and contact with drinking water.

    b) Cook food thoroughly.

    c) Once food is cooked or rehydrated, consume it.

    d) Minimize the use of "leftovers." Food that has been cooked and then cooled to room temperature can promote the growth of bacteria that produce a toxin causing "food poisoning."

e) If you clean as much of the visible remains as possible out of your cooking pot, put it into eating bowls, fill the pot with water, and put it back on the stove or fire right away, the cleaning water will be ready by the time you finish consuming your wilderness meal.

f) Food carried in several small, well-sealed plastic bags has a better chance of remaining intact and uncontaminated than food in one larger bag.

g) Wash and let all community kitchen gear air dry.

h) Keep individual eating utensils out of community dishes.

i) On group trips, try to plan and prepare food in groups of no larger than two to four people.

j) Avoid sharing prepared food between cook groups.

k) Provide individual supplies of things like trail mix and avoid sharing them.

l) Do not share personal utensils, water bottles, etc.

m) Keep anyone with the slightest indications of a cold, flu, or skin infection out of the camp kitchen.

n) On cold-weather trips when the temperature stays below 38°F (2°C), your cooking gear will remain free from germ growth if you allow it to cool off rapidly and then bring your next meal to the boiling point during preparation.

o) Sterilize utensils by immersing them in boiling water for between ten to thirty seconds before using. "Heat . . . does to microbial protein what a hot frying pan does to an egg . . . [It] can no longer perform its germy function" (Tilton and Bennett 1995). A spoon immersed in boiling water will be disinfected, and, if you boil water in a pot, the inside of the pot will be disinfected.

p) Clean water bottles regularly, especially the screw threads in the lid. This and occasional sterilization will keep mold from growing and kill harmful bacteria.

E. Preventing Injury

1. Feet: It is very important to keep feet in good condition as they are the major mode of transportation in the backcountry. Evacuations have occurred because foot care has been neglected. Remember—your feet are "diesel" power. Dies'el get you into the woods, and dies'el get you out of the woods!

a) NO BARE FEET! We recommend that footwear always be worn when in camp and when circumstances dictate (e.g., in stony, rocky, or otherwise unsafe beach areas).

       (1) Sticks, stones, glass, etc., can cut and puncture feet.

       (2) Dirt can easily enter open wounds.

   b) Keep feet as clean and dry as possible.

       (1) Wet, warm environments promote bacterial or fungal growth.

       (2) Irritants such as sand or dirt between toes will encourage blistering.

       (3) Wash and use foot powder when needed.

   c) Treat hot spots immediately. Keep blisters clean and covered. (See chapter 44, Travel Technique: Hiking.)

2. Hands: Hand cream helps prevent dry-skin cracks that are painful and can become infected.

3. Sunburn

   a) In most backcountry situations, it is necessary to carry heavy loads (carrying the backpack or portaging the canoe). People who get sunburn on their back and shoulders endanger the welfare of the group because they may no longer be able to carry their portion of the load. Getting sunburn is an act of selfishness.

   b) The number of people with skin cancer has been increasing rapidly since the 1950s. Skin cancer is the most common form of cancer found in the world today. There are many reasons, but probably the biggest is that people have more leisure time to spend outdoors in the sun. Also, the fashion for tans has meant that people have not been as careful in the sun as they should be. Sun-related skin cancers are the leading cause of death from outdoor recreation.

   c) Avoid potential problems by wearing protective clothing and applying an SPF 30+ sunscreen. For particularly troublesome spots (e.g., the nose and ears) consider using an occlusive cream such as zinc oxide.

   d) Wearing a hat that protects the ears and neck is particularly important.

   e) Remember that the danger of sunburn is higher when on water or snow, or at higher altitudes.

   f) The areas most susceptible to sunburn are face, neck, shoulders, ears, and eyes.

F. Aesthetic concerns for personal hygiene

1. Bathing and washing: Although not bathing regularly is not a health concern in the outdoors, regular bathing certainly goes a long way in promoting good expedition behavior and making one feel good.

   a) Bathe and wash clothes as regularly as possible. The proper techniques are covered in chapter 4, Bathing and Washing.

b) Spot washing can be done when time or weather conditions are not conducive to bathing.

c) Major areas for spot bathing include armpits, crotch, feet, hands, and hair.

2. Brush your teeth regularly: For good dental care and out of consideration for those around you, this is an important activity.

3. Comb or brush your hair: Again, for the sake of personal appearance and for good expedition behavior, caring for your hair is important.

III. Instructional Strategies

A. Timing. This class is best taught early in the trip to set a tone of personal cleanliness and safety.

B. Considerations. A skit can be useful in introducing the subject matter.

C. Activities. See the "Harry Hygiene" challenge at the end of the chapter.

Challenge

Knowledge Outcome	Title	Skill/Disposition Outcome
What do you want them to know? The participants can describe techniques for preventing the most common health problems on a backcountry trip.	"Harry Hygiene" Stays Healthy in the Backcountry	**What skill/disposition do you want them to develop?** Critical thinking: synthesizes ideas and information into a useful whole

Essential Question or Key Issue:

How can we stay healthy in the backcountry?

Description of Challenge/Task/Performance:

With the assistance of your teacher/instructor, create three diverse teams. An overarching question for each group is, "Why is personal hygiene important?" Each team should research one of the following three personal hygiene topic areas for special attention:

- Viruses, fungi and yeast: What are their characteristics, and how do we prevent them from making us ill?
- Bacteria and protozoa: What are their characteristics, and how do we prevent them from making us ill?
- Injury and aesthetics: How do we prevent injury, and what do we do regarding personal hygiene to promote good expedition behavior?

Each team should prepare an entertaining three- to five-minute "Half-Man" skit (see below), in which the team shares the essential information it has learned. After the skit, the performance team should facilitate a debriefing that reinforces the key points of the skit. In the debriefing, be sure to point out very specific practices that expedition members can adopt to apply the basic principles of good hygiene.

Half-Man Skit

The basic "Half-Man" skit is almost always fun and usually messy. The setup is that the arms person (who must agree to love and treat kindly the face/legs person) puts his arms through two slits in an opaque sheet (rain fly or tent entrance), and then through the arms of a large jacket or shirt worn over the shoulders of the face/legs person. The face/legs person has short pants on his arms and shoes and socks on his hands. A tent entrance is an excellent "stage." Helpers are needed to move equipment/props to the table. It is a fun challenge to maximize the improvisational potential of the skit. The more the audience understands that the person in the back really can't see what he's doing, the funnier it is. The face/legs person should intentionally look the wrong way and make sure that things don't go well between hands and mouth or other body parts.

Criteria for Assessment and Feedback:

Form criteria:
- The skit is three to five minutes in length in basic "Half-Man" format.

Content criteria:
- The skit communicates accurate information regarding desirable backcountry hygiene practices that address concerns related to the researched topic.

Knowledge:
- The participants can describe techniques for preventing the most common health problems on a backcountry trip.
- The participants can highlight specific desirable hygiene practices in the debriefing.

Skill: Critical thinking: synthesizes ideas and information into a useful whole
- In debriefing, participants can describe connections between general principles of good hygiene and specific expedition practice.

Developed by Leading EDGE, LLC for The Backcountry Classroom. *For more information log on to www.realworldlearning.info.*

Product Quality Checklist

Date: _____   Class Period: _____

Product Author(s):	Product Title/Name: "Harry Hygiene" Stays Healthy in the Backcountry	Evaluator Name(s):

Observed	Standard/Criteria	Possible Points	Rating
	The skit is three to five minutes in length in basic "Half-Man" format.		
	The skit communicates accurate information regarding desirable backcountry hygiene practices that address concerns related to the researched topic.		
	Total		

Observations:

Elements of Questionable Quality:	Elements of Exceptional Quality:

CHAPTER THIRTY-EIGHT

Rock Climbing: Leadership Considerations for Top Roping

This chapter gives instruction on a potentially dangerous activity. It is not intended to be the only source of information for those wishing to pursue the sport of rock climbing. Supplemental instruction by certified rock-climbing instructors is necessary to safely use this information.

I. Outcomes

A. Outdoor leaders provide evidence of their *knowledge* and *understanding* by:

1. Describing ethical considerations that apply to climbing
2. Describing types of climbing
3. Describing the system used to rate climbs
4. Describing the advantages of top-rope climbing as an instructional activity
5. Describing leadership considerations for programming
6. Describing safety considerations while programming and critiquing the safety system established at a top-rope site
7. Comparing and critiquing various top-rope sites for participant and environmental suitability
8. Critiquing a top-rope site and climbs to determine if they meet the ability level of a group
9. Critiquing the appropriateness of a site for top-rope climbing

B. Outdoor leaders provide evidence of their *skill* by:

1. Critiquing the safety system established at a top-rope site

2. Assessing a climbing site for safety
3. Applying minimum-impact practices when using a top-rope site
4. Implementing safety practices
5. Identifying levels of difficulty associated with an ascent and matching them with the ability level of the participants

C. Outdoor leaders provide evidence of their *dispositions* by:

1. Modeling outdoor-ethics principles when climbing
2. Espousing the programming benefits of top-rope climbing
3. Modeling an attitude of safety throughout the climbing experience
4. Modeling ethical climbing practices

II. Content

A. Institutional climbing. Rock climbing has gained significant popularity as a program offering among a wide variety of organizations. To accommodate that growth in popularity, professional associations have responded by developing accreditation standards, certification programs, or general climbing information.

1. Association for Experiential Education (AEE; www.aee.org): Provides an accreditation service for organizational members that includes accreditation standards for top-rope climbing and bouldering.
2. American Mountain Guides Association (AMGA; www.amga.com): Provides guide certification and program accreditation services. AMGA also offers a five-day top-rope site certification course.
3. In-house training programs: Many outdoor schools, guide services, etc., provide quality, in-house training programs for their staff and occasionally for the general public.
4. The Access Fund (www.accessfund.org): Provides support services and grants to develop and protect natural climbing areas.
5. Leave No Trace (LNT; www.lnt.org): Provides educational materials specific to environmentally friendly climbing practices.
6. American Safe Climbing Association (ASCA; www.safeclimbing.org): Provides information and recommended protocol for safe climbing.
7. Local climbing organizations and clubs: Help communicate the local ethic of a climbing area and may assist in user group self-management.

B. Specific training and experience. To safely facilitate a top-rope climbing experience with a group, specific training and experience are required. An apprenticeship under a more experienced instructor is the prudent approach before taking on the full responsibility as a top-rope site manager. It should be noted that basic rescue skills, such as belay escapes, load releases, and simple raising skills, are standard skills required of top-rope site managers.

C. Types of rock climbing and terminology

1. Free climbing: Using ropes, natural (e.g., trees, boulders, etc.), and artificial protection (e.g., nuts, camming devices, etc.) to ascend rock. Ropes and anchors are not used to support the climber's weight during the ascent of a climb, but to protect the climber in the event of a fall.

2. Aid climbing: Ropes and aids are used to support the climber's weight during an ascent. Specialized gear might include aiders (rope ladders), specialized hooks, nuts, etc.

3. Free soloing: Climbing alone with or without the use of ropes or any means of protection in the event of a fall.

4. Bouldering: Attempting a series of moves without any safety equipment. The climber typically does not stray farther than 10 or 12 feet from the ground, and spotters are used for safety.

5. Lead climbing: An experienced climber begins at the base of a climb, places anchors (camming devices, nuts, or bolts), and runs the ropes through these anchors as he/she advances. Lead climbing requires specialized knowledge and experience to execute safely. (See fig. 38.1.)

6. Traditional climbing: The lead climber places passive (nonbolted) or camming protection (anchors) into the natural features of the rock.

7. Sport climbing: As opposed to traditional climbing, this is generally considered to mean climbing routes that have permanent protection; i.e., bolts already in place.

8. Multipitch climbing: A lead climber climbs a distance of a rope length or less and establishes a belay station (by utilizing traditional or fixed protection) to belay other climbers up. Climbers that follow clean the route by bringing up the gear left by the lead climber. Once another climber has reached the top of this first pitch, a leader climbs a second pitch while being belayed from the station. The climbers continue in this fashion until the summit or the top of the climb is reached.

9. Top-rope climbing: A type of free climbing where the climber is belayed from the top or bottom of the rock face using an anchor at the top of a climb. This is a common technique used for single pitch climbs for beginners and institutional groups. (See fig. 38.1.)

10. Rappelling: Descending a fixed rope (with a single or double rope) by means of a friction (belay/rappel) device attached to the harness. Should be done when possible with a backup belay rope.

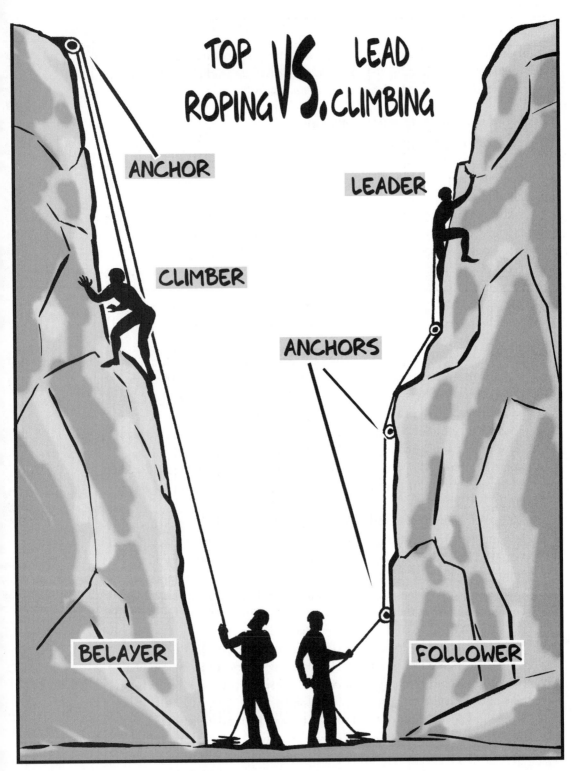

FIGURE 38.1. Top roping versus lead climbing

D. Rock climbing rating systems. There are numerous classification systems used to describe the difficulty and techniques needed to climb a given terrain (e.g., Australian, French, British, or UIAA system). The most common classification system used in the United States is the Yosemite Decimal System (YDS).

1. Description of the YDS (Long 1998, p. 9)
   a) Class 1: Walking.
   b) Class 2: Hiking, mostly on established trails, or perhaps slogging along a streambed.
   c) Class 3: Scrambling; angle is steep enough where hands are used for balance. A rope may be occasionally used as a handline, but it is typically not needed.
   d) Class 4: Climbing is risky enough that a fall could be fatal. Pulling with your arms required. Most mountaineers use a rope, some equipment, and protection techniques.
   e) Class 5: Technical rock climbing. A rope, specialized equipment, and belay techniques are always used to protect against a fall.
2. Class 5 climbing has been further defined as an open-ended scale to accommodate the continuing advances in climbing (Graydon and Hanson 1997).
   a) 5.0–5.7: Easy for experienced climbers; it is where most novices begin.
   b) 5.8–5.9: Where most weekend climbers become comfortable; employs the specific skills of rock climbing, such as jamming, liebacks, and manteling.
   c) 5.10: A dedicated weekend climber might attain this level.
   d) 5.11–5.15: The realm of true experts; demands extensive training and conditioning, often repeated attempts at a route, and excellent natural athletic ability.
3. Class 5 is broken down further using an a, b, c, or d rating beginning at the 5.10 level to better describe the technical difficulty of a climb. For example, a 5.10a is not as demanding as a 5.10d climb. The highest difficulty rating for a climb that has been successfully completed as of the date of this publication is 5.15a. This upper limit will inevitably be surpassed as the sport continues to evolve.

E. Outdoor ethics specific to the sport of climbing. Outdoor leaders who facilitate climbing programs must be aware of ethical standards. The Access Fund has developed protocol and position statements to promote responsible use (www.accessfund.org):

1. Never disturb historically, archaeologically, or environmentally sensitive areas.

2. Don't scar, chisel, glue holds onto, or otherwise deface natural rock.

3. Don't place bolts next to cracks or other features, which afford natural protection. Avoid using colored bolt hangers that contrast with the natural color of the rock.

4. Don't add fixed protection to established routes except to beef up questionable anchors. If you must leave slings at rappel stations or "back off" gear, use colors that blend in with the stone.

5. Don't establish routes in areas of heavy traffic, such as campgrounds or directly above public trails or roads.

6. Don't throw anything—rotten slings, trash, or even human waste—off climbs. It's simple—everything you start up with comes off the climb with you.

7. Accept responsibility, even for the impact of other climbers on the mountain environment, by removing useless slings and garbage from climbs, bivy spots, descent routes, and rope-up areas. Leave the area cleaner than you found it.

8. Know and respect local regulations on climbing and restrictions on bolting, motorized bolting, and chalk usage. Be flexible in your climbing—adapt your style to the accepted style and ethics of each climbing area.

9. Dispose of human waste cleanly and legally. Human waste disposal around climbing areas is a real and growing problem. Follow outdoor-ethics protocol when disposing of waste. When on a route where human waste cannot be buried, dispose of waste in a sturdy plastic bag and carry it out.

10. Use existing trails whenever possible and refrain from cutting across switchbacks. When hiking off trail, take a route that will minimize impacts on native plants or wildlife. Be aware that most damage to soil and vegetation is sustained during descents.

11. Assume complete responsibility for yourself and your party's actions while climbing. Be sure someone (friend or family) has detailed knowledge of your climbing plans and timetable. If you get yourself into difficulties, be prepared to get yourself out of them. Do not rely on a rescue team (or others) to come to your aid. Know and practice what to do in various types of emergencies, including injury, self-rescue rope handling skills, evacuation, unplanned bivouacs, and rapid changes in weather or route conditions.

12. Maintain a low profile. Other users of the land have the same right to undisturbed enjoyment of the area as you do. Remember, climbers can have a highly visible and audible presence and are often a curiosity to tourists and nonclimbers. Whether on the cliffs or in the parking lot, try to minimize this presence.

13. Don't trespass in order to climb. In most places, climbing is a legal and legitimate activity. Should you encounter restrictions or bans on climbing, contact the ACC Access Committee to seek an effective and lasting solution.

14. Respect other climbers in the area, and, above all, be safe while climbing. Remember that courtesy is an element of safety. Falling rock or gear is a serious hazard, so be careful when climbing above another party. Do not create a dangerous situation by passing another party on a route without their consent. If you can't pass safely and easily, don't.

15. Support projects that help all climbers be more aware of and responsive to climber impact issues. In the United States, climbers depend on access to natural areas to pursue their sport. If we care for our public lands and support the agencies that manage them, we further preserve the climbing environment.

16. In addition to the recommendations listed above, top-rope site managers should consult with land managers before altering or rebolting climbs, or establishing new climbs.

17. For a current listing of climbing restrictions that apply to specific climbing areas (organized by state), visit www.accessfund.org/access/access_restrictions.html.

F. Top-rope climbing. Top-rope climbing is the most common type of climbing activity found among outdoor programming providers.

1. Advantages/benefits of using top-rope climbing include:
   a) Top-rope climbing does not require as much technical skill competency as lead climbing and can be done safely with trained leaders.
   b) Many natural rock-climbing areas throughout North America are conducive to top-rope climbing.
   c) Top-rope climbing meets the needs of climbers at all levels—particularly beginners.
   d) Rappelling can be easily integrated into a top-rope site as an additional activity.

2. The following are typical participant outcomes. Participants will:
   a) Improve self-confidence and self-esteem
   b) Develop trust among group members
   c) Develop group cohesion
   d) Develop appreciation for climbing as a lifetime sport
   e) Develop deeper appreciation for the natural environment
   f) Develop decision-making skills

G. Leadership considerations for top-rope climbing

1. Consider using artificial climbing facilities (e.g., climbing gym, outdoor climbing tower, etc.) before bringing a large group to a natural climbing area or a climbing area that is heavily used by others. This will allow climbers to get accustomed to climbing procedures so that, once they get outdoors, they can also focus on protecting the environment.
2. Follow established codes of ethics when facilitating a top-rope climb.
3. Receive proper training (e.g., AMGA certification) and keep current on changes in the industry.
4. Never promise complete safety! Responsibility must be put on the participants to monitor their own safety.
5. Pretrip considerations:
   a) Obtain proper permission and permits to climb at the site
   b) Identify appropriate access to site
   c) Identify potential hazards (e.g., loose rock, bee nests, sharp edges, etc.)
   d) Consider possible impacts on the flora and fauna
   e) Be familiar with potential climbs and the difficulty of each in order to appropriately challenge participants
   f) Know appropriate anchor options for each climb
   g) Preestablish safe zones or helmet-off areas for participants
   h) Know weather patterns of the area
   i) Be aware of history of the area (i.e., the natural and cultural history and local climbing community culture)
   j) Establish emergency response plan in case of an accident or inclement weather
   k) Develop written guidelines for the conduct of the activity (include site-specific protocol in addition to generic climbing protocol)
   l) Develop equipment logs and inspections systems
6. Programming considerations:
   a) Follow the organization's policies and protocols for conducting top-rope climbing with a group.
   b) Provide an appropriate instructor-to-participant ratio (based on factors such as agency policies, group type, instructor skill levels, climbing site characteristics, nature of the activity, etc.).
   c) Assess the ability level of participants. Provide and demonstrate use of fixed lines to assist participants' movement around, or to and from, the climbing site. (For example, there may be a class 3 or 4 climb involved in reaching a climbing site or to access the top of climbs.)
   d) Provide participants with an adequate safety briefing, including:

    (1) Securing long hair

    (2) Removing objects from body, such as rings and other jewelry

    (3) Reviewing hazards

    (4) Reviewing commands

    (5) Reviewing Challenge by Choice (see chapter 24, Group Orienting and Monitoring)

e) Minimize environmental impact at the base and top of climbs by:

    (1) Concentrating group and gear in the most heavily used area at base of climb and establishing boundaries to avoid expanding soil compaction and vegetation damage

    (2) Recommending areas and routes to take when disposing of human waste or bringing a portable latrine for group use in heavily visited areas

    (3) Avoiding the use of natural vegetation as anchors to reduce damage if a suitable alternative exists, and instead using camming devices and passive protection to build anchors in the rock (a more durable surface)

    (4) Employing responsible use of vegetation if used for anchors (i.e., avoid trampling, compacting soil around the base of trees and shrubs; do not allow setups where movement [friction] of climbing gear cuts into bark, etc.)

    (5) Keeping participants on durable surfaces and avoiding fragile vegetation typically found along the edges of climbs

f) Sequence the program to ensure safety and enjoyment. Judgment must be used here; the following is one example of a logical sequence:

    (1) Begin with outcomes for the activity

    (2) Conduct a safety briefing and lead stretching exercises

    (3) Lead a spotting technique discussion and demonstration

    (4) Give a climbing technique discussion and demonstration

    (5) Begin with bouldering, if possible (participants can apply climbing and spotting techniques)

    (6) Facilitate a ground school (e.g., teaching technical skills such as belaying and knot tying)

    (7) Begin top-rope climbing

7. Other safety considerations:

a) Ensure harnesses are correctly fitted and buckled, and implement a double-check system for tie-ins and harness integrity before participants climb

b) Ensure appropriate knots are used for participant tie-ins

c) Ensure helmets are fitted and worn when appropriate

d) Ensure anchor systems are correctly installed

e) Ensure communication system of climbing commands is understood and properly implemented

f) Ensure appropriate belaying techniques are implemented using:

    (1) A standard command system

    (2) Appropriate belay devices

    (3) Adequate and effective protection for belayers

    (4) Policies and procedures for backup belayers

g) Ensure proper care and use of equipment

III. Instructional Strategies

A. Timing. This lesson is intended for individuals who have climbing experience. Therefore, the content of this lesson should be taught after basic climbing skills have been mastered.

B. Activities

1. Facilitate a group discussion on the role of top-rope climbing in an institutional setting. Discuss how this type of programming compares to other types of climbing.

2. Take participants to an unfamiliar climbing site. Break participants up into small groups and have them assess the site. Have each group assess the site for safety and develop a site-specific plan to facilitate a group of beginners.

3. Have participants assess a climbing site based on the environmental impact and document it in their journals.

4. Facilitate a discussion around:

    a) The issue of ethics of group climbing and impact on public lands

    b) Ways to minimize environmental and social impact

C. Materials

1. Accessible climbing site

2. Journals

CHAPTER THIRTY-NINE

Safety: Emergency Procedures

I. Outcomes

A. Outdoor leaders provide evidence of their *knowledge* and *understanding* by:

1. Describing the considerations in the immediate care of the ill or injured beyond the actual administering of emergency medical care
2. Describing criteria for determining which type of evacuation would be most appropriate in a given situation
3. Describing post-accident considerations, including impact of the accident on group dynamics and individual participants

B. Outdoor leaders provide evidence of their *skill* by:

1. Developing a field emergency plan
2. Implementing a field emergency plan

C. Outdoor leaders provide evidence of their *dispositions* by:

1. Modeling cool, calm, and competent thinking and action in an emergency situation

II. Content

A. Emergency procedures

1. Definition: The actions to be performed at the time of an accident or illness.
2. Immediate considerations at the time of the emergency:
   a) Stop and think. Decisions should not be rushed, but rather carefully thought out within the time constraints of the particular emergency.
   b) Delegate authority. The leader should have those who are most qualified take appropriate roles. For example:
      (1) Performance of emergency medical care.
      (2) Secretary: This person should write down times, dates, first aid performed, medicine given the patient, etc.
      (3) Messengers: Those who will request outside assistance if necessary.
      (4) Assistants: Those who may help the rest of the group set up camp or accomplish other tasks as needed.
   c) Miscellaneous care of the patient and the group:
      (1) Creating a calm atmosphere
      (2) Tender, loving, "karmic" care for the patient
   d) Does the patient need to be evacuated?
   e) Is outside assistance required?
3. Considerations in requesting outside assistance
   a) At least three (preferably four) capable "messengers" should be selected to request assistance. (A group of four people is ideal so that if one of the messengers is injured on the way out, one can remain with the injured person and there are still two to continue.) An instructor should ideally be part of the messenger group (for liability reasons).
   b) What to send with the messengers:
      (1) An accident report form.
      (2) An account of total number in group, how much equipment the group has, and the condition of the group overall.
      (3) A detailed description—including a map—of the location of the emergency, with current weather and time of day.
      (4) An evacuation plan with route if a decision has been made to self-evacuate, have rescue personnel meet you at site of emergency, or carry victim to better location for safety or evacuation.
      (5) All requests and information in written form. The spoken word can be easily miscommunicated (especially in an emergency), and written words allow for less interpretation. Ideally, there should be

two copies: One copy should stay with the group, and one copy should go with the messengers.

    c) What is the notification priority?

        (1) Be aware of program policies regarding notification protocols.

        (2) Medical/rescue help will usually be contacted first.

        (3) Trip sponsors (the instructor's supervisor) can contact relatives, news media, etc.

    d) What contingency plans have been made?

B. Evacuation procedures

  1. Evacuation options:

    a) Patient walks out.

    b) Group participants carry patient out.

    c) Rescue group carries patient out (e.g., rangers, rescue squad, etc.).

    d) Helicopter or other mechanical means are used to evacuate patient.

  2. Evacuation considerations:

    a) Condition of the patient

    b) Time issues

    c) Distance

    d) Terrain

    e) Weather

    f) Mental and physical condition of the group

    g) Possible expenses

C. Post-incident considerations

  1. Debrief incident with key participants and program supervisors to assess any future recommendations.

  2. Document all witness statements.

  3. Complete post-accident documentation immediately.

  4. Include all documentation (program application, releases, medical screening, accident form, SOAP note [a standardized way to record medical information that can assist in patient assessment, decision making, and treatment in a backcountry medical emergency; S = subjective "spoken" data, O = objective "observed" data, A = assessment—what you think is wrong with the patient, and P = plan—what you are going to do], witness statements, etc.) in post-accident file.

  5. Inform insurance carrier or risk manager immediately.

  6. Monitor group dynamics:

    a) What has been the impact of the incident on the group?

    b) How should the group be handled?

7. Recommend actions based on the incident.
8. Initiate contact with appropriate land management and rescue agencies to assess any future recommendations or concerns.
9. Implement recommendations.
10. Return personal clothing and equipment.
11. Implement refund policy for the patient.

III. Instructional Strategies

A. Timing. The information in this lesson should be communicated to participants before they go on any small group overnights without staff.

B. Activities. This lesson is usually presented in a lecture/discussion format. Role playing using a simulated accident can also be effectively employed.

C. Materials

1. Accident report form
2. Paper and pencil

CHAPTER FORTY

Safety: Risk Management

I. Outcomes

A. Outdoor leaders provide evidence of their *knowledge* and *understanding* by:

1. Explaining risk management, safety, harm, and disclosure
2. Describing the three phases of risk management
3. Describing the roles of a risk-management committee
4. Explaining the roles of elimination, retention, transfer, and reduction in managing risk
5. Describing and explaining aspects of a risk-management plan
6. Describing communication and documentation considerations

B. Outdoor leaders provide evidence of their *skill* by:

1. Implementing an effective risk-management plan
2. Balancing the potential for risk with the desire for adventure

C. Outdoor leaders provide evidence of their *dispositions* by:

1. Modeling safe outdoor practices
2. Weighing the risks of their actions

II. Content

A. Definitions

1. Risk management: A systematic analysis of risk and a plan for minimizing the risk of harm to clients and staff, as well as the risk of legal liability for harm that does occur.
2. Safety: Freedom from harm.
3. Harm: Physical injury, death, or damage to reputation.
4. Disclosure: The attempt to reduce surprises by informing people of the program's mission, activities, associated risks, and possible outcomes.

B. Three phases of risk management

1. Prevention and planning: What happens *before* there is an accident or disaster, in order to prevent it from happening or to be prepared to handle and control it when it does.
2. Handling: The immediate response to an accident or disaster (see chapter 39, Safety: Emergency Procedures).
3. Documentation and control: The long-term management of the consequences of the accident or disaster, including public relations, legal liability, and interaction with public authorities.

C. Prevention and planning

1. Risk-management committee: Central to the risk-management process is the formation of a risk-management committee, which:
   a) Has primary responsibility for prevention of accidents and planning for emergencies
   b) Has ready access to legal advice
   c) Is prepared to work closely with the program's insurance broker
2. Prediction: One of the functions of the risk-management committee is to predict or think through just what risks there are in your activities. Some of these may be obvious; for example, the risk of drowning while rafting or kayaking, or the risk of falling while rock climbing. Some risks may seem more remote; for example, the risk that a staff member will be accused of sexually molesting a client, or the risk that a noncustodial divorced parent will walk off with a child in your program, or the risk that a client will commit suicide while on your premises. In addition, the committee should consider more general risks of fire, flood, and weather, including tornadoes or hurricanes, which may pose risks to your clients, staff, or property.
3. Managing risk

a) Elimination: When you discontinue or avoid activities that have been determined to be too great a risk. For example, you no longer have a rock-climbing program because it is too hard to hire qualified staff and the activity puts your organization at too great a risk.

b) Retention: When you decide to do something even though it is determined to place your organization at risk. For example, you can't afford insurance to take campers to Siberia but decide to do it anyway because the opportunities and benefits appear to outweigh the risks.

c) Transfer: When you transfer the risk to another entity. For example, you obtain liability insurance or certify your staff through an outside agency.

d) Reduction: When you minimize your risk by:
   (1) Maintaining facilities and equipment
   (2) Providing additional training for staff

4. The risk-management plan: Below is a possible outline for a risk-management plan, along with considerations for specific aspects of the plan (Cline 1999).

a) Risk-management mission statement

b) Risk-management goals

c) Risk-management oversight: Who is responsible for risk management within your organization?

d) Risk-management committee and its role

e) Medical screening: What is your policy, and how do you determine who can and can't attend your program?

This might be an appropriate time to have participants discuss their medical histories within the group. It should be mentioned that this is confidential information, but that it is to everyone's benefit to share as much about his or her medical history as possible. Medical histories, although sometimes embarrassing, are of great educational value.

f) Waivers: How do you plan to use them?

g) Disclosure: Is your information regarding medical and physical requirements, expectations regarding behavior issues, program policies, and risks sufficient to minimize surprises to both the participant and the provider?

h) Administration
   (1) Is your organization too bureaucratic or too understaffed?
   (2) What is the chain of command?
   (3) How are you determining whether your administrative needs are being met?

(4) Are you getting feedback from all levels of your organization regarding the administration of programs?

i) Statement of compliance: What accreditations, certifications, or nationally recognized protocols does your organization have or follow?

j) Outside professionals: What outside professionals do you consult (e.g., doctor to review medical protocols and review medical screening, risk-management consultants, etc.)?

k) Internal and external risk-management audits

(1) What do you do within your program and whom do you invite from outside your program to audit your risk?

(2) Are reports accurate and acted on? For example, if a report recommends replacing personal flotation devices, are they replaced in a reasonable amount of time?

l) Incident review: What incidents should be recorded, and how do you record and review incidents that occur within your program?

m) Practice and policies/rules and regulations: Are practices and policies written, clear, and concise, and do both staff and clients understand them and the consequences if they are not followed?

(1) What are the minimum rules and regulations you need to run your program?

(2) "Only those rules and regulations which are essential for the safety and well being of the participants should be established. Too many rules and regulations cause problems for both leadership and the participants—no participant can abide by all the rules if too many, nor can the leadership enforce so many" (Van der Smissen 1997).

n) Insurance

(1) You owe it to yourself, your program, and your clients to carry sufficient liability insurance to cover foreseeable risks.

(2) It is advisable for the risk-management committee to do an insurance audit with your broker and, ideally, with an attorney. Such an audit has two purposes:

(a) To make sure that there is sufficient primary and excess liability coverage for the level of risk in your program.

(b) To review any exclusions from that coverage that may be part of your policy. For example, some commercial general liability policies may exclude coverage for allegations of sexual assault or abuse, or for injuries incurred while playing sports. It is important to be aware of any gaps in your liability coverage and to take steps to obtain any additional coverage necessary. In addition, you should determine whether your program's liability coverage extends to your staff and to the officers and directors of your organization. Some insurance companies provide coverage specifically designed for schools or outdoor programs, and you should investigate these with your broker.

    (c) As a course instructor, you should know what kind of insurance coverage your employer provides, including workmen's compensation.

o) Equipment

    (1) Are you letting your participants know what gear to bring with them and what your program will be providing?

    (2) Is your outfitting state-of-the-art and in good condition?

    (3) Are you maintaining records of the use and condition of critical equipment; e.g., personal floatation devices, climbing ropes, etc.?

p) Food

    (1) Are your rations varied and nutritious?

    (2) Are your food storage and handling practices and procedures up to local health-department standards?

q) Transportation: What are your training and maintenance protocols, and are they being followed?

r) Emergency procedures plan: What is your plan, are your staff trained to implement it, and are your clients prepared and informed regarding how to implement it should the occasion arise? (See chapter 39, Safety: Emergency Procedures.)

    (1) Preemergency

        (a) Are your staff members trained as Wilderness First Responders or higher?

        (b) Do you have medical histories of participants and staff?

        (c) Have you implemented your risk-management plan?

        (d) Do you have an appropriate emergency medical kit? This might be an appropriate time to review the group's medical kit and explain why different things are brought and how they can be used in an emergency.

        (e) Emergency communication protocols: How are you going to communicate with the appropriate parties in an emergency (cell phone, satellite phone, pay phone, etc.)?

        (f) Emergency contacts: In an emergency, who are you going to contact, and in what order?

                    i)   Rescue personnel
                    ii) Organization supervisors
                    iii) Relatives of the group participants
                    iv) Others
                (g) Evacuation routes: Have you anticipated potential evacuation routes?
            (2) Emergency action: See chapter 39, Safety: Emergency Procedures.
            (3) Post-emergency: See chapter 39.
    s) Screening and supervision of staff
        (1) How do you screen potential employees?
        (2) Do you check references?
        (3) What kind of staff training do you have?
        (4) Are staff jobs clearly defined?
        (5) How do you supervise employees and document their performance?
        (6) Are there appropriate mechanisms in place for all employees to provide feedback to each other?
        (7) How do you conduct and review staff evaluations and use them to increase program effectiveness?
    t) Environment: Where are you running your trips?
        (1) Are the clients appropriately educated regarding the demands of the environment in the relevant season of travel so they can properly prepare to participate?
        (2) Are the staff trained in the environment and season that you will be taking clients?
    u) Activities
        (1) Skill and skill sets
        (2) Sequencing
        (3) Curriculum
        (4) Equipment
        (5) Trip planning
        (6) Supervision of participants
    v) Public relations/communication: How are you going to communicate with all parties, including the media, regarding the emergency? (See section E, below.)

D. Handling. This phase is how your organization responds to an accident or disaster. It is covered in section r, above, and in chapter 39.

E. Communication and documentation

1. Communication: When something has gone wrong, you will have to communicate with clients, staff, parents, public officials, and the general public. Under stressful circumstances, it is tempting to circle the wagons. This is often a mistake. It is better to try to provide accurate information, maintain your credibility, avoid confrontation, and seek consensus on ways to solve problems.

2. Documentation: Above all, documentation of the accident or disaster must be clear and accurate. Remember that your documentation will almost inevitably be available to a plaintiff if a lawsuit is filed against you or your program. Where documentation is necessary, it should carefully record the facts that are known at the time. The documentation should not lay blame, make judgments, guess, speculate, embellish, or in any way appear callous or unfeeling. Proceed on the assumption that your documentation of the accident or disaster will become public, either to the press or in litigation.

III. Instructional Strategies

A. Timing. A philosophy of effective risk management and the modeling of that philosophy starts with the first communication with group participants. The grasshopper approach (see chapter 1, Teaching and Learning, for more about the grasshopper approach) is an effective way to share much of the contents of this chapter. It is important to have a formal learning experience regarding risk management before students go on any small group adventures without staff.

B. Materials. See Wilderness Risk Managers Committee forms at the end of the chapter.

Wilderness Risk Managers Committee

Incident Reporting Project
Instructions

This project and these reporting forms were designed to collect useful information about incidents in adventure programming. The Incident Report Form can be used both to track information for your organization's use and to submit incident data to the committee. The Program Day Report Form that accompanies this material is used to calculate rates of incidents. Please try to use the format provided; it will allow us to generate statistics by type of incident, type of injury, type of illness, type of environment, and by activity. However, if this format does not meet your needs, you may modify it to better suit your organization's operations.

Please take the time to complete these forms carefully. Write *legibly* to ensure the incident is recorded accurately in the database. Illegible reports will be discarded. Complete and accurate information is essential to the strength of the Wilderness Risk Managers Committee (WRMC) database. **Both the Program Day Report Form and copies of the Incident Reports should be submitted together annually.** We recommend that the data be collected by calendar year; for example, from January 1st through December 31st. Program Day Report Forms and Incident Reports should be sent to:

Incident Data Reporting Project
Association for Experiential Education
2305 Canyon Boulevard, Suite 100
Boulder, CO 80302-5651
(303) 440–8844, ext. 16
(303) 440–9581 (fax)

Questions about completing the Incident Report Form or Program Day Report Form should be directed to WRMC member Drew Leemon at NOLS (307–332–8800, ext. 2256 or drew_leemon@nols.edu).

Definitions

Incident: An unplanned for or unintended, potentially dangerous occurrence or condition that results in injury, illness, property damage, near miss, or other loss (or potential loss).

Motivational or behavioral incident: Any incident that arises from the actions, responses, or behaviors of individuals or groups of individuals. Examples include reluctance or unwillingness to participate, verbally or physically abusive utterances or acts, running away, alcohol or drug use, suicidal or homicidal ideation, or any emotional or psychological situation or condition that compromises the students' ability to participate in the program.

Injury: Any harm that impairs normal functioning or causes wounds or damage to a person.

Illness: Any ailment, sickness, or unhealthy condition that interferes with normal functioning or causes distress.

Near miss: A "close call." A potentially dangerous situation where safety was compromised but that did not result in injury. An unplanned for and unforeseen event. A situation where those involved express relief when the incident ends without harm.

Property damage: Any loss of or harm to material goods that results in replacement or repair of those goods.

Program days (user days): A measure of program size. The product of multiplying the number of participants and staff in an activity by the number of days of participation. (Note: Any portions of days should be counted as a full day.)

Risk: The possibility (probability) of injury or other loss.

Risk management: The process of analyzing exposure to risk and determining how to best address the exposure. Practices vary by industry and location, but common strategies include acceptance, avoidance, elimination, and transfer.

Incident Report Form Instructions

As defined above, an incident includes any unplanned for or unintended occurrence or condition that resulted in, or could have resulted in, a significant injury, illness, or other loss. A *reportable* incident, injury, or illness, for the purpose of this project, meets one or more of the following criteria:

- Requires more than simple first aid (i.e., a Band-Aid)
- Requires more than cursory staff attention
- Requires follow-up care by staff in the field
- Requires follow-up care by a medical professional
- Requires follow-up care by a therapist, psychologist, or social worker
- Requires use of prescription medications
- Interferes with the student's or client's active participation

- Requires evacuation from the field
- Requires the loss of a day or more of participation in the program (i.e., a lost-day case)
- Results in a near miss

Incidents that do not meet these criteria should not be included in the submitted data. If you are in doubt about whether an incident is reportable or not, please report it.

Affiliate: The name of the organization (confidential).

Program type: The type of program offered. For example, environmental education, adventure education, therapeutic program, adjudicated youth, etc.

Course name or designation: Your name or designation for this course (confidential).

Name: The name (or names) of the person(s) involved in the incident. The identity of persons involved in incidents will be kept confidential.

Age, gender, and staff or participant: Self-explanatory.

Incident date and time: Self-explanatory.

Day of course incident occurred: The number of days the participant was in the field when the incident occurred; e.g., day seven of a nine-day trip.

Type of environment: Choose the most appropriate description from the list.

Surface condition: Choose the two most significant or appropriate descriptions from the list.

Type of incident: An incident may result in injury, illness, motivation/behavioral outcome, or a near miss. Choose the most appropriate description from the list.

Lost-day case: A lost-day case occurs if a participant or staff missed one or more days of activity, beginning with the day following the incident.

Near miss: Please rule out situations such as routine top-rope falls, failure to roll a kayak for a beginning student, or a fall on the trail with no injury.

Did the patient leave the field?: Evacuations occur when a person leaves the field as a result of an incident. There are several levels of definition that aid in determining the seriousness of the incident:

- Participants or staff who leave the field
- Participants or staff who seek medical care
- The type of evacuation (unassisted, assisted but ambulatory, litter carry, helicopter, etc.)
- If hospitalization was required

Evacuation method: Choose the most appropriate method from list. Describe the method if the category of other was chosen.

Medical facility visit: Choose "yes" if the patient received treatment at a hospital, clinic, doctor's office, etc.

Property damage: Self-explanatory.

Type of injury: Choose the most significant illness from the list. Please describe the illness if the category "other" is checked.

Anatomical location of injury: Choose the most appropriate.

Type of illness: Choose the most significant illness from the list. Please describe the illness if the category "other" is checked.

Type of activity: Choose the most appropriate activity from the list to describe the activity the person was engaged in at the time of the incident.

Contributing factors: This is a list of common incident factors or in adventure programming. Prioritize the applicable categories 1, 2, 3, etc.

Narrative: Describe the incident and provide details (distances, times, sizes, sequence of events, etc.) to present a clear picture of the incident.

Analysis: Include any suggestions, observations, or recommendations regarding the incident. Why did it happen? Describe follow-up care and any diagnosis or other outcome.

Names and signatures: Please provide the name of the person who completed the form and the name of the administrator who reviewed the form.

Wilderness Education Association
Wilderness Risk Managers Committee Incident Report Form

If you have any questions regarding how to complete this form properly, please consult the accompanying instruction sheet.

Affiliate: _____

Program type: NSP   PSC   WSP   WEW (circle one)

Course name: _____

Name: _____

Age: _____   ☐ Male   ☐ Female   ☐ Staff   ☐ Student/client

Incident date: _____ / _____ / _____   Time _____:_____ A.M./P.M.

Total days of course: _____   Day incident occurred: _____

Type of environment. Check all that apply:

☐ River   ☐ Lake   ☐ Ocean   ☐ Forest   ☐ Mountain   ☐ Cliff

☐ Glacier   ☐ Snow/ice   ☐ Desert   ☐ Cold environment

Surface condition. Check the two most significant:

☐ Wet   ☐ Dry   ☐ Snow   ☐ Ice   ☐ Trail   ☐ Rock   ☐ Uneven   ☐ Flat   ☐ Sloped

Type of incident. Check most significant:

☐ Injury   ☐ Illness   ☐ Motivation/behavioral   ☐ Near miss   ☐ Fatality

Is this a lost-day case?   ☐ No   ☐ Yes   Number of days lost _____

Did the patient leave the field?   ☐ No   ☐ Yes   Date: _____ / _____ / _____

Evacuation method: ☐ Unassisted   ☐ Walking assisted   ☐ Litter carry   ☐ Vehicle

☐ Helicopter   ☐ Other _____

Did the patient visit a medical facility?   ☐ No   ☐ Yes   If yes: ☐ Outpatient?   ☐ Admitted?

Victim returned to the course?   ☐ No   ☐ Yes   Date: _____ / _____ / _____

Property damage: ☐ No   ☐ Yes   If yes: ☐ Vehicle   ☐ Equipment   ☐ Other: _____

Wilderness Risk Managers Committee Incident Report Form

Type of injury. Choose the most significant:

- ☐ Blister(s)
- ☐ Burn
- ☐ Dental
- ☐ Dislocation
- ☐ Eye injury
- ☐ Fracture
- ☐ Frostbite

- ☐ Head injury (change in level of consciousness)
- ☐ Head injury (no change in level of consciousness)
- ☐ Immersion/submersion
- ☐ Ligament sprain
- ☐ Muscle strain

- ☐ Near drowning or immersion
- ☐ Soft tissue (bruise, wound, abrasion)
- ☐ Sunburn
- ☐ Tendonitis
- ☐ Other (explain) _____

_____

Anatomical location of injury. Choose most appropriate:

- ☐ Abdomen
- ☐ Ankle
- ☐ Chest
- ☐ Elbow
- ☐ Eye
- ☐ Face

- ☐ Foot
- ☐ Forearm
- ☐ Hand/fingers
- ☐ Head
- ☐ Hip
- ☐ Knee

- ☐ Lower back
- ☐ Lower leg
- ☐ Neck
- ☐ Pelvis
- ☐ Shoulder
- ☐ Thigh

- ☐ Toe
- ☐ Upper arm
- ☐ Upper back
- ☐ Wrist

Type of illness. Choose most significant:

- ☐ Abdominal pain
- ☐ Allergic reaction
- ☐ Altitude illness
- ☐ Apparent food-related illness
- ☐ Chest pain or cardiac condition

- ☐ Dehydration
- ☐ Diarrhea
- ☐ Eye or ear infection
- ☐ Flu symptoms/"cold"
- ☐ Heat illness
- ☐ Hypothermia
- ☐ Nausea or vomiting

- ☐ Nonspecific fever illness
- ☐ Skin infection
- ☐ Upper respiratory illness
- ☐ Urinary tract infection
- ☐ Other (explain) _____

_____

Type of activity. Check the activity at the time of the incident:

- ☐ Backpacking
- ☐ Camping
- ☐ Canoeing
- ☐ Caving
- ☐ Cooking
- ☐ Cycling
- ☐ Dog sledding
- ☐ Glacier travel
- ☐ Hiking (no pack)

- ☐ Horseback riding
- ☐ Independent travel
- ☐ Initiative game
- ☐ Mountaineering
- ☐ Portage
- ☐ Rafting
- ☐ Rappelling
- ☐ River crossing
- ☐ River kayaking

- ☐ Rock climbing
- ☐ Ropes course
- ☐ Running
- ☐ Sailing
- ☐ Sea kayaking
- ☐ Service project
- ☐ Ski (telemark/ downhill)
- ☐ Ski touring

- ☐ Snowboarding
- ☐ Snow/ice climbing
- ☐ Snowshoeing
- ☐ Solo
- ☐ Swim/dip
- ☐ Transportation
- ☐ Other (explain)

Wilderness Risk Managers Committee Incident Report Form

Contributing factors. Prioritize the applicable categories 1, 2, 3, etc.

- ☐ Altitude
- ☐ Avalanche
- ☐ Animal encounter
- ☐ Carelessness
- ☐ Cold exposure
- ☐ Dehydration
- ☐ Equipment
- ☐ Exceeded ability
- ☐ Exhaustion
- ☐ Fall on rock
- ☐ Fall on snow
- ☐ Fall/slip on trail
- ☐ Falling tree/branch
- ☐ Fitness/ability

- ☐ Hygiene
- ☐ Immersion/submersion
- ☐ Instruction
- ☐ Inattention
- ☐ Loose rock (not rockfall)
- ☐ Misbehavior
- ☐ Missing/lost
- ☐ Not following instructions
- ☐ Overuse injury
- ☐ Plant poisoning/toxicity/ contact
- ☐ Preexisting medical condition
- ☐ Psychological issue

- ☐ Rock fall
- ☐ Screening
- ☐ Sunburn
- ☐ Supervision
- ☐ Technical systems failure
- ☐ Technique
- ☐ Unknown
- ☐ Visibility
- ☐ Weather
- ☐ Other (explain) _____
  _____
  _____
  _____

Narrative: Describe the incident and provide details (distances, times, sizes, sequence of events, etc.) to present a clear picture of the incident.

_____

_____

_____

_____

_____

Analysis: Include any suggestions, observations, or recommendations regarding the incident. Why did it happen? Describe follow-up care and any diagnosis or other outcome.

_____

_____

_____

_____

_____

Prepared by: _____   Position: _____

Signature: _____   Date: _____ / _____ / _____

Reviewed by: _____   Position: _____

Signature: _____   Date: _____ / _____ / _____

CHAPTER FORTY-ONE

Safety: Waterfront Safety in the Backcountry

I. Outcomes

A. Outdoor leaders provide evidence of their *knowledge* and *understanding* by:

1. Describing safety considerations involved in identifying and inspecting an appropriate swim site
2. Critiquing a swim site for safety and appropriateness for swimming ability of participants
3. Describing a process for identifying swimming competency
4. Describing considerations in providing adequate supervision of a swim site
5. Describing safety considerations regarding use of personal flotation devices (PFDs)
6. Developing a response plan for potential emergencies

B. Outdoor leaders provide evidence of their *skill* by:

1. Applying backcountry waterfront-safety practices
2. Checking a swim site for obstructions and hazards
3. Using a PFD when appropriate
4. Implementing a response plan that will adequately address potential emergencies

C. Outdoor leaders provide evidence of their *dispositions* by:

1. Modeling an attitude of safety at all times when around water

II. Content

A. Water safety

1. Why practice water safety?
   a) It is better to be "safe than sorry."
   b) Water-safety practices reduce overall risk of the trip.
   c) An evacuation could take several days, be costly, and even end an expedition.

2. Swim-site considerations
   a) The needs of the group should be considered when selecting a swim site. While a group of nonswimmers might be uncomfortable in a natural pool that is 10 feet (3 meters) deep with rock sidewalls, a group of strong swimmers need not be limited to waist-high water.
   b) An ideal swim site would be sandy; gradually sloping; clear of grass, trees, and vegetation; and with no strong current. However, such a site is rarely found in the wilderness.
   c) Inspecting potential swim sites is an important precaution that should not be overlooked.

3. Inspecting the site
   a) Before allowing anyone to enter a swimming area, check the site for obstructions. Potential hazards might include:
      (1) Water features
         (a) Current
         (b) Tides
         (c) Water temperature
         (d) Turbidity
      (2) Physical features
         (a) Rocks
         (b) Logs
         (c) Drop-offs
         (d) Broken glass and other man-made hazards
      (3) Animals and plants
         (a) Snakes
         (b) Leeches
         (c) Jellyfish
         (d) Sea urchins

4. Identifying swimming ability
   a) Before allowing swimming in the backcountry, the trip leader or assigned waterfront-safety person should identify the swimming ability

of each group member. Completion of a simple 100-yard swim followed by a three-minute float will allow the leader to determine whether participants have adequate swimming ability.

    b) Identifying swimming ability gives qualified staff an opportunity to offer instruction to weaker swimmers.

5. Adequate supervision

    a) Qualified (certified) staff with knowledge of reaching and throwing rescue techniques and the potential hazards of a swim area should be assigned to supervise any swimming activity.

    b) This "lifeguard" should know how many people are in the water at all times. One method is to have swimmers leave a shirt in a designated place while they are in the water. The number of shirts would correspond with the number of swimmers in the water.

    c) A moonlit swim can be a refreshing sensory experience, but the added dimension of darkness can lead to disorientation. Adequate supervision and judgment are necessary to conduct this activity safely.

6. Adequate knowledge

    a) Make no assumptions. Carefully observe each participant's swimming ability.

    b) Anyone leading groups in, on, or around water should be skilled in life-saving techniques.

    c) Identify hazards and take steps to avoid problems (e.g., mark hazards and have participants wear proper aquatic footwear).

    d) Stay well away from water during lightning storms—water is a great conductor of electricity.

B. Backcountry waterfront considerations

1. Number of bathers: In the backcountry setting, group sizes are usually small enough that this isn't an issue.

2. Disbursement of bathers: Consider the distance the bathers will go from shore, how far apart they will be, and the location of water access sites.

3. Water conditions

    a) Water depth

    b) Water visibility: Clarity/turbidity, presence of foreign matter, color

    c) Water currents: Types and strength

    d) Waves: Size, type, location, and type of break line

4. Bottom conditions

    a) Amount of slope: Is slope smooth or uneven?

    b) Sandbar locations

    c) Rocks

    d) Holes

    e) Seashells, clamshells

    f) Vegetation

    g) Debris (e.g., glass, fish hooks, cans, etc.)

5. Waterfront size

    a) Size of beach area

    b) Size of designated supervised area

    c) Visibility

        (1) Fog

        (2) Sight lines

6. Weather conditions

    a) Air temperature

    b) Prevailing winds

    c) Amount of sun

    d) Chance of violent weather (e.g., thunderstorms, high winds, tornadoes, etc.)

7. Equipment: PFDs and improvised rescue tubes

    a) Condition

    b) Availability and placement

8. Waterfront personnel

    a) Training

    b) Awareness of Emergency Response Plan (see chapter 39, Safety: Emergency Procedures)

9. Emergency response

    a) Emergency response time: Access to medical care

    b) Emergency Response Plan

10. Special considerations

    a) Separation of incompatible activities

        (1) Will multiple activities exist?

        (2) Should activities be separated?

    b) Restriction of activities

    c) Use of site by other groups

        (1) Will other groups use the site for swimming?

        (2) Will other groups use the site for other compatible or noncompatible activities (e.g., boat or canoe launch, portage, sailboarding, etc.)?

III. Instructional Strategies

A. Timing

1. A pretrip discussion of waterfront safety considerations is advisable.
2. At the first swim site, describe the process for selecting a proper swim area and the safety considerations that are involved.

B. Activities

1. Ask students to discuss specific safety considerations.
2. Assign a different person each day to be responsible for swim site selection.
3. Include safety concerns as part of daily debriefings. Were there any potential problems?

CHAPTER FORTY-TWO

Stove Operation

I. Outcomes

A. Outdoor leaders provide evidence of their *knowledge* and *understanding* by:

1. Describing, comparing, and critiquing common stove types and their advantages and disadvantages
2. Describing proper stove terminology
3. Describing considerations in maintaining and safely using liquid-gas stoves and handling stove fuel
4. Describing environmental considerations for stove use
5. Describing principles of stove operation
6. Comparing stove types to meet a group's specific needs
7. Critiquing appropriate safety procedures for stove use

B. Outdoor leaders provide evidence of their *skill* by:

1. Starting and operating a variety of backpacking stoves
2. Practicing safety considerations in stove use and fuel handling
3. Caring for and maintaining stoves
4. Properly packing stoves and fuel for transport

C. Outdoor leaders provide evidence of their *dispositions* by:

1. Modeling outdoor-ethics principles related to stove use
2. Modeling the safe use and maintenance of stoves and their volatile fuels
3. Implementing preventive stove-maintenance measures

A. Environmental considerations. In order to minimize campfire impacts, it is recommended that stoves be used instead of fires. Even if you are in an area where fires are permitted, use a stove when:

1. Firewood is scarce (i.e., dead and down firewood cannot be readily found).
2. Available wood is not small enough to break with your hands.
3. The area is heavily camped and there is concern that the firewood supply will not readily replenish itself.
4. A site to build a minimum-impact fire is not available (e.g., fire ring, fire pan, or materials for a mound fire).
5. Land management agencies indicate high fire danger, a fire ban is in place, or if students are not capable of safely managing fires.
6. There is any doubt about safety or what the environmental impact might be.

B. Choosing a stove and fuel

1. Butane stoves
   a) Description: Stoves operate using fuel in pressurized canisters.
   b) Advantages:
      (1) Require no priming and are easy to use
      (2) Flame is easy to regulate
      (3) Used internationally
   c) Disadvantages:
      (1) Performance declines in cold weather
      (2) Disposal of the canisters is an environmental issue
   d) Examples:
      (1) MSR Superfly
      (2) Brunton Crux Foldable Butane Canister Stove
2. Propane/butane stoves
   a) Description: Propane stoves are comparable to butane stoves, but they perform better because they use heavier cartridges to accommodate higher pressures. They tend to be heavy, so for backpacking you are more likely to see stoves that use a blend of propane and butane.
   b) Advantages:
      (1) Double-burner propane stoves and refillable propane tanks can be used in water-based programs such as rafting when weight is not a consideration.

(2) Temperature is less of a factor in their operation.

(3) They are easy to use.

c) Disadvantages:

(1) Propane fuel is available on a limited basis internationally.

(2) Pressurized canister stoves tend to cost more to operate per hour compared to liquid-fuel stoves.

(3) Disposal of the canisters is an environmental issue.

d) Examples:

(1) Peak 1 Expedition Stove

(2) Turbo Bleuet 270 Stove

3. Denatured alcohol stoves

a) Description: Stoves have a small alcohol burner usually accompanied by a windshield.

b) Advantages:

(1) Burn clean and quietly

(2) Not highly flammable compared to other gas stoves

(3) Lightweight

c) Disadvantages: Stoves generate less heat, which increases cooking time.

d) Examples:

(1) Trangia Mini-Trangia 28-T

(2) Hike 'N' Light Alcohol Stove

4. Kerosene stoves

a) Description: Burn kerosene, a fuel readily available around the world.

b) Advantages: Once the kerosene is hot enough to burn efficiently, the stove puts out a hot flame equal to a white-gas stove.

c) Disadvantages:

(1) Difficult or tricky to prime and light

(2) Flame does not burn clean and leaves black soot on pots

d) Examples:

(1) Optimus 00

(2) Manaslu No. 96

5. White gas stoves

a) Description: One of the most commonly used stoves in outdoor programs in the United States.

b) Advantages: Stoves are efficient, hot, clean burners.

c) Disadvantages: The liquid is highly flammable and, while readily available throughout the United States, is not readily available internationally.

d) Examples:
    (1) Peak 1 Feather 400
    (2) MSR Whisperlite Shaker

6. Multifuel stoves
  a) Description: Stoves that have the ability to burn a variety of liquid fuels, such as white gas, kerosene, unleaded gas, or leaded gas.
  b) Advantages: Ideal for international travel when fuel sources are unknown.
  c) Disadvantages: Some stove types require more care and cleaning when using fuels other than white gas.
  d) Examples:
    (1) Coleman Feather 442 Duel-Fuel
    (2) MSR Dragonfly

C. General stove safety for white-gas or multifuel stoves with priming pumps.
We have chosen to highlight safety considerations in the use of these stoves because they are the most widely used in the backcountry of North America.

1. Using a stove is probably the second most dangerous thing done on the course. (Probably the most dangerous aspect of an expedition is traveling in vehicles.) As long as some basic safety considerations are followed, problems are minimized.
2. Considerations for stove location (see chapter 15, Food: Introduction to Cooking, for additional information):
  a) Place stove on the ground in a level, stable area.
  b) Nonflammable surroundings: Be sure there are no flammable materials around the stove, or place the stove on a fire-retardant cloth such as Nomax to prevent ground fires.
  c) Protect the stove from the wind (wind screens help to increase fuel efficiency and decrease cooking times).
  d) Do not use the stove in a tent unless there are no other options.
    (1) If you must cook in a tent, do not start the stove in the tent.
    (2) Be sure there is adequate ventilation, since carbon dioxide fumes can reach dangerous levels in the close quarters of a tent.
    (3) Check with the agency sponsoring the group; policies will vary regarding stove use in tents.
    (4) Cooking in tents should be considered a last-resort, extreme-weather-only activity.
3. If the stove should flare up and/or burst into flames:
  a) If possible, turn the stove off.

b) Smother the stove by putting a large pot or another appropriate object over the stove. The object must fit completely over the entire stove, cutting off all oxygen to extinguish the fire. The results are immediate. Nomax cloth can also be used to smother the flame.

c) Do not use water to extinguish the flame—this will only help spread the fire. Fuel is lighter than water and will stay on top of it.

d) As a last resort, throw sand or dirt on the stove to extinguish the flame. While this method works, the stove will have to be cleaned thoroughly.

4. General stove maintenance

a) Be sure to check for loose nuts and bolts, especially around fuel valves. This should be done before entering the field. Carry pliers (e.g., a multitool) for stove repair and maintenance while in the field.

b) Make sure gaskets on fuel caps are secure and not compromised in any way (e.g., cracked).

c) Pack extra parts that tend to need replacement or be lost in the field; e.g., pump leathers, generators, O-rings, gaskets, and extra fuel caps.

d) Make sure the fuel pump remains lubricated (vegetable oil can be used in a pinch).

D. Safety considerations for fueling liquid-fuel stoves

1. Judgment dictates the following considerations when filling a stove:

a) The stove should be cool before filling.

b) No open flame should be nearby (e.g., other lit stoves, matches, lighters, candles, cigarettes, etc.).

c) Consider establishing a fuel station for the group approximately 50 feet from any kitchen area. Fill the stove in a different location than where it will be lit and used. Any fuel that may have been spilled when the stove was filled could ignite when the stove is operating.

d) Gas vapors are heavier than air and float along the surface of the ground, and they will ignite if they come into contact with open flame. This is another reason to establish a fuel station away from the cooking area.

e) When taking off the stove's fuel cap, keep the stove away from your face to prevent pressurized gas from spraying into the eyes. (If gas enters the eyes, flush immediately and thoroughly for several minutes.)

2. The fuel bottle

a) Be careful not to lose any washers to the fuel bottle cap, or the bottles will leak.

b) Be careful not to cross thread the fuel bottle cap threads.

c) Be careful not to lay the fuel cap on the ground, where it will pick up debris that may eventually work its way into a stove and clog fuel lines.

d) When opening a fuel bottle, hold it far away from the face to prevent pressurized fuel from getting into the eyes.

3. The stove

a) Be careful not to lose the stove fuel-tank cap. Place it where you can easily find it and where it will not pick up dirt and debris.

b) Follow the manufacturer's directions to determine how much to fill the stove. Most stoves should be filled three-quarters full. Overfilling a stove does not allow enough space for the fuel to vaporize, creating a hazard in which pure fuel could ignite rather than fuel vapors.

c) Once the stove has been filled, securely replace the stove fuel-tank cap and the fuel bottle cap.

d) It is expedient to fill the stove before each use so that:

(1) The fuel won't run out in the middle of cooking a meal

(2) The stove can be filled without having to wait for it to cool

E. Stove terminology

This would be an appropriate time to explain all the parts of the stove and their function.

F. Stove operation

1. Liquid-gas stoves must be primed. This is the process of pressurizing the stove so that the liquid fuel becomes vapor.

a) Vaporized fuel burns hotter and cleaner (this ensures a hot, blue flame as opposed to a yellow flame).

b) Some stoves require that fuel be poured directly on the stove and then lit to prime it. Others are equipped with pumps to pressurize the stove. (Be sure to read the operating instructions.)

2. Starting the stove

a) Have a pot of water or food ready to go before lighting the stove. Valuable fuel is wasted if a stove runs without the pot or pan on top.

b) Explain and demonstrate how to start the stove using the manufacturer's operating instructions.

(1) Light the match before turning on the gas. This allows the vapors to ignite as soon as the valve is turned, preventing vapor buildup and a sudden dangerous flame.

(2) Light the stove in the "light to go" position. (The "light to go" position means on your feet, but in a squatting position with head back away from the stove—do not sit or kneel to light a stove.) This

position keeps the user on his or her feet so he or she can quickly spring out of the way if the stove produces a large, unexpected burst of flame. Keeping the face and head back prevents losing body hair. Long hair, loose clothing, etc., should be pulled back.

(3) Hold the match upside down so it will burn more efficiently.

(4) Once the match is completely out, do not lay it on the ground. Once the stove is lit, the match can be incinerated by carefully placing it on the burner. Matches placed on the ground tend to disappear in leaves and dirt and will likely be left behind as litter.

(5) Don't leave a lit stove unattended.

3. Once the stove has heated up, wearing gloves will:

   a) Minimize the chance of getting burned

   b) Prove handy as potholders

   c) Prove helpful when turning the stove off

G. Packing the stove

1. Let the stove cool before packing it.

2. Release fuel pressure by loosening the cap, but be sure to retighten it securely. Make sure the on/off valve is in the "off" position.

3. Be sure the stove is protected so it won't get damaged or damage other items in the pack.

4. Pack the stove upright to minimize the chance of fuel leakage.

5. Pack the stove well away from food items to prevent potential contamination.

III. Instructional Strategies

A. Timing

1. Stove use is usually taught before the first meal is cooked. Participants should bring the stoves and fuel bottles to class so they can learn the parts and their function as the instructor demonstrates proper stove use. An organized, step-by-step demonstration is recommended when teaching stove use. The leader's goal should be to role-model appropriate stove use and safety so that participants mimic appropriate behaviors immediately. It is recommended that leaders check each participant's stove-lighting technique after the initial lesson. Sometime during the first part of a trip, each participant should call the instructor over to her/his kitchen to observe. Participants should not light stoves independently until they have demonstrated competency. After the class, participants start their stoves and cook

breakfast while instructors monitor their activity.

2. This class is usually taught in conjunction with the first cooking class so participants can immediately put their knowledge into practice.

3. Stove maintenance is taught using teachable moments (see chapter 1, Teaching and Learning) or later in the course.

B. Activities. Initiate a discussion of the advantages and disadvantages of stoves versus fires.

C. Materials

1. Stove
2. Stove operating instructions
3. Fuel bottle with fuel
4. Matches
5. Stove storage container (stuff sack, etc.)
6. Stove repair kit
7. Pot or billy can to extinguish stove if necessary
8. Pot of food or water ready to go
9. Gloves
10. Pot grips

CHAPTER FORTY-THREE

Travel Technique: An Introduction to Travel

I. Outcomes

A. Outdoor leaders provide evidence of their *knowledge* and *understanding* by:

1. Describing the basic concepts of travel technique so they may travel efficiently, comfortably, and safely while minimizing the chances of encountering major problems
2. Explaining the concept of energy conservation and why it is important
3. Describing the importance of group organization and communication while traveling
4. Defining the roles of leader, scout, smoother, logger, and sweep and describing their adaptation for both water and land travel
5. Explaining the concept of a Time Control Plan
6. Describing the role of physical fitness in backcountry travel

B. Outdoor leaders provide evidence of their *skill* by:

1. Traveling efficiently, comfortably, and safely
2. Using principles of energy conservation
3. Utilizing the roles of leader, scout, smoother, logger, and sweep
4. Practicing the skill of rhythmic breathing
5. Implementing accurate Time Control Plans
6. Keeping the group within communicating distance at all times

II. Content

A. The energy-conservation concept

1. What is energy conservation?
    a) The use of as little energy as possible to accomplish the task as efficiently and comfortably as possible (e.g., the tortoise and the hare).
    b) The concept involves coordinating the heartbeat and breathing to regulate the pace rather than the reverse (for example, determining that a group wants to be able to talk without gasping for breath would dictate a slow pace). The degree to which energy conservation should be practiced is related to the objectives of the outing (e.g., if physical challenge is a primary objective, then energy conservation techniques may be used less).
2. What activities require energy conservation? Any activity that requires above-average physical demands (e.g., high-altitude climbing, backpacking, day hiking, canoeing, kayaking, cross-country skiing, and snowshoeing).
3. Why is it important to practice energy conservation?
    a) Energy conservation minimizes changes in body temperature by decreasing perspiration.
    b) Elimination of fast starts and prolonged rests minimizes the fluctuation of heartbeat rates.
    c) It increases the chance of arriving in camp without being exhausted.
    d) Energy is saved for emergency needs.
    e) It minimizes the chance of emotional outburst due to exhaustion and frustration.
    f) It decreases the impact of less oxygen at higher altitudes that may affect the brain, and therefore judgment.
4. How are the components of energy conservation used?
    a) Rhythmic breathing
        (1) Synchronize motions (e.g., steps or paddle strokes) with breathing.
        (2) If breathing rate increases from increased effort, slow down the pace.

(3) Develop a rhythm by coordinating the number of steps (or strokes) with the number of breaths.

    (a) For example, on level terrain with a moderate load, take three large steps for every breath.

    (b) As the terrain gets steeper, the load heavier, or the oxygen thinner, shorten the length of each step and the number of breaths between steps.

    (c) Similarly, when paddling against the current or into the wind, shorten your strokes and vary the number of breaths to match the output of energy.

(4) The objective is to maintain a comfortable pace and still make forward progress.

(5) With concentration and practice, rhythmic breathing will eventually become second nature.

b) Pace

(1) Pace is one of the most difficult things for a leader or scout to master. There is a tendency to travel too fast, which tires group members. A good leader exhibits patience and has the ability to travel at a pace appropriate for the whole group.

(2) The pace is probably appropriate if:

    (a) A conversation can be held at all times while traveling.

    (b) The group can travel all day with occasional short rests and not be exhausted at the end of the day.

c) Rest breaks

(1) The objective should be resting in order to prevent exhaustion, not because of exhaustion.

(2) If it is difficult to make it from rest break to rest break, either:

    (a) The pace is too fast

    (b) The time between breaks is too long

(3) How often and for how long should the group break?

    (a) Establish travel/resting times (e.g., travel thirty minutes, rest five) and stick to them for a couple of hours. Modify if necessary.

    (b) Be sure to communicate to the group when and how long break times will be and stick to them. This gives struggling members of the group a goal to work toward and something to look forward to.

    (c) Depending on certain factors, such as the group's physical condition, the trip objectives, and the hiking terrain, hiking and resting times range from hiking twenty minutes and resting five to hiking an hour and resting five to ten minutes. Again, remember to rest before becoming tired, not when the group is already tired.

(4) Length of break: Five-minute breaks will minimize lactic acid buildup, a waste product of muscle activity. While this is a worthy goal, it is difficult to achieve. Whatever length of time is decided on, try to stick to it unless judgment dictates otherwise.

(5) Where to break

    (a) Have the scout pick a site that is reasonably comfortable with an available water source. It is usually worth hiking an extra ten minutes or taking a break five minutes early to have a good rest break location.

    (b) Have the group rest on one side of the trail and well out of the way of others who may come down the trail. It is ideal from an outdoor-ethics perspective to get far enough off trail to go unnoticed by passersby.

(6) Starting and ending the break

    (a) Start the break when the last person gets to the break location.

    (b) Be sure to communicate clearly how long the break will be.

    (c) Announce to the group when one minute is left. Be sure group members understand that they should start putting on packs at this time.

(7) Eating and drinking at breaks: Encourage the intake of fluids and calories during breaks to replenish lost water and burned-up energy.

(8) Flexibility: Be sure to remain flexible. If a break needs to be taken early, take it. If the group needs extra time, give it to them. Don't be so tied to a schedule that the fun is taken out of the hike.

B. Travel logistics and organization

1. Assigning travel responsibilities: Stress the importance of trail organization. Groups that practice poor communication are a contributing cause of lost hikers.

2. Group size: Optimal group size should be determined using the following considerations:

a) Safety: How many people can be safely organized and monitored?
b) Environmental impact: What group size will have the least amount of impact on the area?
c) Social carrying capacity: What group size will have minimal aesthetic and psychological impact on the group and other users?
d) Managing agency policies: Does the managing agency have regulations that will determine or influence group size?

3. Group roles
   a) Leader: The leader may want to travel back and forth among the group to stay aware of how participants are feeling. The leader has overall responsibility for the group and ultimate decision-making responsibility.
      (1) The leader may determine:
          (a) Rest stop times and locations (with the logger's input)
          (b) Lunch stop time and location
          (c) When and where the campsite should be established
      (2) Stress the importance of communication between the leader and the group.
   b) Scout: The scout sets the pace and consults with the leader to determine the route. The scout is, of course, at the front of the line.
   c) Smoother: When traveling in areas in which the travel is not in a direct line, the smoother improves the route that the scout selects.
      (1) The smoother must stay far enough behind the scout to make this effective.
      (2) Judgment can dictate when and where a smoother is necessary.
   d) Logger
      (1) The logger notes all times of the day's activities.
      (2) This information can be used to develop a Time Control Plan (TCP).
      (3) Generally, these times are reviewed during debriefings. The logger is responsible for having the times available at debriefings.
   e) Sweep: The sweep is the last person in the expedition.
      (1) The sweep makes sure no one gets behind and that the pace is appropriate for the group.
      (2) The sweep makes sure the group does not get too spread out on land and water.
      (3) Communication with the scout and leader is an essential aspect of the sweep's role.

C. Slower travelers

1. If the weakest or slowest travelers (hikers, climbers, paddlers, skiers, snowshoers) are left at the end of the group to constantly worry about catching up, it will likely create a negative emotional mood for them—and the rest of the participants.
2. Try putting slower travelers near the front of the group and have the scout set a pace that they can keep up with, or try having slower travelers scout. Sometimes it may be best for a leader to set the pace for the group in order to demonstrate an appropriate pace.
3. The responsibility of being scout may take a slower traveler's mind off the physical effort of the hike.
4. Eliminating weight to unburden slower travelers may enable them to travel a bit faster. This offer should be made diplomatically to avoid hurt feelings.
5. On paddling trips, it may help to make some changes in paddling partners.
6. Help slower travelers by providing encouragement or engaging them in conversation or activities to take their minds off the physical effort. Remind them that they will get stronger as the days go by.

D. The Time Control Plan. A detailed itinerary of the day's travel, known as a Time Control Plan or TCP, is extremely helpful in encouraging participants to closely examine the potential route, anticipate what the day is going to be like, and determine how long it will take to get to the day's destination.

1. We encourage students individually (or in pairs) to create their own TCP, and then the instructor collects them. At the end of the day, the leader gives them back out and perhaps rewards the "winning" TCP; i.e., the one that is closest to predicting the actual time while still being comprehensive.
2. Effective TCPs are developed with consideration for:
    a) Knowledge of the country: It is important to know the country well. If this is not possible, be conservative in planning.
    b) Need for flexibility: Once a plan has been developed and is instituted, be sure to continuously reevaluate progress and, if necessary, modify the objectives. If progress is not satisfactory, don't be afraid to turn back or camp at a different location.
3. TCPs are very useful:
    a) On small group day hikes for emergency purposes
    b) In learning to anticipate travel times in various environments
    c) In developing map interpretation skills
    d) In developing judgment and decision-making skills

4. TCPs usually include:
   a) Group information
      (1) Group leader and names of group members
      (2) Number in group
      (3) Group gear to be carried
   b) Starting point
      (1) Geographical description
      (2) Common name of location
      (3) Longitude and latitude or UTM (Universal Transverse Mercator; see chapter 36, Navigation: An Introduction to GPS) data if possible
   c) Destination point
      (1) Geographical description
      (2) Common name of destination
      (3) Longitude and latitude or UTM data if possible
   d) Distance to travel: An estimate of the distance in miles from the starting point to the destination point. This estimate should be accurate to approximately ¼ mile.
   e) Elevation gain
      (1) Measure the total elevation that will be gained and the total that will be lost, and determine the net gain or loss in elevation. This is an excellent activity for practicing the reading of contour lines. We frequently have a volunteer participant count out loud each contour line, whether it is going uphill or downhill, as the group looks on. A recorder tallies the number of "up" contour lines and the number of "down" contour lines. When the exercise is complete, the participants know how many feet or meters they will be ascending or descending and the net gain or loss in elevation. All three figures are then included in the TCP.
   f) Estimated travel time: This estimate should also include time of departure and time of arrival.
   g) Estimated rest time: Try to determine what the hiking/rest ratio will be (e.g., hike thirty minutes and rest ten minutes) and anticipate the group's total rest time.
   h) Description of the route: This should give a description of the trails to be traveled, intersections to be encountered, and major physical features. Descriptions should be very specific and include elevations and distances.

i) Contingency plan: In case your group is unable to make it to camp, it is necessary to have an alternate plan so that others will know where to look.

j) Obstacles and hazards: Describe all the hazards and obstacles that the group may encounter.

5. Travel-time guidelines:

a) On a flat trail with a relatively heavy pack, most groups can travel at about 2 miles per hour.

b) When off-trail hiking, most groups can travel at about 1 mile per hour.

c) At altitudes up to 7,000 feet, add one hour of travel time for every 1,000 feet of elevation gained.

d) At altitudes between 7,000 feet and 11,000 feet, add one and a half hours of travel time for every 1,000 feet of elevation gained.

e) For every 1,000 feet of elevation lost, add thirty minutes of travel time.

f) Many factors should be considered, including:

(1) How heavy are the packs?

(2) Is there any illness, or are there any injuries?

(3) Will there be any river crossings?

(4) How difficult does the terrain look on the map?

(5) For water travel, what is the (likely) wind direction and speed, and, if applicable, what is the amount and direction of river current?

g) For water-based travel, compute the effects of wind and current and adjust for average paddling speed. If you know that the group's average paddling speed is 3 knots and you have a 2-knot head wind, your rate of travel could be reduced to 1 knot. Over a number of days of travel, the plan can be more accurately compiled since the group will be able to better estimate based on past attempts to predict progress.

6. Build on experience: As you gain experience in wilderness travel, use that experience in developing a TCP.

E. The role of physical fitness

1. Values of physical fitness. Physical fitness:

a) Allows for more enjoyment because fatigue doesn't occur as quickly

b) Helps to minimize frustration and interpersonal conflict

c) Avoids injuries and illnesses

d) Provides an extra margin of safety in emergency situations

2. The importance of physical fitness for the leader

a) The leader has a responsibility to be at least as physically fit as the average person in the group, and preferably to be as fit as the strongest person in the group. This allows the leader to plan and lead trips that are physically challenging for the whole group.

b) Individuals participating in a wilderness experience have a right to expect their leader to be knowledgeable and physically fit.

c) A fit leader insures an extra margin of safety in case of emergency.

III. Instructional Strategies

A. Timing

1. An introduction and overview of the topics in this lesson are appropriate on a morning early in the trip. Most of the material can be taught and reinforced while traveling by using teachable moments (see chapter 1, Teaching and Learning).

2. Debriefings are an important means of reinforcing these concepts and gaining an indication of how well participants understand them and can practice them. The importance of debriefing the day's experiences cannot be overemphasized.

3. The material on TCPs can be introduced as a daily part of planning and debriefing. This information should be taught along with the leadership roles. An important aspect of the daily debriefing is to review the accuracy of the TCP.

B. Considerations

1. Time Control Plans

a) It is recommended that the leadership team for the next day's travel (leader, scout, logger, sweep, and, if used, smoother) prepare (or at least jointly review) the TCP for the next day's travel.

b) At the daily debriefing, the TCP should be compared to the logger's official times. This activity allows participants to start creating an experience base that can aid in estimating how long a given trip will take.

c) This activity can be turned into a game by having each person complete a TCP for the day and then giving an "award" to the individual with the most accurate TCP.

2. Assessment strategies: One of the most effective assessment strategies is to use the daily debrief to discuss the accuracy of the TCP, as well as each leader's role during the day's travel. The accuracy of the TCP can be compared to the logger's official record for the times, distances, and amount of time required to reach specific locations. This information can then be used in constructing the TCP for the following day. The debriefing usually

involves an evaluation of the leaders' roles during the day. This is often started by having each person in turn reflect on his or her role for the day (e.g., sweep) in terms of what he or she did well and what he or she would change if he or she were to do it again. Afterward, other participants are invited to give positive feedback and then constructive criticism to the individual. This evaluation is an effective way of determining one's effectiveness in various leadership roles.

C. Materials

1. Maps (at least one for every two people)
2. TCP forms
3. Paper and pencil
4. Watch

CHAPTER FORTY-FOUR

Travel Technique: Hiking

I. Outcomes

A. Outdoor leaders provide evidence of their *knowledge* and *understanding* by:

1. Describing outdoor-ethics principles as they relate to hiking
2. Describing the concepts of travel technique as applied to hiking
3. Describing the importance of foot care

B. Outdoor leaders provide evidence of their *skill* by:

1. Implementing outdoor-ethics principles when hiking
2. Implementing basic hiking trail technique practices
3. Dealing with situations and concerns that arise on the trail
4. Knowing the group's location at all times within ¼ mile

C. Outdoor leaders provide evidence of their *dispositions* by:

1. Modeling hiking practices that lead to safe, organized, efficient travel with minimum energy expenditure and maximum enjoyment
2. Practicing hiking techniques that rely on teamwork, cooperation, and good communication

II. Content

A. Practice outdoor-ethics principles. Travel damage occurs when surface vegetation or communities of organisms are trampled beyond recovery. The resulting barren area is susceptible to soil erosion. Undesired trails are also likely to develop as a result of damage to vegetation and soil impaction. Whether backcountry travel involves travel over trails or in off-trail areas or some combination of the two, the goal is to move through the backcountry while avoiding damage to the land and ecosystem.

1. Trail hiking versus off-trail hiking
   a) Land management agencies construct trails in backcountry areas to provide routes that concentrate traffic. Constructed trails are themselves an impact on the land; however, they are necessary if we are to allow people to use the backcountry and protect its overall integrity. When traveling, concentrate travel on trails in order to reduce the likelihood that multiple routes will develop and scar the landscape.
   b) Use one well-designed route rather than many poorly chosen paths.
   c) Stay on trails whenever possible. Hikers should stay within the width of the trail and not cut switchbacks (i.e., hike directly up or down a hill and not follow the zigzags of the maintained trail).
   d) Travelers should leave room for other hikers when taking breaks along the trail.
   e) Off-trail travel: Try to spread use and impact in pristine areas (except in some desert areas).
2. Respect others. Avoid shouting to communicate while hiking. Loud noises usually are not welcome in natural areas.
3. Keep group size small. Frequency of use and large group size both increase the likelihood that a large area will be trampled or that a small area will be trampled multiple times.
4. Durability refers to the ability of surfaces or vegetation to withstand wear or remain in a stable condition and varies in different types of environments. The following surfaces allow different amounts of use:
   a) Rock, sand, and gravel: These surfaces are highly durable and can tolerate repeated trampling (the lichens that grow on rocks, however, are vulnerable to hiking traffic and should be avoided).
   b) Ice and snow: Ice and snow are good choices for travel. Any impact is temporary as long as the snow layer is of sufficient depth to prevent damage to vegetation. Safety is a separate issue, and appropriate precautions should be taken.

c) Vegetation: The resistance of vegetation to trampling varies. Careful decisions must be made when traveling across vegetation. In general:
   (1) Try to select areas of durable vegetation, or sparse vegetation that is easily avoided.
   (2) Hike on dry grasses as they tend to be resistant to trampling.
   (3) Avoid wet meadows and other fragile vegetation as they quickly show the effects of trampling.
   (4) If you must venture off trail, spread out to avoid creating paths that encourage others to follow. Creating one obvious route will likely ensure that new travelers take the same route and lead to the formation of undesirable trails.
   (5) Avoid vegetation whenever possible, especially on steep slopes where the effects of off-trail travel are magnified.
d) Cryptobiotic soil: Cryptobiotic soil is a living soil dominated by cyanobacteria, but it also includes lichens, mosses, green algae, micro-fungi, and bacteria. These crusts, frequently found in desert environments, play an important role in the ecosystems in which they occur and are extremely vulnerable to foot traffic.
   (1) Cryptobiotic soil can be identified by a blackish and irregular raised crust upon the sand.
   (2) This crust retains moisture in desert climates and provides a protective layer that inhibits erosion.
   (3) One footstep can destroy cryptobiotic soil. It is important to use developed trails in these areas.
   (4) Travel across cryptobiotic soil only when absolutely necessary. Walk on rocks or other durable surfaces if you must travel off trail.
   (5) In broad areas of cryptobiotic soil where damage is unavoidable, it is best to follow in one another's footsteps so the smallest possible area of crust is destroyed. This is exactly the opposite rule from travel through most environments.
e) Desert puddles and mud holes: Water is a preciously scarce resource for all living things in the desert.
   (1) Don't walk through desert puddles or mud holes, and don't disturb surface water in any way.
   (2) Leave potholes alone as they are home to tiny desert animals.

B. Tips for following marked trails

1. Understand the importance of knowing where the group is at all times. Make sure the trail goes where it is expected to go. Keep comparing the map with the terrain.

2. Learn to follow trail markers, blazes, and cairns (cairns are piles of rocks that mark a trail). Trails can give a false sense of security and may not go where expected.
   a) A season's growth of vegetation may cover up trail blazes.
   b) Missing just one marker can be misleading and throw hikers off a marked trail.

C. Tips for following rarely hiked trails

1. Pay careful attention to map, compass, and terrain since the trail may be overgrown with vegetation and not clearly identifiable.
2. Watch carefully for trail markers since they may be covered or missing.

D. Trail courtesy

1. Move to one side and let other groups go by.
2. Come to a complete stop and stand to the downhill side of the trail when encountering horses. Horses are very easily spooked by humans wearing backpacks. Speak softly to the horse packers and make the horses aware of the group's presence.

E. Miscellaneous hiking considerations

1. Hiking uphill
   a) Stand straight to maintain balance or improve the chances of being able to recover quickly if footing is lost. It is important to keep your weight over your feet; don't lean too far forward—your feet can slip out from under you more easily.
   b) The "rest step" can ease muscle tension caused by always putting weight on a leg bent at the knee. To use the rest step, straighten your leg after taking a step. This locks your knee, giving the muscles a chance to relax for a short period of time. This step puts body weight on bone structure for a moment and makes a difference at the end of the day.
   c) Smaller steps conserve energy.
   d) If obstacles are too large to step over easily, go around them. (Raising your foot and using the leg muscle uses more energy.)
2. Hiking downhill
   a) Injuries may be more likely to occur while walking downhill.
   b) Bend the knees slightly and use small, controlled steps to help resist the force of gravity that pulls the body forward. Try not to lean backward. Again, keep your weight over your feet. This helps with balance, especially on loose dirt and gravel where feet have a tendency to slide out from under you.

c) Try different ways of tying boots to help minimize friction and maximize comfort.

3. Contouring

   a) A less direct route with fewer elevation changes will help conserve energy, and it may also be easier and safer.

   b) Judgment should determine whether contouring is the best option.

F. Clothing. Rest breaks should be used to add or shed clothing and maintain a constant and comfortable body temperature. (See chapter 7, Clothing Selection, for a more detailed discussion of climate control.)

G. Off-trail hiking

1. Thick forest cover

   a) Everyone has the responsibility to stay a safe distance behind the person in front of him or her to avoid getting a branch slapped in the face.

   b) Minimize the "accordion effect" by being sure group members keep some space between themselves and the person in front of them.

   c) Use of game trails

      (1) Game trails are natural trails formed by animals traveling through the area.

      (2) They often provide the best route when hiking off trail since they usually follow a path of least resistance.

      (3) It is still advisable to keep track of the route with map and compass since the path may not lead to the group's destination.

2. Talus and scree slopes

   a) Talus and scree are rock fragments that have broken off cliffs or peaks.

   b) Talus ranges in size from rocks the size of cobblestones to small boulders. Talus is often sharp edged, increasing the risk of dangerous falls and injury.

   c) Descending talus slopes can be more difficult than ascending since downward momentum increases the risk of falling more often and farther.

   d) Hiking on talus requires precise footing and quick, light steps to move from rock to rock.

   e) Scree ranges from the size of sand to the size of a fist. Ascending scree is more difficult than descending because it slips easily underfoot.

   f) Keep the group close together on either talus or scree so that rocks that are loosened by one hiker don't pick up too much speed before hitting the next hiker.

g) Group members should avoid walking beneath the fall line of those ahead in case rocks are loosened.

h) If a rock is loosened and/or falls, hikers should shout "Rock!" to warn those below of the danger.

H. Blister prevention and care

1. Prevention
   a) Socks
      (1) Wearing two pairs of socks will help minimize blisters, which are caused by the friction of a boot or sock against the foot. Two socks will rub against each other and the boot, minimizing friction against the foot.
      (2) Adjusting socks and bootlaces can help prevent blisters or minimize discomfort once they develop.
   b) Walking technique: Walking flat-footed will help minimize blisters because the foot will do less bending, thereby generating less friction.
   c) Hot spots: It is important to stop and care for feet before a blister occurs. Learn to feel hot spots and take preventive measures without delay.
   d) Feet
      (1) Applying moleskin at the trailhead may prevent further troubles down the trail.
      (2) Using foot powder or Vaseline on the feet can help prevent blisters.
   e) Checking on the group: Leaders should frequently check with the group during the early part of the trip to see how their feet are doing. In some cases, foot checks in which all hikers bare their feet for inspection may be necessary.

2. Care: Moleskin, Molefoam, Second Skin
   a) Use on hot spots.
   b) Use once a blister has formed.
   c) Moleskin reduces friction and, because it is thin, fits easily inside a boot.
   d) Molefoam provides more cushioning, but it may take up more room inside a boot because it is thicker.
   e) Second Skin is a thin layer of gel that has a cooling effect on hot spots and blisters, relieving soreness. It practically eliminates friction. It is a more expensive alternative, however, and, because it has no adhesive, additional tape is necessary to secure it.

III. Instructional Strategies

A. Timing. This lesson should be taught using teachable moments (e.g., when a participant gets a blister) and after participants have gained some experience on the trail.

B. Activities

1. These activities build on the Time Control Plan (TCP) lesson developed in chapter 43.
   a) Time Control Plans
      (1) It is recommended that each participant write up a TCP on a daily basis and hand it in to the group leader.
      (2) At the next debriefing, the TCPs can be compared to the logger's official times.
   b) Contour counting
      (1) If hiking on terrain that involves increases or decreases in elevation, each morning one participant is asked to count the contours to the destination before participants write up their TCP.
      (2) The individual counts each contour as either an "up contour" or a "down contour."
      (3) The logger keeps a count and adds up the total number of "up contours" and the total number of "down contours."
      (4) The elevation in feet that the group will ascend and descend is then used as an aid in computing the TCP.
      (5) This activity accomplishes two objectives:
         (a) It develops map-reading skills.
         (b) It stresses the role that elevation change has in determining how long it takes to get to the group's destination.

C. Materials

1. Maps (at least one for every two people)
2. Pencil or pen
3. Paper
4. Watch

CHAPTER FORTY-FIVE

Travel Technique: Canoeing and Sea Kayaking

I. Outcomes

A. Outdoor leaders provide evidence of their *knowledge* and *understanding* by:

1. Describing the concepts of travel technique as they apply to canoeing and sea kayaking expeditions
2. Describing the importance of special considerations for water travel

B. Outdoor leaders provide evidence of their *skill* by:

1. Dealing with situations and concerns that arise on the water
2. Making a Time Control Plan (TCP) for water travel
3. Implementing outdoor-ethics practices when traveling
4. Knowing the group's approximate location at all times

C. Outdoor leaders provide evidence of their *dispositions* by:

1. Practicing canoeing and sea kayaking travel techniques that lead to safe, organized, efficient travel with minimum energy expenditure and minimal impact
2. Practicing canoeing and sea kayaking travel techniques that rely on teamwork, cooperation, and good communication

II. Content

A. General considerations for water travel

1. Practice water safety
   a) Participants should demonstrate their swimming ability in water or wear their personal flotation devices (PFDs) when around water.
   b) Make sure that participants wear their PFDs when in their boats.
   c) Use the "buddy system" of pairing up when around the water.
2. Practice minimal impact
   a) In addition to packing out whatever was brought in, participants should be encouraged to pack out any other litter that is found along the way. This is a good way to express stewardship and avoid hypocritical practices.
   b) There are special outdoor-ethics considerations for certain water environments that should be taken into account. For example, some marine environments may require that you pack out feces or even deposit them in certain tidal zones.
3. Make sure that all equipment is in good working order and fits properly.
4. Have backup equipment (e.g., paddles).
5. Practice deploying rescues and using emergency gear in the conditions in which they may be utilized. It may only be of limited help to practice rescues in a pool if a rescue may be necessary in cold-water conditions.
6. Clothing
   a) Special clothing is essential for paddling, although many adaptations from hiking gear may do.
      (1) Wet suits or dry suits may be essential for cold-water travel.
      (2) Rain gear may work for canoeing or sea kayaking if it does not restrict vision and is not so bulky that it impedes rescues or swimming.
   b) Rest breaks should be used to add or shed clothing and maintain a constant and comfortable body temperature. (See chapter 7, Clothing Selection, for a more detailed discussion of climate control.)
7. Slower paddlers
   a) If the weakest or slowest paddlers are left at the end of the group to constantly worry about catching up, it will likely have a negative psychological effect on them.
   b) Try putting slower paddlers near the front of the group and have the scout set a pace that they can keep up with. Try having slower paddlers scout.

8. As conditions get rougher or windier, have the group "pod" (travel closer to one another) with the goal of staying within shouting distance of the paddlers in front and behind.

9. As with other specialized forms of travel, leaders should have specialized training prior to leading trips on water. Organizations that offer instruction and certification include the American Canoe Association (www.acanet.org), the British Canoe Union (www.bcu.org.uk), and the Canadian Recreational Canoe Association (www.crca.ca).

B. Instruction for water-based travel. A typical outline of information to cover:

1. Orientation to paddling
   a) Participants should be introduced to paddling with an overview and a discussion of safety issues.
   b) Review the water to be traveled and what is required of participants.
   c) Review equipment:
      (1) Acquaint participants with gear and help them select equipment.
      (2) Review group gear and rescue gear.
      (3) Review clothing needed for paddling, including layers and dry clothes in case of immersion.
      (4) Discuss the basics of biomechanics—the effective use of the body. Include stretching exercises.
2. Canoe or kayak nomenclature
3. Carrying and launching the watercraft
4. Boarding and sitting in the watercraft
5. Basic rescue skills
6. Paddles:
   a) Types
   b) Nomenclature
   c) Selection
7. Effective paddling considerations:
   a) Hand position
   b) Watercraft moves through the water versus paddle
   c) Body and shoulder rotation
   d) Pushing versus pulling water
   e) Parts of the stroke:
      (1) Ketch
      (2) Stroke
      (3) Exit
      (4) Recovery
   f) Relaxation during the recovery

g) Basic strokes:
    (1) Forward/power stroke
    (2) Back/reverse stroke
    (3) Draw
    (4) Push-a-way
    (5) Pry
    (6) Sweeps: forward and reverse
    (7) Stern rudder
    (8) J-stroke
    (9) Bracing strokes: high and low braces

h) Advanced strokes:
    (1) Cross draw
    (2) Pivot turns
    (3) Sideslipping

8. Knots
9. Watercraft construction and design
10. Portaging considerations
11. Practice sites: Choose sites that allow for safety and for rescues to be set up.
    a) Sites should approximate the type of water to be paddled on the trip but not be as challenging as the most difficult water to be paddled.
        (1) This allows for practice under controlled circumstances.
        (2) This permits paddlers to gain practice prior to launching for the trip.
        (3) This promotes safety and comfort.
    b) If paddling on moving water, the practice site should have slow-moving water. Progress to water that mirrors the conditions likely to be paddled only after competence has been demonstrated on less challenging water.
    c) While basic levels of paddling should be practiced prior to leaving base camp, more advanced skills (e.g., lining a canoe) can be taught while the expedition is in progress.

C. Float plans. Specialized trip plans for use on the water. (See the sample at the end of this chapter.)

D. Getting under way
1. Boat trim: Make sure that your boat is level in the water—before and aft, starboard and port.
2. Make sure that gear is secure, with easy access to essential items:
    a) Snacks
    b) Rain gear

c) Maps and compasses

d) Emergency and rescue equipment

3. Clarify leadership roles

    a) The "scout" or "lead boat":

        (1) Selects the general course and communicates this to the other boats

        (2) Scouts rapids or other potentially dangerous areas

        (3) Carries extra rescue gear, especially on river travel, so as to set up safety equipment as subsequent craft negotiate the rapid (or other area of travel)

    b) The "sweep":

        (1) Is the last boat and makes sure that all other paddlers are in front

        (2) Carries extra gear, often helping with rescues and first aid

        (3) Helps to keep the group together

    c) The navigator:

        (1) Sets the direction of travel and makes sure that the group is on course

        (2) Coordinates with the group leader and others in a leadership role

        (3) Knows the location of the group relevant to the map or chart, as well as the plan for the day

    d) These roles are to be used in conjunction with other leadership roles (Leader of the Day, etc.).

4. Establish and use a set of signals. See figures 45.1, 45.2, 45.3, and 45.4, from the American Whitewater Association. (An alternate set of signals agreed upon by the group may be substituted for these signals.)

III. Instructional Strategies

A. Timing. This lesson should be taught prior to leaving the base camp area and prior to leaving for a trip. More specialized skills, such as lining a canoe or portaging, can be taught once the trip is under way.

B. Activities

1. For this instructional activity the map and Float Plan for Cape Lookout National Seashore at the end of the chapter can be used. Participants are given a task, for which they must complete a Float Plan. The exercise for this activity is to develop a plan for travel from the visitor center on Harker's Island to the ranger station in Portsmouth Village. This activity accomplishes two objectives:

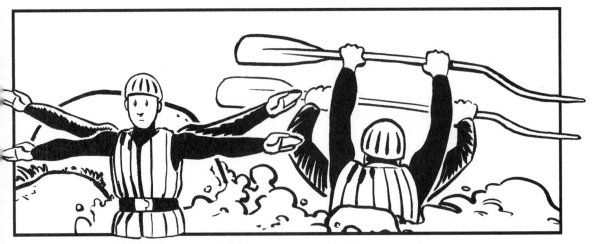

FIGURE 45.1. Stop: Potential hazard ahead. Wait for "all clear" signal (see fig. 45.3) before proceeding, or scout ahead. Form a horizontal bar with your outstretched arms. Those seeing the signal should pass it back to others in the party.

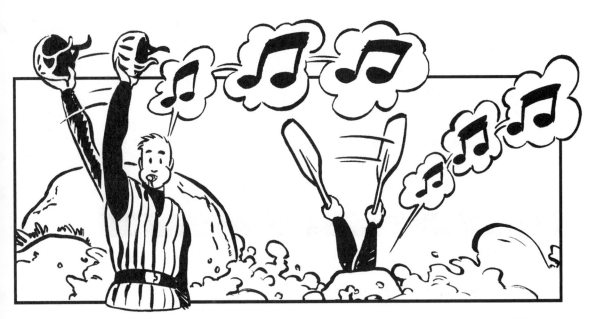

FIGURE 45.2. Help/emergency: Assist the signaler as quickly as possible. Give three long blasts on a police whistle while waving a paddle, helmet, or life vest over your head. If a whistle is not available, use the visual signal alone. A whistle is best carried on a lanyard attached to your life vest.

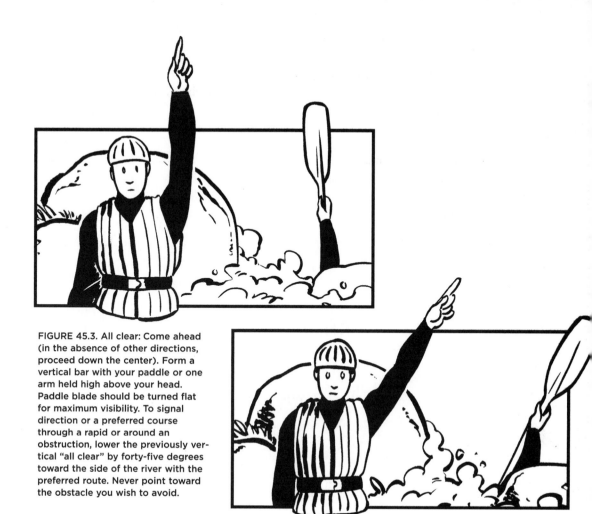

FIGURE 45.3. All clear: Come ahead (in the absence of other directions, proceed down the center). Form a vertical bar with your paddle or one arm held high above your head. Paddle blade should be turned flat for maximum visibility. To signal direction or a preferred course through a rapid or around an obstruction, lower the previously vertical "all clear" by forty-five degrees toward the side of the river with the preferred route. Never point toward the obstacle you wish to avoid.

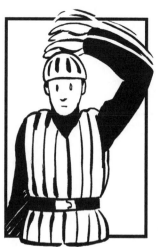

FIGURE 45.4. I'm okay: I'm okay and not hurt. While holding the elbow outward toward the side, repeatedly pat the top of your head.

a) It develops map-reading skills.

b) It introduces the notion of Float Plans and their use for water-based travel activities.

C. Materials

1. Cape Lookout map
2. Cape Lookout Float Plan
3. Pencil or pen
4. Ruler

Cape Lookout National Seashore Float Plan

Name: _____

Address: _____

City/state: _____

Phone number: _____

Emergency contact: _____

Name: _____

Phone number: _____

Departure date: _____   Return date: _____

Time: _____   Time: _____

Place: _____   Place: _____

Proposed route: _____

_____

_____

Alternate route: _____

_____

_____

Conditions that would cause use of alternate route: _____

_____

_____

Escape route: _____

_____

_____

Conditions that would cause use of escape route: _____

_____

_____

Proposed destination: _____

_____

_____

Alternate destination: _____

_____

_____

Group members (list names, addresses, phone numbers, boat description, and safety equipment list): _____

_____

_____

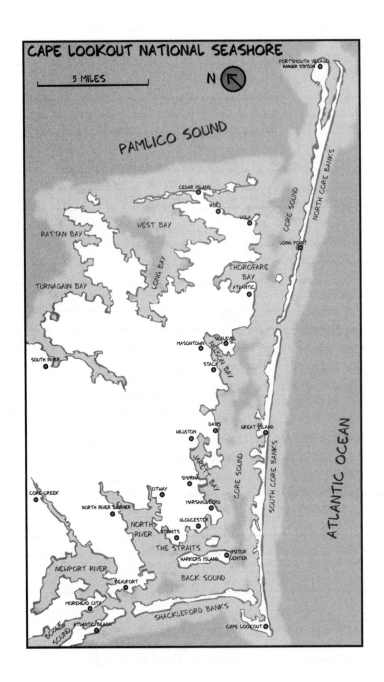

CHAPTER FORTY-SIX

Trip Planning

I. Outcomes

A. Outdoor leaders provide evidence of their *knowledge* and *understanding* by:

1. Describing how to plan safe, enjoyable, and environmentally sound wilderness trips of various lengths
2. Describing and critiquing guidelines of trip planning
3. Describing and critiquing various trip-planning considerations

B. Outdoor leaders provide evidence of their *skill* by:

1. Planning and implementing a wilderness trip

C. Outdoor leaders provide evidence of their *dispositions* by:

1. Modeling trip-planning procedures
2. Modeling an appreciation of and need for effective planning

II. Content

A. Trip-planning guidelines

1. Organization: Use an organizational structure so that group members know to whom they are responsible and what their responsibilities are.
2. Lists: Make lists and utilize them. Possible lists include:
   a) Tasks to accomplish
   b) Items to purchase
   c) Equipment and clothing
   d) Food
   e) Recommendations for future trips
3. Anticipate
   a) Plan ahead and anticipate what may happen and what can be done.
   b) Have contingency plans. For example, what will be done if certain equipment doesn't arrive in time?

B. Trip-planning considerations

1. Outcomes
   a) Without clear outcomes/objectives, individuals seek personal outcomes that may clash and result in an unsuccessful trip or even disaster.
   b) Insuring that everyone knows and agrees to the trip outcomes contributes to the success of the trip.
   c) Once an individual agrees to the trip outcomes, that person then has a vested interest and a responsibility to see that objectives are met. (See chapter 24, Group Orienting and Monitoring, for more information on trip goals and objectives.)
2. Leadership
   a) Is a feeling of trust, comfort, and safety communicated by the person in the leadership role; i.e., is he or she qualified?
   b) Is there someone assuming overall responsibility for what happens? If the leader gets hurt, is it clear who is in charge?
3. Itinerary: The itinerary should be made in conjunction with and in consideration of:
   a) Trip outcomes. (For example, on trips with primarily educational outcomes, plan on traveling fewer miles; on trips with the outcome of reaching a destination, plan on longer days on the trail; for recreational trips build in many options for play and exploration.)
   b) Physical abilities and limitations of group members (physical limitations, knowledge and skill limitations, ability to evacuate, etc.).

c) Permit restrictions.

d) Environmental: Implementing outdoor-ethics practices.

4. Emergency planning (See chapter 39, Safety: Emergency Procedures, and chapter 40, Safety: Risk Management)

　a) Develop a plan that includes:

　　(1) Copies of the planned itinerary and a list of group members

　　(2) Emergency procedures in an emergency situation

　　(3) Evacuation options and routes

　　(4) Emergency telephone numbers and contact persons

　　(5) Post-emergency plans

　b) Have the proper forms, including:

　　(1) Those to be taken on the trip

　　(2) Those to remain on file

5. Liability and risk management (see chapter 40, Safety: Risk Management)

　a) Does the program have an overall risk-management plan?

　b) Is there adequate liability insurance coverage?

　c) Is there an assumption of risk form?

　　(1) Waiver of claims

　　(2) Liability releases

　　(3) Photo release

　d) Do participants have medical insurance?

　e) Do you have health forms and medical information for all participants?

　f) Do you have medication information, backup medication, know where is it stored, etc.?

6. Land management rules and regulations

　a) Is there knowledge of rules and regulations?

　b) Are permits needed, where is camping legal, etc.?

7. Food and nutrition (see chapter 21, Food: Nutrition, Rations Planning, and Packaging)

　a) How will food be selected?

　b) How will amounts and nutritional balance be determined?

　c) Who will purchase and pack food?

　d) If food drops are needed, how will they be coordinated?

8. Equipment and clothing (see chapter 7, Clothing Selection)

　a) Develop a master equipment and clothing list.

　b) What needs to be purchased?

　c) Who is responsible for clothing and equipment acquisition?

　d) How and when will equipment and clothing be issued?

e) If participants provide their own clothing and equipment, when and how will it be inspected to make sure it meets program requirements? If it is inadequate, what provisions are there to make sure that proper gear is obtained?

9. Skills and knowledge
   a) What skills and knowledge do individuals have (e.g., medical training and certifications, technical skills, etc.)?
   b) Have participants been told what skills and knowledge they should have prior to the trip?
   c) What skills and topics should be reviewed before the trip?
   d) Who will teach specific skills and topics during the trip?

10. Expedition behavior
   a) What steps have been taken to insure that group members will get along and that objectives will be met?
   b) Do the leaders have a model for conflict resolution that will help them mediate disputes?

11. Water sources
   a) Where is potable water available?
   b) How will water be purified?
   c) Is there a backup system?
   d) Are there containers for carrying water?

12. Finances
   a) Is there a budget?
   b) Who is responsible for the expenses, and how much money is needed?
   c) Who will handle the finances, and how will it be documented?
   d) How much cash is needed on the trip?
   e) How will phone calls and other miscellaneous expenses be handled and paid?

13. Weather
   a) What are the historical weather patterns in the area?
   b) What is the short-term weather forecast?
   c) What is the long-term weather forecast?
   d) Who will keep a log of the weather during the trip?

14. Transportation
   a) Who will provide vehicles?
   b) What are vehicles needed for specifically?
      (1) Shopping
      (2) Transportation to and from the trailhead
      (3) Laundry and/or showers after the trip

c) Are they in properly maintained condition?

d) Who is responsible for the cost of the vehicles (e.g., fuel, oil, and maintenance)?

e) Who will drive the vehicles?

    (1) Do the drivers have appropriate licenses, organizational approval, and training?

    (2) Is there a backup driver?

f) Will drivers know when and where to meet the group, and the route and destination?

    (1) When possible, have a driver orientation to review specific issues unique to the trip (e.g., meeting times and locations, where food and equipment is to be stored, etc.)

    (2) Provide drivers with written instructions that include procedures for accessing vehicles and resupply items, meeting dates and times, maps to trailheads and reration locations, emergency contacts, etc.

g) Is auto insurance current and documented?

15. Resources

a) Human

    (1) Is there anyone who has been to the planned trip area before who can provide firsthand information (e.g., rangers, locals, guides, etc.)?

    (2) Who will visit or contact land agency administrative offices for available information?

b) Written: Are there books, brochures, magazine articles, or other written materials available about the area?

c) Photographic: Are there photographs available of the area?

d) Maps

    (1) Are there new or old maps available of the area?

    (2) Are there sufficient copies of maps for the instructors and course participants?

e) Online resources: Frequently a search for the aforementioned resources can be initiated on the Internet.

16. Post trip

a) Are shower or laundry facilities available?

b) Where and when will the group debrief the overall trip, and when will participant and course assessments take place?

c) Who will inventory the leftover food, and how will extra food be disposed of?

d) How will equipment be inventoried, repaired, or replaced (including how these expenses will be covered)?

e) Who will write thank-you notes for anyone who helped out?

f) Who will make arrangements for a party or banquet?

g) How will toilet systems (if used) be cared for?

17. Public relations

a) Who will arrange for press releases for participants' hometown newspapers?

b) Who will organize photographs for participants to share, for press releases, or for future promotion?

c) Will T-shirts, patches, pins, and other memorabilia be available for group participants?

III. Instructional Strategies

A. Timing. When this lesson is taught is dependent on whether or to what extent participants are involved in the planning of the course. If participants are involved in the actual planning of the trip, then this becomes a high-priority lesson at the outset. If participants are not involved in the planning of the trip, then this becomes a lower-priority lesson that can be taught later in the course. See the Trip Planning Annotated Timeline challenge at the end of the chapter.

B. Considerations

1. Different programs involve participants in trip planning to varying degrees. Options include:

a) The participants plan nearly every aspect of the expedition.

b) An alternative to the outline used in this chapter is to make a list of all the things that have to be done and categorize the items according to the acronym TRIP PLANS:

T = Transportation
R = Risk-management issues (liability, forms, emergency procedures, etc.)
I = Itinerary
P = Purpose (outcomes)

P = Permits, public relations, post trip
L = Leadership
A = Abilities, skills, knowledge
N = Nature (weather, the environment, water sources, etc.)
S = Supporting resources (equipment, clothing, maps, human, money)

c) The participants get involved in certain aspects of the expedition (e.g., food planning and itinerary).

d) The participants do not get involved in the direct planning of their first trip but get involved in subsequent expeditions. For example, some programs have staff do all the logistics for participants on their first trip but give veteran participants nearly total responsibility for planning a subsequent expedition.

2. Assessment strategies

a) Have the participants get involved in specific phases of trip planning (whether a short trip or an extended trip). It is important to assess their planning process and give them specific feedback.

b) Debrief the experience to determine how to improve future trips. This is invaluable.

C. Materials

1. Maps, pictures, and guidebooks of the area
2. Equipment, food, clothing, and other lists
3. Guidelines for risk management and other forms

Challenge

Knowledge Outcome	Title	Skill/Disposition Outcome
What do you want them to know? The participants can discuss various considerations in planning a safe, enjoyable, and environmentally sound wilderness trip.	Trip Planning Annotated Timeline	**What skill/disposition do you want them to develop?** Critical thinking: synthesizes ideas and information into a useful whole

Essential Question or Key Issue:

What must we consider when planning a safe, environmentally responsible, and personally enjoyable back-country trip?

Description of Challenge/Task/Performance:

Your guide service has earned a well-deserved reputation for planning and implementing very successful backcountry expeditions that are safe, environmentally responsible, and enjoyable to the participants. A YMCA in your area has hired you to submit a proposal for a ten-day trip in the coming summer season for some of their members. The Y group is a mix of six males and four females ranging in age from sixteen through twenty-eight. All are in reasonably good health, and none are physically challenged. Two of the males are overweight, and one of the women is a vegetarian. A few of them have their own packs and sleeping bags. One of the males has had some National Outdoor Leadership School training, while the rest indicate they have had some "camping" experience with family and friends. They have expressed an interest in learning the skills of backcountry living, overland navigation, elementary rock climbing, fishing, and plant identification. They want you to give them a fairly detailed understanding of what the experience will be like if they accept your proposed plans.

Your task: Create an informative, clear, and concise trip proposal for this group. A major feature of your proposal should be an annotated timeline that charts in reasonable detail what will happen from the time the group members start preparing for the trip until the final closing activity at the end of the trip. You will be expected to use this annotated timeline as the primary visual reference when you present your proposal to the representatives of the YMCA.

As you put together your proposal and design your timeline, please address the following:
- What are the "key questions" your participants will want answered by your proposal/timeline? How will you answer them?
- How will you keep the presentation interesting and concise while providing sufficient detail to satisfy curiosity?
- What opportunities will there be on the trip for participants to pursue the interests mentioned above?
- How will you ensure that the trip is safe, environmentally responsible, and enjoyable for all the participants?

Criteria for Assessment and Feedback:

Form criteria:
- The presentation and timeline are informative; i.e., they provide essential information that satisfies curiosity and provides a sense of what the trip will be like.
- The timeline is annotated; i.e., it has written comments clarifying or adding detail to the events depicted.

Content criteria:
- The presentation and timeline clearly indicate when and how the participants will be able to pursue their interests.
- All of the participant "key questions" are addressed directly and adequately.

Knowledge:
- The participants can discuss various considerations in planning a safe, enjoyable, and environmentally sound wilderness trip
- All of the participant "key questions" are addressed directly and adequately.

Skill: Critical thinking: synthesizes ideas and information into a useful whole
- The participants can describe how the specific choices they made reflect the application of the accepted principles of high-quality trip planning.

Developed by Leading EDGE, LLC for **The Backcountry Classroom.** *For more information log on to* www.realworldlearning.info.

Product Quality Checklist

Date: _____ Class Period: _____

Product Author(s):	Product Title/Name:	Evaluator Name(s):
	Trip Planning Annotated Timeline	

Observed	Standard/Criteria	Possible Points	Rating
	The presentation and timeline are informative; i.e., they provide essential information that satisfies curiosity and provides a sense of what the trip will be like.		
	The timeline is annotated; i.e., it has written comments clarifying or adding detail to the events depicted.		
	All of the participant "key questions" are addressed directly and adequately.		
	Total		

Observations:

Elements of Questionable Quality:	Elements of Exceptional Quality:

CHAPTER FORTY-SEVEN

Water Treatment

I. Outcomes

A. Outdoor leaders provide evidence of their *knowledge* and *understanding* by:

1. Describing when water should be treated
2. Explaining why water should be treated
3. Describing, comparing, and critiquing three methods of water treatment

B. Outdoor leaders provide evidence of their *skill* by:

1. Competently using at least two methods of treating water

C. Outdoor leaders provide evidence of their *dispositions* by:

1. Modeling careful, consistent treatment of water to avoid illness in the backcountry

II. Content

A. First things first

    1. The evidence is becoming clearer that, in the backcountry, most infectious illnesses are transmitted by poor hygiene. Typically, someone will defecate, not clean his or her hands properly, and then communicate illnesses from hand to mouth. There is considerable evidence that infections originating in the backcountry are spread through this mechanism rather than by the consumption of contaminated water.

    2. When someone has an infectious illness and he or she handles water bottles or other containers, or shares bags of trail food, the infection can be spread to others who touch these items. Thus, it is even more important to practice good personal hygiene (i.e., wash your hands!) than to treat the water.

    3. If one is concerned about the quality of a specific water source, the concern is that it could be contaminated with human feces. Thus *any* of the diseases that can be spread through feces must be considered, and treatment that is effective against all of those should be put into practice.

B. Why does water need to be treated?

    1. Microorganisms in North American waters that may cause illness (see chapter 37, Personal Hygiene, for a more extensive discussion of this topic):

        a) Viruses

            (1) Extremely tiny microorganisms that can only reproduce in living animals and tend to be species specific. (For example, usually viruses found in humans are not found in other animals and vice versa.)

            (2) They can be killed by either:

                (a) Boiling the water

                (b) Treating it with a halogen (chlorine- or iodine-based chemicals)

            (3) Viruses are generally too small to be filtered out of the water with conventional backpacking filters.

        b) Bacteria

             (1) Microscopic single-cell plants that can grow and reproduce, unlike viruses, outside of a host.

            (2) Bacteria can be killed by:

                (a) Boiling the water

                (b) Treating it with a halogen (chlorine- or iodine-based chemicals)

                (c) Filtration

c) Protozoan
  (1) A phylum of very simple, single-celled microorganisms
  (2) Protozoa can be killed by:
    (a) Boiling the water.
    (b) Filtration.
    (c) Treating it with a halogen (chlorine- or iodine-based chemicals). But while halogen treatments are effective against virtually all bacterial and viral pathogens likely to be encountered in the backcountry of North America, protozoa are another question. "Giardia lamblia in the adult active form is mostly sensitive to halogens; the quiescent oocyst form is moderately resistant to halogens. The pathogen Cryptosporidium parvum in its common oocyst form in surface waters, on the other hand, is very resistant to halogens even at high concentrations. Do not trust a halogen to rid your water of Cryptosporidium" (Tilton and Bennett 2002; e-mail correspondence with Thomas Welch, September 30, 2004). On the other hand, there is no evidence that Cryptosporidium has ever been a problem for healthy users of North American backcountry water.
  (3) Giardia lamblia: A case study
    (a) What is Giardia lamblia?
      i) Giardia lamblia is a protozoan.
      ii) It is of considerable concern in wilderness travel today.
      iii) It is a parasite that causes giardiasis, a gastrointestinal illness.
      iv) It occurs throughout the world.
      v) In the United States, the vast majority of cases of giardiasis are caused by hand-to-mouth spread. There have been a few outbreaks associated with community water supplies. No studies have shown that consumption of backcountry water in North America is an important cause of this disease.
    (b) Symptoms of giardiasis include:
      i) Diarrhea
      ii) Abdominal cramps
      iii) Flatulence

iv) Nausea

v) An eventual nutritional deficiency due to malabsorption

(c) Diagnosis and treatment

    i) Diagnosis is through examination of fecal smears or fluid from the upper intestine.

    ii) It is most commonly treated with the antibiotic metronidazole, sold under the brand name Flagyl.

(d) Other facts about Giardia

    i) Giardia is carried and spread by all mammals. It is not at all clear, however, whether subspecies affecting one mammal can cause disease in other types of mammals.

    ii) One stool can contain up to 300 million cysts, which are infectious forms of Giardia.

    iii) Surface waters in which Giardia has been isolated typically have one cyst per liter or less.

    iv) Ten cysts is the minimum number that must be ingested to cause disease.

    v) The length of illness ranges from a few days to three months.

    vi) Most infected individuals (75 percent) experience no symptoms and never realize they have had it (Bloch and Patzkowsky 1985).

    vii) All backpackers must consider themselves carriers of giardiasis and dispose of their feces appropriately and practice good personal hygiene. (See chapter 6, Catholes and Latrines: Proper Disposal of Human Waste.)

    viii) Should symptoms of diarrhea, flatulence, and/or nausea persist, a physician should be consulted.

(e) How big a problem is giardiasis or Cryptosporidium? Some noted physicians feel giardiasis is blown out of proportion because:

    i) Most people won't even know they have ingested cysts.

    ii) A few people will get an intestinal upset similar to a nasty hangover.

    iii) Fewer still will get a troublesome illness that responds well to therapy.

iv) As one doctor put it, "This . . . places Giardiasis in the category of blisters and mosquito bites: a nuisance reminder of a trip in the wilderness for some, with an occasional hiker developing a more serious complication" (Welch 1986).

v) "Virtually all of the interest in Cryptosporidium as a water-borne pathogen has been with community drinking water; people should be more worried about their TAP WATER than wilderness streams if this is the organism which concerns them! This resonates with a fact about this whole issue which is seldom recognized. No one is likely to be unlucky enough to catch something from a single swig of any water source. The risk relates to continued consumption from the same source over an extended period of time. This was nicely shown by the NYS health department in the giardiasis outbreak in Long Lake, NY. It was the residents, drinking the water day-in, day-out, who got the disease, not the tourists who stopped at the local restaurants and had a glass of water with their lunch. There was a direct correlation between how much water residents drank per day and the likelihood of their becoming sick. This is why I rarely, if ever, treat water I come across on the trail and intend to 'slurp and run.' On the other hand, if I am going to be at a busy base camp for a few days, and will be drinking lots of water from the same place, I am more likely to treat" (e-mail correspondence with Thomas Welch, September 30, 2004).

C. Methods of treating water

1. Boiling
   a) All waterborne microorganisms found in the backcountry of North America are sensitive to heat.
   b) Research clearly indicates that water in the North American backcountry that has reached a full boil is safe to drink. Additional boiling time is not necessary.
   c) Advantages of boiling:
      (1) It is inexpensive—the only expense is the fuel.
      (2) It is completely effective when the water reaches a full boil.

(3) Boiling does not affect the taste of the water.

(4) When the boiling point is reached in the cooking process, food is safe for consumption.

d) Disadvantages of boiling:

    (1) It takes time and consumes fuel.

    (2) It is inconvenient for treating drinking water along the trail.

2. Filtration

    a) Filters are commercially available that will filter out Giardia and bacteria.

    b) Advantages of filtration:

        (1) It is easy to filter drinking water along the trail.

        (2) Filtration does not affect the taste of the water.

    c) Disadvantages of filtration:

        (1) Filters are generally slow (one to three minutes per liter).

        (2) Filters are often ineffective against viruses.

        (3) Filtration is a more expensive method due to the cost of filters ($30 to $175).

        (4) Filters require maintenance and can be cumbersome.

3. Chemical treatment

    a) Crystalline iodination: Commercial brands are available, such as Polar Pure.

        (1) A small amount of water is added to iodine crystals. After a period of time (how long it takes depends on water temperature), this creates a saturated solution of iodine. The saturated solution is then added to the water to be treated.

        (2) Advantages of crystalline iodination:

            (a) If used correctly, it appears to be completely effective, although some question remains as to its effectiveness in killing Cryptosporidium.

            (b) It is inexpensive.

            (c) It is easy to use.

            (d) Its shelf life is unlimited.

        (3) Disadvantages of crystalline iodination:

            (a) Water must sit for thirty minutes or longer (up to several hours if it is cold water) before consumption.

            (b) It has some effect on the taste of the water.

            (c) As with any chemical, large concentrated doses have the potential to be toxic.

b) Iodine tablets: Commercial brands are available, such as Potable Aqua and Globaline.
    (1) A tablet that releases an iodine solution is added directly to the water.
    (2) Advantages of iodine:
        (a) It is readily available.
        (b) It is easy to use.
        (c) If used properly, it is usually effective, although some question remains as to its effectiveness in killing Cryptosporidium.
    (3) Disadvantages of iodine:
        (a) Water must sit for thirty minutes or longer (up to several hours if it is cold water) before consumption.
        (b) Iodine affects the taste of the water.
        (c) Tablets have a limited shelf life and lose effectiveness from frequent exposure to air.
        (d) As with any chemical, large concentrated doses have the potential to be toxic.
c) Chlorination: Commercial brands are available, such as chlorine-based SweetWater ViralStop, and Katadyn Micropur MP and Aquamira, which are chlorine dioxide products.
    (1) Advantages of chlorination:
        (a) It is readily available.
        (b) It is inexpensive.
        (c) It is easy to use.
        (d) A small amount treats a large amount of water.
    (2) Disadvantages of chlorination:
        (a) It is not always effective against Giardia lamblia (0.5 percent chlorine concentrations commonly used by municipal water systems do not assure effectiveness).
        (b) Water must sit for thirty minutes or longer (up to several hours if it is cold water) before consumption.
        (c) Chlorine affects the taste of the water, although chlorine dioxide products are not supposed to have an adverse effect on taste.
        (d) Chlorine-based products generally have a shorter shelf life, ranging from a few months to three years. Its effectiveness is reduced if it is stored at higher temperatures or exposed to air.

(e) As with any chemical, large concentrated doses have the potential to be toxic.
4. Special filters/purifiers: A few purifying systems that are available are virtually as effective as boiling. Two are listed below:
   a) Katadyn Exstream Water Purifier: A water-bottle purification system with a "ViruStat" purification cartridge that purifies water on demand. It removes bacteria and protozoa (Giardia, Cryptosporidium) and, in addition, is said to kill more than 99.99 percent of waterborne viruses.
   b) MSR MIOX Purifier: Modeled after a high-tech, municipal water-treatment system, the MIOX Purifier works by creating brine out of untreated fresh water and salt, and then passing a small electrical charge through the solution, which results in a powerful dose of mixed oxidants (MIOX). This "cocktail" is poured into untreated water, inactivating all viruses, bacteria, Giardia, and Cryptosporidium (which even iodine doesn't kill) and leaving you with safe, purified water.

D. The final word

1. Remember: Washing hands is the number-one step in preventing illness in the backcountry and is probably more important than treating your water.
2. If you are worried enough about a water source to treat it, you should treat for all three types of microorganisms: protozoa, bacteria, and viruses.
3. Giardia myths: The following are myths because it takes at least ten cysts to make a person ill, yet even in highly contaminated water there is rarely more than one cyst per liter. There is virtually no chance of getting giardiasis from:
   a) Water trapped in the threads of a water bottle cap
   b) A single swig of untreated spring water
   c) A few drops of water on the outside of a filter

III. Instructional Strategies

A. Timing. This topic should be introduced immediately and course policy communicated as to what types of treatment will be used.

B. Considerations

1. It is essential that, if water is to be treated, instructors set a consistent example.
2. When teaching this class, it is important to demonstrate at least one means of water treatment.

a) Filtration or chemical treatments are preferable methods of water treatment to demonstrate.

b) Use the water source as a classroom setting and demonstrate the whole sequence from water acquisition to treatment and consumption.

C. Materials

1. Equipment for at least one type of water treatment
2. Water container
3. Water source (stream, lake, or spring)

CHAPTER FORTY-EIGHT

Weather

I. Outcomes

A. Outdoor leaders provide evidence of their *knowledge* and *understanding* by:

1. Describing how to predict weather in the field using the physical senses, a compass, an altimeter, and a barometer
2. Explaining why weather is difficult to predict accurately
3. Explaining how to identify wind direction and its role in predicting weather
4. Describing how different cloud formations are helpful in predicting weather
5. Describing how various kinds of weather lore can be helpful in predicting weather

B. Outdoor leaders provide evidence of their *skill* by:

1. Using their physical senses, a compass, an altimeter, and a barometer to predict weather in the field
2. Identifying wind direction and using this information to predict weather
3. Identifying cloud formations and using this information to predict weather
4. Identifying weather lore and using it to help predict weather

C. Outdoor leaders provide evidence of their *dispositions* by:

1. Modeling competency in using a compass, a barometer, and an altimeter to predict weather in the field
2. Modeling use of the physical sensations to make observations useful in predicting weather in the field
3. Consistently using weather prediction skills in decision making to ensure the group has a safe, enjoyable, and environmentally sound trip

II. Content

A. Weather is difficult to accurately predict.

1. Atmospheric movements are mostly random in nature.
2. No two weather systems, masses, or fronts are alike.
3. Weather observers and weather stations are too far apart to get an accurate reading of regional weather.
4. Some weather phenomena are very localized (e.g., thunderstorms and snow squalls).

B. Barometric pressure

1. Barometric pressure is the pressure created by the weight of air above us.
   a) Because the molecules are farther apart, warm air is less dense than cold and holds more moisture.
   b) Warm air rises; cold air sinks.
2. As air cools and sinks, it becomes increasingly dense, and the atmospheric pressure rises. This denser air keeps other systems away; therefore, skies in a high-pressure system remain clear.
3. Air in a low-pressure system is less dense than in a high, which causes it to draw winds (which are often moist) into the system. Therefore, low-pressure systems often bring cloudy, stormy weather.

C. Barometer/altimeter. With the advent of reasonably priced altimeter watches with built-in altimeters/barometers, field-based weather prediction is more convenient than ever.

1. A barometer or altimeter can be used to determine elevation.
   a) Barometers or altimeters are affected by changes in elevation.
   b) Pressure drops about 1 inch (actually 1.05 to 1.10 inches/2.66 cm to 2.79 cm) or 25.4 mm, 33.86 mb (millibars) of mercury for each 1,000 feet/305 meters of elevation gained.
2. A barometer or altimeter can be used to predict weather.
   a) The following guidelines are usually dependable, although exceptions occur:
      (1) Steady or zero change in pressure: More of the same weather and often not windy.
      (2) Rising pressure: Clearing, but watch for instability that may mean showers in the mountains.
      (3) Falling pressure: Clouding over and precipitation may follow unless the storm passes over far enough away.

(4) Rapid change, up or down: A rapid change in the weather, usually windy.

b) The average pressure adjusted to sea level is 30.00 inches (762 mm, 1,016 mb). Always adjust the barometer to sea level readings. Before using the barometer in the field, it is necessary to set it at home based on a weather report. Once in the field, it needs to be calibrated daily based on your elevation.

    (1) General rule:

        (a) High pressure: Above 30.00 (adjusted to sea level)

            i)   Summer = clear weather

            ii) Winter = clear and cold weather

        (b) Low pressure: Below 30.00 (adjusted to sea level)

            i)   Summer = rainy, stormy weather

            ii) Winter = rain or snow

Inches (in)	Millimeters (mm)	Millibars (mb)
31.00	787	1,050
30.00	762	1,016
29.92	760	1,013
29.53	750	1,000
29.00	737	982
28.00	711	948
27.00	686	914

1 in = 25.4 mm = 33.86 mb
1 mm = 1.333 mb

FIGURE 48.1. Barometer scales compared

D. Wind. It is virtually impossible for the weather to change without wind. It is the wind, at varying elevations, that blows in different weather. It is extremely important, therefore, to understand the prevailing winds in the area you travel and the implications of any changes in wind direction. The following examples show how weather is affected by wind in three different regions of the United States.

1. Northeastern United States
    a) South or southwest air usually comes from the south Atlantic Ocean or Gulf of Mexico, bringing above-normal temperatures, warm nights, humidity, frequent showers, partly cloudy skies in between showers, and poor visibility. When south or southwest winds strengthen, a cold front may be approaching.
    b) North or northwest winds bring cooler, drier air from the Canadian interior and colder than normal temperatures, instability, flurries, and showers. These winds are most severe from November through January.
    c) West winds usually bring fair weather with normal temperatures.
    d) Southeast, east, or northeast winds frequently mean a coastal storm is approaching, with accompanying rain or snow if the storm is close enough. Winds normally shift to northwest after the storm.
    e) North to northeast wind brings Canadian maritime air with cold, cloudy, and wet conditions. This is rare.
    f) No wind, high pressure at center of air mass means fair, warm days and cold nights with low humidity.

2. Rocky Mountains, Colorado
    a) West is the most common direction from which wind blows in the Rockies—it usually means fair weather with normal temperatures. Wind from this direction often brings air masses capable of producing lightning storms and rainsqualls on summer afternoons between June and August.
    b) Northwest winds bring cooler, wetter air from the Pacific Northwest, colder than normal temperatures, heavy snow in the winter, and heavy rain in the summer. Wind from this direction often brings air masses capable of producing lightning storms and rainsqualls on summer afternoons between June and August.
    c) North winds bring arctic air down from the extreme north that is dry and very cold. It usually accompanies a southern dip in the jet stream.
    d) South or southwest air from the Gulf of Mexico or the Gulf of California, usually called an upslope condition, brings above-normal tempera-

tures, warm nights, increased humidity, and frequent snow in the winter and rain showers in the summer.

e) Southeast, east, or northeast winds are extremely rare in the Colorado Rockies, except along the Front Range north of Denver, where a cyclonic effect made by mixing air masses from the plains and larger systems coming from the west or northwest can bring thunderheads from the east in the summer months. Without this effect, wind rarely comes from an easterly direction.

f) No wind, high pressure at center of air mass means fair, warm days and cold nights with low humidity.

g) Note: At high elevations in the Rockies, snow can fall any day of the year.

3. Sierra Nevada range in California, southern California, and Baja California

a) Normal patterns of wind for the eastern Sierra Nevada range:

(1) Up-canyon "valley" winds in the morning

(2) Down-canyon flow by midafternoon

b) Normal patterns of wind for the western Sierra Nevada range: Wind on the west side of the Sierra Range "is not well understood"; i.e., it isn't a big factor in predicting the weather.

c) For the southwestern desert region, especially southern California and Baja California: "Santa Ana winds" develop when high pressure builds over the high desert or the Great Basin in Nevada. The clockwise rotation forces the desert air from Nevada toward the Pacific coast. These winds gain speed as they funnel through canyons along the southern California coastal ranges and deserts. October through March are the most common months for Santa Anas, with wind speeds from 35 to 100 knots. Typically the strongest winds occur at night, when the daily wind blowing in from the Pacific Ocean can't suppress it. Telltale signs include warm, dry weather with little humidity; clear skies all the way to the coast; and no dew point at night. Wind comes from the northeast and may or may not start slowly; i.e., it can come "from nowhere" and rip the kayak paddle out of your hand.

E. Temperature changes occur with change in elevation. Temperature changes can be used as a guide to determine changes in barometric pressure. If the temperature changes (over at least several hours) more than the degrees given below for every 1,000 feet (305 m) of elevation gained or lost, then this would indicate that the barometric pressure is changing.

1. 3°F (6°C) drop in temperature per 1,000 feet (305 m) of ascent is average.
2. 2°F (4°C) drop in temperature per 1,000 feet (305 m) of ascent when wet and/or windy indicates a low-pressure system.
3. 4°F (8°C) drop in temperature per 1,000 feet (305 m) of ascent when dry and/or calm indicates a high-pressure system.
4. 5°F (11°C) drop in temperature per 1,000 feet (305 m) of ascent is the theoretical maximum possible, with 0 percent relative humidity and absolutely still air, rarely realized in nature.

F. Clouds

1. Types of clouds: The types of clouds are classified according to how they are formed in the atmosphere.
    a) Cumulus (see fig. 48.2)
        (1) Formed by rising air currents at almost any altitude.
        (2) Classic puffy, white clouds.
        (3) Appear in the middle of a high-pressure air mass, mainly building up in the afternoon. Clouds with flat bottoms above mountains indicate fair weather.

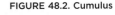

FIGURE 48.2. Cumulus

    b) Stratus (see fig. 48.3)
        (1) *Stratus* refers to the word *layer*.
        (2) Sheets or horizontal layers formed when air cools to the dew point (the point at which air becomes saturated and reaches 100 percent humidity).
2. Families of clouds: Families of clouds are classified according to their altitude.
    a) High clouds:
        (1) 20,000 to 25,000 feet above the earth

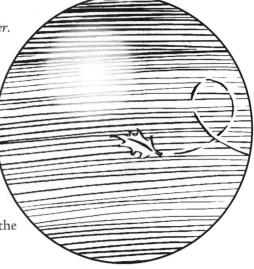

FIGURE 48.3. Stratus

(2) Consist of ice crystals

(3) Types of high clouds:

(a) Cirrus (*cirrus* refers to the word *streak*): Thin, wispy, and delicate. These don't contain precipitation but may indicate precipitation within the next twenty-four hours. These so-called mares' tails (scattered and wispy) often consist of ice crystals and indicate approaching precipitation. (See fig. 48.4.)

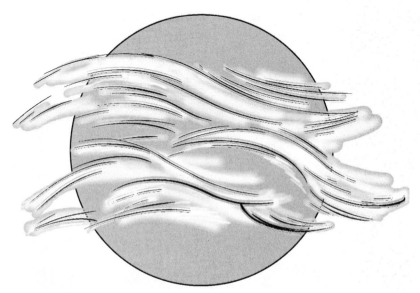

FIGURE 48.4. Cirrus

(b) Cirrocumulus: Rippled and thin. These often consist of ice crystals that reflect light and create a "halo" around the sun or moon. These are also known as a "mackerel sky." They often indicate fair weather but may also bring brief showers. (See fig. 48.5.)

b) Middle clouds

(1) 10,000 to 6,500 feet above the earth, but sometimes as high as 20,000 feet

(2) Consist of water and may contain some ice crystals

(3) Types of middle clouds:

(a) Altocumulus (*alto* refers to the middle range): Puffy, white, or gray; indicate fair weather with precipitation likely within eight to ten hours (see fig. 48.6)

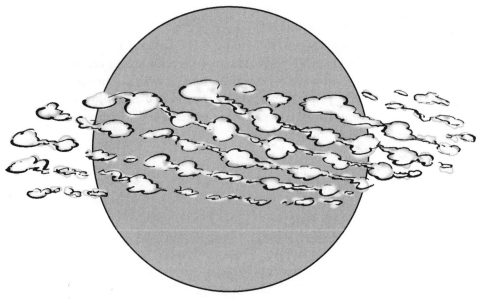

FIGURE 48.5. Cirrocumulus

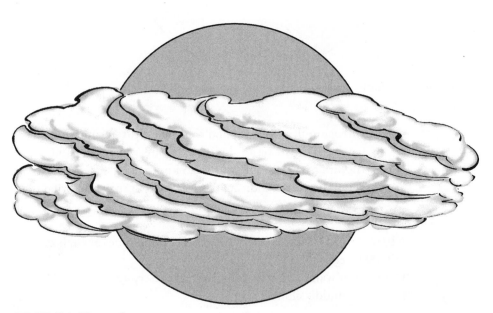

FIGURE 48.6. Altocumulus

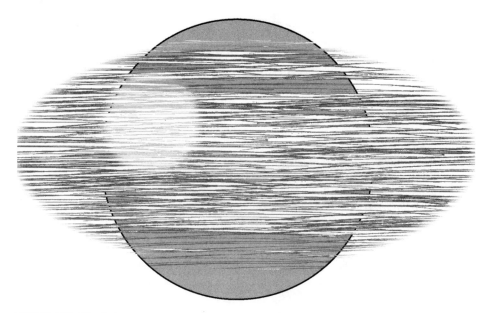

FIGURE 48.7. Altostratus

        (b) Altostratus: Gray or blue; usually bring light rain or snow (see fig. 48.7)

  c) Low clouds

    (1) About 6,500 feet or less above the earth

    (2) Types of low clouds:

        (a) Stratus: Low, uniform, and thin; consist of water droplets; may produce a fine drizzle but not a rain (see fig. 48.3)

        (b) Nimbostratus: Low, thick, and dark gray; yield steady rain or snow (see fig. 48.8)

        (c) Stratocumulus: Thick, gray, and irregular; don't produce precipitation, but often change into nimbostratus (see fig. 48.9)

  d) Towering

    (1) Range from low altitudes up to 40,000 feet

    (2) Cumulonimbus: Cauliflower-shaped with flat, anvil-like tops; classic thunderheads that produce heavy thunderstorms, rain, snow, or hail (see fig. 48.10)

3. Ground fog and/or dew

  a) Fog

    (1) Morning fog is the result of moisture in damp air that condenses

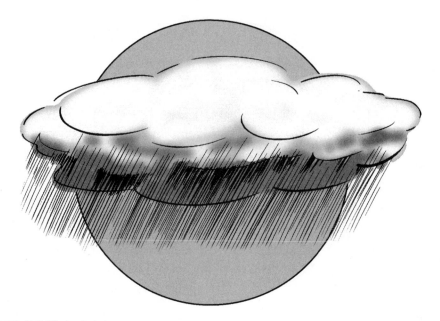

FIGURE 48.8. Nimbostratus

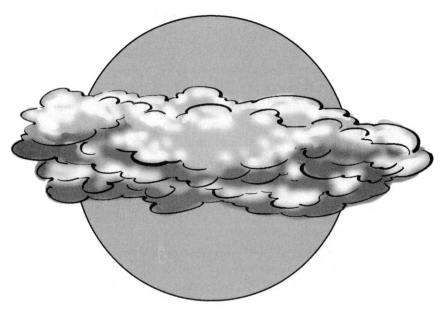

FIGURE 48.9. Stratocumulus

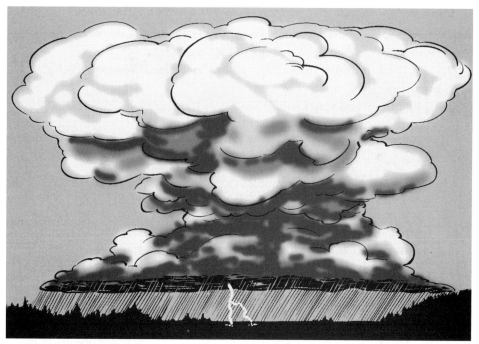

FIGURE 48.10. Cumulonimbus

in the cold of the night and is usually burned off by the heat of the morning sun.

(2) Late-afternoon or evening fog is usually formed as moisture falls through warmer air and often indicates a coming storm.

b) Dew

(1) Warm air holds more moisture than cold air, so the relative humidity increases as the air cools until the moisture in it reaches the maximum that it can hold at that temperature (this is called the dew point). If the air continues to cool, some moisture in it has to condense and may be deposited as dew.

(2) At night, the air near the surface of the earth cools. If it cools below its dew point, dew forms on the ground.

(3) Dew is most common on calm, cloudless, cool nights. Since both wind and clouds reduce the cooling rate of air near the surface of the earth, temperatures drop more slowly, and the air may not reach its dew point before the sun rises again in the morning.

(4) No dew at night may indicate rain by morning. No dew in the morning may indicate rain by the next day.

G. Other factors to consider when forecasting weather

1. Season: Various factors related to seasons (e.g., rainy or dry seasons in some regions) or the change of seasons impact weather.
2. Local conditions (e.g., mountains and valleys, large lakes, frost pockets, aspect, elevation, microclimate)
   a) Mountain and valley winds: Since wind (moving air) takes the path of least resistance, winds can be quite strong in lower elevations such as valleys and mountain passes. As the wind "squeezes" through these narrow areas, it picks up speed.
   b) Deserts: Very hot air quickly rises, creating "heat lows" such as dust devils (small whirlwinds) when surrounding air rushes in and fills the void.
   c) It is of utmost importance to be aware of extreme weather patterns and phenomena that may occur (tornadoes, hurricanes, possible summer snowstorms at high altitude, spring and fall snowfall at high altitude even in temperate regions, etc.), particularly if planning a trip in a distant region of the United States that may be unfamiliar or new territory.
3. Weather forecasts, average weather conditions, and historical weather patterns for the area can be obtained from a variety of sources, particularly National Weather Service publications. The following is a sampling of agencies that publish weather statistics and can provide weather forecasts or climatological summaries of regional weather.
   a) National Weather Service (Weather Radio): National Oceanic and Atmospheric Administration (NOAA), 1325 East West Highway, Silver Spring, MD 20910; www.nws.noaa.gov/
   b) Storm Prediction Center: NOAA/National Weather Service, 1313 Halley Circle, Norman, OK 73069; www.spc.noaa.gov/
   c) Archived Weather Information: NOAA National Climatic Data Center, www.noaa.gov/pastweather.html
   d) Climate reports and data: Natural Resources Conservation Service, Attn: Conservation Communications Staff, P.O. Box 2890, Washington, DC 20013; www.wcc.nrcs.usda.gov/climate/
   e) United States Regional Climate Centers: www.wrcc.dri.edu/rcc.html
   f) Tides Online: www.tidesonline.nos.noaa.gov/
   g) Great Lakes Online: www.glakesonline.nos.noaa.gov/
   h) Coastal marine forecasts by zone: www.nws.noaa.gov/om/marine/zone/usamz.htm

H. The facts about weather lore. Weather lore frequently has a basis in fact. Below are some examples of common weather lore and their connection to science. Remember to use judgment when applying weather lore.

1. Animals
    a) Cat: "If cats lick themselves, fair weather."
        (1) During fair weather, when the relative humidity is low, electrostatic charges (static electricity) can build up on a cat as it touches other objects. Cat hair loses electrons easily, so cats become positively charged.
        (2) When a cat licks itself, the moisture makes its fur more conductive so the charge can "leak" off the cat.
        (3) In fair weather during high pressure, dry air sinks from above. Relative humidity is low, and cat hair becomes a better insulator.
    b) Crickets as a thermometer (*Old Farmer's Almanac* 2005)
        (1) Crickets tend to chirp faster in warmer weather. You can estimate what temperature it is by counting the number of chirps in fifteen seconds and adding forty.
        (2) This will give the approximate temperature in degrees Fahrenheit (accurate about three-quarters of the time).
    c) Cow: "A cow with its tail to the west makes weather the best; a cow with its tail to the east makes weather the least."
        (1) This New England saying has some truth in it, for an animal grazes with its tail to the wind.
        (2) This is a natural instinct so the animal may face and see an invader; an invader from the opposite side would carry out its scent to the cow in the wind.
        (3) Inasmuch as an east wind is a rain wind and a west wind is a fair wind, the grazing animal's tail becomes somewhat of a weather sign.
    d) Humans: "If your corns all ache and itch, the weather fair will make a switch."
        (1) Studies have shown that some people experience increased pain when the barometric pressure falls.
        (2) This is not the case with everyone, but changes in air pressure do seem to cause aches and pains to increase for some folks, particularly those with arthritis or old injuries.
2. Dew: "When the dew is on the grass, rain will never come to pass. When grass is dry at morning light, look for rain before the night."
    a) Meaning, if there is no dew on the grass, it means the sky is cloudy or the breeze is strong, both of which may mean rain.
    b) The formation of dew requires nighttime cooling, which usually occurs only on very clear, calm nights. Such a night is usually followed by fair, sunny daytime weather, so inclement weather would be unlikely.

c) A weather system moving very rapidly could arrive during the day, however, thus interfering with this proverb.

3. Clouds
   a) "Mares' tails and mackerel scales make lofty ships carry low sails."
      (1) The "mares' tails" refer to trails of ice crystals blown in streaks from cirrus clouds. They are called mares' tails because they sometimes resemble the flowing tail of a horse in the wind.
      (2) The mackerel sky is composed of cirrus and cirrocumulus clouds (which resemble scale patterns on a mackerel's back). Mackerel scales are altocumulus clouds. They appear broken and scaly.
      (3) Neither of these cloud types will bring rain or snow themselves. They do, however, precede an approaching storm front by a day or two.
   b) "If fleecy white clouds cover the heavenly way, no rain should mar your plans that day."
      (1) Woolly fleece or fleecy white clouds refer to cumulus clouds with little vertical development (fair-weather cumulus).
      (2) This is sound folklore (as long as the clouds remain flat and do not grow vertically later on).
   c) "The higher the clouds, the finer the weather."
      (1) Clouds are formed by moisture that condenses out of rising air currents.
      (2) The higher the air must rise before condensation begins, the drier it was to begin with.
   d) "When clouds appear like rocks and towers, the earth will be washed by frequent showers."
      (1) Towering clouds, lofted high by strong updrafts, are cumulonimbus clouds.
      (2) These are the thunderstorm clouds that produce heavy showers, wind, and lightning. They are not, however, associated with steady rain.
   e) "Mountains in the morning, fountains in the evening."
      (1) The mountains refer to high, billowing cumulus clouds, indicative of instability and possible development of cumulonimbus clouds and a late-afternoon or evening thunderstorm.

4. Leaves: "When leaves turn their back 'tis a sign it's going to rain."
   a) Some trees, such as oak and maple, have leaves that will curl when the humidity is very high and the wind is blowing strongly.
   b) Both the above conditions indicate an approaching storm.

5. Moon: "If a circle forms 'round the moon, 'twill rain soon."
   a) The circle that forms around the sun or moon is called a halo. Halos are formed by the light from the sun or moon refracting (bending) as it passes through the ice crystals that form high-level cirrus and cirrostratus clouds.
   b) These clouds do not produce rain or snow, but they often precede an advancing low-pressure system that may bring bad weather.
6. Smoke: "If smoke hovers low near the ground, it is likely to rain."
   a) Smoke particles tend to absorb moisture from the air. The more moisture present in the air, the more a particle of smoke will absorb, and the heavier it gets.
   b) Heavy, moisture-laden smoke particles do not disperse as easily as the lighter, dry ones do.
7. Sound: "When sounds travel far and wide, a stormy day will betide."
   a) Sound travels at different speeds through different substances. It travels faster through a solid substance than it does through air, for instance.
   b) Sound travels better in air that is heavily laden with moisture than it does in dry air.
8. Stars: "Cold is the night when the stars shine bright."
   a) The more moisture there is in the sky, the more the light from the sun, moon, and stars is dimmed or reddened.
   b) A very clear sky permits more starlight to penetrate, thus the stars appear brighter. Moisture tends to hold in the day's heat, like a blanket.
   c) The less moisture there is in the air at night, the more the temperature tends to fall. Thus, the brighter the stars appear, the cooler is the night.
9. Sun: "Red sky at night, sailors delight; red sky in the morning, sailors take warning."
   a) A red sunset indicates that tomorrow's weather may be dry.
   b) Dry air refracts red light.
   c) This indicates that clear, dry air is to the west, which is often the direction from which storms come.
   d) Red sunrises are caused by reflections in moist air that may indicate rain later in the day.
10. General: The following ditty summarizes a variety of weather lore. Although they all have some basis in truth, don't rely too much on them for accurate weather forecasting.

> When the sky is red in the morning,
> And sounds travel far at night;
> When fish jump high from the water
> And flies stick tight, and bite;

When you can't get salt from your shaker,
And your corn gives you extra pain,
There's no need to consult an almanac,
You just know it's going to rain.

III. Instructional Strategies

A. Timing. Individual elements of this lesson can be effectively communicated using teachable moments (see chapter 1, Teaching and Learning) when changes in weather occur.

B. Considerations

1. Participants can choose a "weatherperson" to record temperature highs and lows and weather patterns during the course. These patterns can be studied to better understand weather systems.
2. This is a good lesson for students who have a special interest in meteorology to instruct.

C. Activities

1. The weather rock: A fun tongue-in-cheek activity that can be used to start or wrap up a lesson on weather is to find a small stone and, with a piece of cord and some small sticks, create a small tripod from which you can hang it. Explain how this "weather rock" can be a weather indicator.
   a) If it's dry and you can see it, then the weather is clear
   b) If it's wet, then it is raining
   c) If it's white, then it has been snowing
   d) If it is swinging, then it is windy
   e) If it's gone, then a tornado or hurricane has been through
   f) If you can't see it, then perhaps it is night

D. Materials

1. Barometer
2. Altimeter
3. Compass
4. Thermometer

References and Recommended Reading

1: Teaching and Learning

Bloom, B. S., B. B. Mesia, and D. R. Krathwohl. 1964. *Taxonomy of educational objectives.* 2 vols. New York: David McKay.

De Bono, E. 1999. *New thinking for the new millennium.* New York: Penguin Books.

Education By Design/The Critical Skills Program. 1999. *Level I coaching kit: Support for educators getting started with EBD.* 3rd ed. Antioch, NH: Antioch New England Graduate School.

Gardner, H. 1993. *Frames of mind: The theory of multiple intelligences.* New York: Basic Books.

Gookin, J., and D. Wells, eds. 2002. *Environmental education notebook.* Lander, WY: National Outdoor Leadership School.

Hartman, H. 2002. Search on cooperative learning. http://candor.admin.ccny .cuny.edu/~eg9306/candy%20research.htm.

Marzano, R. J., D. J. Pickering, and J. E. Pollock. 2001. *Classroom instruction that works: Research-based strategies for increasing student achievement.* Alexandria, VA: Association for Supervision and Curriculum Development.

Mobilia, W. 1995. *The Critical Skills classroom.* 5th ed. Antioch, NH: Antioch New England Graduate School.

National Outdoor Leadership School. 1999. *Wilderness educator notebook.* Lander, WY: National Outdoor Leadership School.

Petzoldt, P. 1984. *The new wilderness handbook.* 2nd ed. New York: W. W. Norton & Company.

Rohnke, K., and S. Butler. 1995. *Quicksilver: Adventure games, initiative problems, trust activities and a guide to effective leadership.* Hamilton, MA: Project Adventure.

Schoel, J., D. Prouty, and P. Radcliffe. 1988. *Islands of healing: A guide to adventure-based counseling.* Hamilton, MA: Project Adventure.

Tucker-Ladd, C. E. 1996–2000. *Psychological self-help.* Mental Health Net. www.mentalhelp.net/psyhelp.

Wiggins, G., and J. McTighe. 1998. *Understanding by design.* Alexandria, VA: Association for Supervision and Curriculum Development.

2: Backpacks: Pack Fitting

Drury, J. K., and E. R. Holmlund. 1997. *The camper's guide to outdoor pursuits: Finding safe, nature-friendly and comfortable passage through wild places.* Champaign, IL: Sagamore Publishing.

Harvey, M. 1999. *The National Outdoor Leadership School's wilderness guide: The classic handbook, revised and updated.* 2nd ed. New York: Simon & Schuster.

Keay, W. 1996. *Expedition guide.* 3rd ed. Wellingborough, Northamptonshire, UK: Sterling Press.

Manning, H. 1986. *Backpacking one step at a time.* 4th ed. New York: Vintage Books.

3: Backpacks: Pack Packing

Drury, J. K., and E. R. Holmlund. 1997. *The camper's guide to outdoor pursuits: Finding safe, nature-friendly and comfortable passage through wild places.* Champaign, IL: Sagamore Publishing.

Keay, W. 1996. *Expedition guide.* 3rd ed. Wellingborough, Northamptonshire, UK: Sterling Press.

National Outdoor Leadership School. 1999. *Wilderness educator notebook.* Lander, WY: National Outdoor Leadership School.

4: Bathing and Washing

Keay, W. 1996. *Expedition guide.* 3rd ed. Wellingborough, Northamptonshire, UK: Sterling Press.

National Outdoor Leadership School. 1997. *Leave no trace: Outdoor skills and ethics.* Lander, WY: National Outdoor Leadership School.

———. 1999. *Wilderness educator notebook.* Lander, WY: National Outdoor Leadership School.

Petzoldt, P. 1984. *The new wilderness handbook.* 2nd ed. New York: W. W. Norton & Company.

Schatz, C., and D. Seemon. 1994. *A basic guide to minimum impact camping.* Cambridge, MN: Adventure Publications, Inc.

Tilton, B., and R. Bennett. 1995. *Camping healthy: Hygiene for the outdoors.* Merrillville, IN: ICS Books.

5: Campsite Selection

Drury, J. K., and E. R. Holmlund. 1997. *The camper's guide to outdoor pursuits: Finding safe, nature-friendly and comfortable passage through wild places.* Champaign, IL: Sagamore Publishing.

Harvey, M. 1999. *The National Outdoor Leadership School's wilderness guide: The classic handbook, revised and updated.* 2nd ed. New York: Simon & Schuster.

Keay, W. 1996. *Expedition guide.* 3rd ed. Wellingborough, Northamptonshire, UK: Sterling Press.

National Outdoor Leadership School. 1997. *Leave no trace: Outdoor skills and ethics.* Lander, WY: National Outdoor Leadership School.

———. 1999. *Wilderness educator notebook.* Lander, WY: National Outdoor Leadership School.

Peacock, D. October 1990. A practical guide to grizzly country. *Backpacker* 18 (6): 80–85.

Petzoldt, P. 1984. *The new wilderness handbook.* 2nd ed. New York: W. W. Norton & Company.

Schatz, C., and D. Seemon. 1994. *A basic guide to minimum impact camping.* Cambridge, MN: Adventure Publications, Inc.

6: Catholes and Latrines: Proper Disposal of Human Waste

Drury, J. K., and E. R. Holmlund. 1997. *The camper's guide to outdoor pursuits: Finding safe, nature-friendly and comfortable passage through wild places.* Champaign, IL: Sagamore Publishing.

Hampton, B., and D. Cole. 1995. *Soft paths.* Revised ed. Mechanicsburg, PA: Stackpole Books.

Hart, J. 1977. *Walking softly in the wilderness.* San Francisco: Sierra Club Books.

Keay, W. 1996. *Expedition guide.* 3rd ed. Wellingborough, Northamptonshire, UK: Sterling Press.

Meyer, K. 1989. *How to shit in the woods.* Berkeley, CA: Ten Speed Press.

———. 1994. *How to shit in the woods: An environmentally sound approach to a lost art.* 2nd ed. Berkeley, CA: Ten Speed Press.

National Outdoor Leadership School. 1997. *Leave no trace: Outdoor skills and ethics.* Lander, WY: National Outdoor Leadership School.

——. 1999. *Wilderness educator notebook.* Lander, WY: National Outdoor Leadership School.

Petzoldt, P. 1984. *The new wilderness handbook.* 2nd ed. New York: W. W. Norton & Company.

Schatz, C., and D. Seemon. 1994. *A basic guide to minimum impact camping.* Cambridge, MN: Adventure Publications, Inc.

Simer, P., and J. Sullivan. 1983. *The National Outdoor Leadership School's wilderness guide.* New York: Simon and Schuster.

7: Clothing Selection

Drury, J. K., and E. R. Holmlund. 1997. *The camper's guide to outdoor pursuits: Finding safe, nature-friendly and comfortable passage through wild places.* Champaign, IL: Sagamore Publishing.

Forgey, W. W. 1991. *The basic essentials of hypothermia.* Merrillville, IN: ICS Books, Inc.

Gonzalez, R. 1987. Biophysical and physiological integration of proper clothing for exercise. *Exercise and Sport Science Reviews* 15: 261–95.

Harvey, M. 1999. *The National Outdoor Leadership School's wilderness guide: The classic handbook, revised and updated.* 2nd ed. New York: Simon & Schuster.

Hodgson, M. 1999. Waterproof/breathable jackets: Making the functional choice. www.adventurenetwork.com/cgi-bin/adventurenetwork/Waterproof_Breathable_Jackets.html?id=6M5LSnCz.

Jordan, R., ed. 2004. *Lightweight backpacking: A field guide to wilderness hiking equipment, technique, and style.* Bozeman, MT: Beartooth Mountain Press.

Keay, W. 1996. *Expedition guide.* 3rd ed. Wellingborough, Northamptonshire, UK: Sterling Press.

Koehler, K. R. 1996. Body temperature regulation. In *College physics for students of biology and chemistry.* www.rwc.uc.edu/koehler/biophys/8d.html.

Manning, H. 1986. *Backpacking one step at a time.* 4th ed. New York: Vintage Books.

National Outdoor Leadership School. 1999. *Wilderness educator notebook.* Lander, WY: National Outdoor Leadership School.

Petzoldt, P. 1984. *The new wilderness handbook.* 2nd ed. New York: W. W. Norton & Company.

The Virtual Naval Hospital Project. 1991. Thermal stresses and injuries: Thermal equilibrium. In *United States naval flight surgeon's manual*. www.vnh.org /FSManual/20/02ThermalEquilibrium.html.

———. 1997–2005. Ventilation and thermal stress ashore and afloat, section 1: Definitions and instrumentation. In *Manual of naval preventive medicine*. www.vnh.org/PreventiveMedicine/Chapter3/3.02.html.

8: Collaboration: How We Approach Teamwork

Adizes, I. 1991. *Mastering change: The power of mutual trust and respect*. Santa Monica, CA: Adizes Institute Publications.

9: Crisis Management in the Backcountry

American Psychiatric Association. 1994. *Diagnostic and statistical manual of mental disorders*. 4th ed. Washington, DC: American Psychiatric Association.

Caraulia, A., and L. Steiger. 1997. *Nonviolent crisis intervention: Learning to defuse explosive behavior*. Brookfield, WI: Crisis Prevention Institute Publishing.

Dixon, S. 1979. *Working with people in crisis: Theory and practice*. St. Louis, MO: Mosby.

Mitchell, J., and G. Everly. 1995. Critical incident stress debriefing (CISD) and the prevention of work-related traumatic stress among high risk occupational groups. In *Psychotraumatology: Key papers and core concepts in post-traumatic stress*, ed. G. Everly and J. Lating. New York: Plenum.

10: Decision Making

Adams, J. N. n.d. Critical thinking, problem solving, and decision making. http://home.att.net/~juddadams/critical_thinking.htm.

Buell, L. 1983. *Outdoor leadership competency: A manual for self-assessment and staff evaluation*. Greenfield, MA: Environmental Awareness Publications.

Chesterton, G. K. 1935. *The scandal of Father Brown*. Cassell, London, UK: House of Stratus.

Cockrell, D., ed. 1991. *The wilderness educator: The Wilderness Education Association curriculum guide*. Merrillville, IN: ICS Books, Inc.

De Bono, E. 1999. *New thinking for the new millennium*. New York: Penguin Books.

Ford, P., and J. Blanchard. 1993. *Leadership and administration of outdoor pursuits*. 2nd ed. State College, PA: Venture Publishing.

Gookin, J., M. Doran, and R. Green, eds. 2001. *2001 NOLS leadership education toolbox*. Lander, WY: National Outdoor Leadership School.

Graham, J. 1997. *Outdoor leadership: Technique, common sense & self-confidence*. Seattle: The Mountaineers.

Grube, D., M. Phipps, and A. Grube. 2004. Practicing leader decision making through a systematic journal technique: A single case analysis. *Journal of Experiential Education* 25 (1).

Hersey, P., and K. H. Blanchard. 1982. *Management of organizational behavior: Utilizing human resources*. 4th ed. Englewood Cliffs, NJ: Prentice Hall, Inc.

Hughes, R. L., R. C. Ginnett, and G. J. Curphy. 1993. *Leadership: Enhancing the lessons of experience*. Burn Ridge, IL: Richard D. Irwin, Inc.

Petzoldt, P. 1984. *The new wilderness handbook*. 2nd ed. New York: W. W. Norton & Company.

Priest, S., and M. A. Gass. 1997. *Effective leadership in adventure programming*. Champaign, IL: Human Kinetics.

Sessoms, H. D., and J. L. Stevenson. 1981. *Leadership and group dynamics in recreation services*. Boston: Allyn and Bacon, Inc.

Tucker-Ladd, C. E. 1996–2000. Methods for developing skills: Decision-making and problem-solving. In *Psychological self-help*. Mental Health Net. www.mentalhelp.net/psyhelp.

Weiss, R. 1987. How dare we?: Scientists seek the sources of risk-taking behavior. *Science News* 132 (4): 57–59.

11: Environmental Ethics

Brill, N. I. 1998. *Working with people*. 6th ed. New York: Longman.

Cockrell, D., ed. 1991. *The wilderness educator: The Wilderness Education Association curriculum guide*. Merrillville, IN: ICS Books, Inc.

Cordell, H. K., B. L. McDonald, R. J. Teasley, J. C. Bergstrom, J. Martin, J. Bason, and V. R. Leworthy. 1999. Outdoor recreation participation trends. In *Outdoor Recreation in American Life*, H. K. Cordell et al. Champaign, IL: Sagamore

Publishing. Retrieved from www.srs.fs.usda.gov/pubs/viewpub.jsp ?index=767.

Dustin, D. L. 1993. *The wilderness within: Journeys in self-discovery*. San Diego: Institute for Leisure Behavior.

Egan, G. 1990. *The skilled helper: A systematic approach to effective helping*. 4th ed. Pacific Grove, CA: Brooks/Cole.

Ford, P., and J. Blanchard. 1993. *Leadership and administration of outdoor pursuits*. 2nd ed. State College, PA: Venture Publishing.

Gookin, J., and D. Wells, eds. 2002. *Environmental education notebook*. Lander, WY: National Outdoor Leadership School.

Harvey, M. 1999. *The National Outdoor Leadership School's wilderness guide: The classic handbook, revised and updated*. 2nd ed. New York: Simon & Schuster.

Hendee, J., and C. Dawson. 2002. *Wilderness management: Stewardship and protection of resources and values*. 3rd ed. Golden, CO: Fulcrum Publishing.

Johnson, D. W., and F. Johnson. 1987. *Joining together: Group theory and group skills*. 3rd ed. Englewood Cliffs, NJ: Prentice-Hall, Inc.

Keay, W. 1996. *Expedition guide*. 3rd ed. Wellingborough, Northamptonshire, UK: Sterling Press.

Leopold, A. 1966. *A Sand County almanac*. New York: Ballantine Books.

Manning, R. 2003. Emerging principles for using information/education in wilderness management. *International Journal of Wilderness* 9 (1): 20–21.

Matthews, B. E., and C. K. Riley. 1995. *Teaching and evaluating outdoor ethics education programs*. Vienna, VA: National Wildlife Federation, Educational Outreach Department.

Nash, R. F. 1989. *The Rights of nature: A history of environmental ethics*. Madison, WI: University of Wisconsin Press.

———. 2001. *Wilderness and the American mind*. 4th ed. New Haven: Yale University Press.

National Outdoor Leadership School. 1997. *Leave no trace: Outdoor skills and ethics*. Lander, WY: National Outdoor Leadership School.

———. 1999. *Wilderness educator notebook*. Lander, WY: National Outdoor Leadership School.

Petzoldt, P. 1984. *The new wilderness handbook*. 2nd ed. New York: W. W. Norton & Company.

Sax, J. L. 1980. *Mountains without handrails: Reflections on the National Parks.* Ann Arbor: University of Michigan Press.

Schatz, C., and D. Seemon. 1994. *A basic guide to minimum impact camping.* Cambridge, MN: Adventure Publications, Inc.

Wilderness Education Association. 1989. *The WEA affiliate handbook: For current and prospective affiliate members.* Saranac Lake, NY: Wilderness Education Association.

12: Expedition Behavior

Brill, N. I. 1998. *Working with people.* 6th ed. New York: Longman.

Drury, J. K., and E. R. Holmlund. 1997. *The camper's guide to outdoor pursuits: Finding safe, nature-friendly and comfortable passage through wild places.* Champaign, IL: Sagamore Publishing.

Egan, G. 1990. *The skilled helper: A systematic approach to effective helping.* 4th ed. Pacific Grove, CA: Brooks/Cole.

Ford, P., and J. Blanchard. 1993. *Leadership and administration of outdoor pursuits.* 2nd ed. State College, PA: Venture Publishing.

Gookin, J., M. Doran, and R. Green, eds. 2001. *2001 NOLS leadership education toolbox.* Lander, WY: National Outdoor Leadership School.

Harvey, M. 1999. *The National Outdoor Leadership School's wilderness guide: The classic handbook, revised and updated.* 2nd ed. New York: Simon & Schuster.

National Outdoor Leadership School. 1999. *Wilderness educator notebook.* Lander, WY: National Outdoor Leadership School.

Petzoldt, P. 1984. *The new wilderness handbook.* 2nd ed. New York: W. W. Norton & Company.

Silvester, S. 2003–4. Inspiring communication: Using more than words. 5.12 Solutions. www.512solutions.com/article2.html.

13: Fire Site Preparation and Care

Boy Scouts of America. 1984. *Fieldbook.* 3rd ed. Irving, TX: Boy Scouts of America.

Cole, D. N. 1986. *NOLS conservation practices.* Lander, WY: National Outdoor Leadership School.

Drury, J. K., and E. R. Holmlund. 1997. *The camper's guide to outdoor pursuits: Finding safe, nature-friendly and comfortable passage through wild places.* Champaign, IL: Sagamore Publishing.

Hammitt, W. E., and D. N. Cole. 1987. *Wildland recreation: Ecology and management.* New York: John Wiley & Sons.

Hampton, B., and D. Cole. 1988. *Soft paths.* Harrisburg, PA: Stackpole Books.

Harvey, M. 1999. *The National Outdoor Leadership School's wilderness guide: The classic handbook, revised and updated.* 2nd ed. New York: Simon & Schuster.

Jacobson, C. 1986. *The new wilderness canoeing and camping.* Merrillville, IN: ICS Books, Inc.

Keay, W. 1996. *Expedition guide.* 3rd ed. Wellingborough, Northamptonshire, UK: Sterling Press.

Mason, B. S. 1939. *Woodcraft.* New York: A. S. Barnes & Company.

National Outdoor Leadership School. 1997. *Leave no trace: Outdoor skills and ethics.* Lander, WY: National Outdoor Leadership School.

——. 1999. *Wilderness educator notebook.* Lander, WY: National Outdoor Leadership School.

Pearson, C. 1997. *NOLS cookery.* 4th ed. Mechanicsburg, PA: Stackpole Books.

Petzoldt, P. 1984. *The new wilderness handbook.* 2nd ed. New York: W. W. Norton & Company.

Phillips, J. 1986. *Campground cookery: Outdoor living skills series* (instructor manual). 2nd ed. Jefferson City, MO: Missouri Department of Conservation.

Schatz, C., and D. Seemon. 1994. *A basic guide to minimum impact camping.* Cambridge, MN: Adventure Publications, Inc.

Simer, P., and J. Sullivan. 1983. *The National Outdoor Leadership School's wilderness guide.* New York: Simon and Schuster.

14: Fire Building

Boy Scouts of America. 1980. *Lifesaving.* Irving, TX: Boy Scouts of America.

——. 1984. *Fieldbook.* 3rd ed. Irving, TX: Boy Scouts of America.

——. 1989. *Canoeing.* Irving, TX: Boy Scouts of America.

Drury, J. K., and E. R. Holmlund. 1997. *The camper's guide to outdoor pursuits: Finding safe, nature-friendly and comfortable passage through wild places.* Champaign, IL: Sagamore Publishing.

Keay, W. 1996. *Expedition guide.* 3rd ed. Wellingborough, Northamptonshire, UK: Sterling Press.

National Outdoor Leadership School. 1999. *Wilderness educator notebook*. Lander, WY: National Outdoor Leadership School.

Pearson, C. 1997. *NOLS cookery*. 4th ed. Mechanicsburg, PA: Stackpole Books.

Petzoldt, P. 1984. *The new wilderness handbook*. 2nd ed. New York: W. W. Norton & Company.

Simer, P., and J. Sullivan. 1983. *The National Outdoor Leadership School's wilderness guide*. New York: Simon and Schuster.

15: Food: Introduction to Cooking

Drury, J. K., and E. R. Holmlund. 1997. *The camper's guide to outdoor pursuits: Finding safe, nature-friendly and comfortable passage through wild places*. Champaign, IL: Sagamore Publishing.

Gisslen, W. 1999. *Professional cooking*. 4th ed. New York: Wiley & Sons.

Harvey, M. 1999. *The National Outdoor Leadership School's wilderness guide: The classic handbook, revised and updated*. 2nd ed. New York: Simon & Schuster.

Keay, W. 1996. *Expedition guide*. 3rd ed. Wellingborough, Northamptonshire, UK: Sterling Press.

National Outdoor Leadership School. 1999. *Wilderness educator notebook*. Lander, WY: National Outdoor Leadership School.

Pearson, C. 1997. *NOLS cookery*. 4th ed. Mechanicsburg, PA: Stackpole Books.

Petzoldt, P. 1984. *The new wilderness handbook*. 2nd ed. New York: W. W. Norton & Company.

Richard, S., D. Orr, and C. Lindholm, eds. 1988. *The NOLS cookery: Experience the art of outdoor cooking*. 2nd ed. Lander, WY: National Outdoor Leadership School.

Simer, P., and J. Sullivan. 1983. *The National Outdoor Leadership School's wilderness guide*. New York: Simon and Schuster.

16: Food: Granola Preparation

Pearson, C. 1997. *NOLS cookery*. 4th ed. Mechanicsburg, PA: Stackpole Books.

Petzoldt, P. 1984. *The new wilderness handbook*. 2nd ed. New York: W. W. Norton & Company.

Richard, S., D. Orr, and C. Lindholm, eds. 1988. *The NOLS cookery: Experience the art of outdoor cooking.* 2nd ed. Lander, WY: National Outdoor Leadership School.

Simer, P., and J. Sullivan. 1983. *The National Outdoor Leadership School's wilderness guide.* New York: Simon and Schuster.

17: Food: Waste Disposal

Hampton, B., and D. Cole. 1995. *Soft paths.* Revised ed. Mechanicsburg, PA: Stackpole Books.

Hart, J. 1977. *Walking softly in the wilderness.* San Francisco: Sierra Club Books.

Keay, W. 1996. *Expedition guide.* 3rd ed. Wellingborough, Northamptonshire, UK: Sterling Press.

Petzoldt, P. 1984. *The new wilderness handbook.* 2nd ed. New York: W. W. Norton & Company.

Simer, P., and J. Sullivan. 1983. *The National Outdoor Leadership School's wilderness guide.* New York: Simon and Schuster.

18: Food: Identification, Organization, and Preparation Tips

Drury, J. K. 1986. Idea notebook: Wilderness food planning in the computer age. *Journal of Experiential Education* 9 (3): 36–40.

National Outdoor Leadership School. 1999. *Wilderness educator notebook.* Lander, WY: National Outdoor Leadership School.

Pearson, C. 1997. *NOLS cookery.* 4th ed. Mechanicsburg, PA: Stackpole Books.

Petzoldt, P. 1984. *The new wilderness handbook.* 2nd ed. New York: W. W. Norton & Company.

Simer, P., and J. Sullivan. 1983. *The National Outdoor Leadership School's wilderness guide.* New York: Simon and Schuster.

19: Food: Quick-Bread Making

Drury, J. K., and E. R. Holmlund. 1997. *The camper's guide to outdoor pursuits: Finding safe, nature-friendly and comfortable passage through wild places.* Champaign, IL: Sagamore Publishing.

Gisslen, W. 1999. *Professional cooking.* 4th ed. New York: Wiley & Sons.

Harvey, M. 1999. *The National Outdoor Leadership School's wilderness guide: The classic handbook, revised and updated.* 2nd ed. New York: Simon & Schuster.

National Outdoor Leadership School. 1999. *Wilderness educator notebook.* Lander, WY: National Outdoor Leadership School.

Pearson, C. 1997. *NOLS cookery.* 4th ed. Mechanicsburg, PA: Stackpole Books.

Petzoldt, P. 1984. *The new wilderness handbook.* 2nd ed. New York: W. W. Norton & Company.

Richard, S., D. Orr, and C. Lindholm, eds. 1988. *The NOLS cookery: Experience the art of outdoor cooking.* 2nd ed. Lander, WY: National Outdoor Leadership School.

Simer, P., and J. Sullivan. 1983. *The National Outdoor Leadership School's wilderness guide.* New York: Simon and Schuster.

20: Food: Yeast Baking

Drury, J. K., and E. R. Holmlund. 1997. *The camper's guide to outdoor pursuits: Finding safe, nature-friendly and comfortable passage through wild places.* Champaign, IL: Sagamore Publishing.

Gisslen, W. 1999. *Professional cooking.* 4th ed. New York: Wiley & Sons.

National Outdoor Leadership School. 1999. *Wilderness educator notebook.* Lander, WY: National Outdoor Leadership School.

Pearson, C. 1997. *NOLS cookery.* 4th ed. Mechanicsburg, PA: Stackpole Books.

Richard, S., D. Orr, and C. Lindholm, eds. 1988. *The NOLS cookery: Experience the art of outdoor cooking.* 2nd ed. Lander, WY: National Outdoor Leadership School.

21: Food: Nutrition, Rations Planning, and Packaging

Drury, J. K., and E. R. Holmlund. 1997. *The camper's guide to outdoor pursuits: Finding safe, nature-friendly and comfortable passage through wild places.* Champaign, IL: Sagamore Publishing.

Harvey, M. 1999. *The National Outdoor Leadership School's wilderness guide: The classic handbook, revised and updated.* 2nd ed. New York: Simon & Schuster.

Howley, M. 2002. *NOLS nutrition field guide*. Lander, WY: National Outdoor Leadership School.

National Outdoor Leadership School. 1999. *Wilderness educator notebook*. Lander, WY: National Outdoor Leadership School.

Pearson, C. 1997. *NOLS cookery*. 4th ed. Mechanicsburg, PA: Stackpole Books.

Petzoldt, P. 1984. *The new wilderness handbook*. 2nd ed. New York: W. W. Norton & Company.

Richard, S., D. Orr, and C. Lindholm, eds. 1988. *The NOLS cookery: Experience the art of outdoor cooking*. 2nd ed. Lander, WY: National Outdoor Leadership School.

Simer, P., and J. Sullivan. 1983. *The National Outdoor Leadership School's wilderness guide*. New York: Simon and Schuster.

22: Food: Protection

Boy Scouts of America. 1984. *Fieldbook*. 3rd ed. Irving, TX: Boy Scouts of America.

Drury, J. K., and E. R. Holmlund. 1997. *The camper's guide to outdoor pursuits: Finding safe, nature-friendly and comfortable passage through wild places*. Champaign, IL: Sagamore Publishing.

Harvey, M. 1999. *The National Outdoor Leadership School's wilderness guide: The classic handbook, revised and updated*. 2nd ed. New York: Simon & Schuster.

National Outdoor Leadership School. 1997. *Leave no trace: Outdoor skills and ethics*. Lander, WY: National Outdoor Leadership School.

———. 1999. *Wilderness educator notebook*. Lander, WY: National Outdoor Leadership School.

Schatz, C., and D. Seemon. 1994. *A basic guide to minimum impact camping*. Cambridge, MN: Adventure Publications, Inc.

23: Group Development

Caple, R. B. 1978. The sequential stages of group development. *Small Group Behavior* 9 (3): 470–76.

Ewert, A., and J. Heywood. 1991. Group development in the natural environment: Expectations, outcomes, and techniques. *Environment and Behavior* 23 (5): 592–615.

Ford, P., and J. Blanchard. 1993. *Leadership and administration of outdoor pursuits.* 2nd ed. State College, PA: Venture Publishing.

Johnson, D. W., and F. Johnson. 1987. *Joining together: Group theory and group skills.* 3rd ed. Englewood Cliffs, NJ: Prentice-Hall, Inc.

Jones, J. E. 1973. A model of group development. In *The annual handbook for group facilitators,* eds. J. E. Jones and J. W. Pfeiffer. La Jolla, CA: University Associates.

———. 1974. A model of group development. In *Book for group facilitators,* eds. J. E. Jones, J. W. Pfeiffer, and L. D. Goodstein. San Diego, CA: University Associates.

Jones, J. E., and W. L. Bearley. 1994. *Group development assessment: Facilitator guide.* King of Prussia, PA: HRDQ.

Jordan, D. J. 1996. *Leadership in leisure services: Making a difference.* State College, PA: Venture Publishing, Inc.

Kalisch, K. 1979. *The role of the instructor in the Outward Bound process.* Three Lakes, WI: Wheaton College.

National Outdoor Leadership School. 1999. *Wilderness educator notebook.* Lander, WY: National Outdoor Leadership School.

Rohnke, K., and S. Butler. 1995. *Quicksilver: Adventure games, initiative problems, trust activities and a guide to effective leadership.* Hamilton, MA: Project Adventure.

Schoel, J., D. Prouty, and P. Radcliffe. 1988. *Islands of healing: A guide to adventure-based counseling.* Hamilton, MA: Project Adventure.

Schoel, J., and R. Maizell. 2002. *Exploring islands of healing: New perspectives on adventure-based counseling.* Hamilton, MA: Project Adventure.

Shaw, M. 1981. *Group dynamics: The psychology of small group behavior.* 3rd ed. New York: McGraw-Hill Books.

Shutz, W. C. 1966. *The interpersonal underworld.* Palo Alto, CA: Science and Behavior Books.

Tuckman, B. 1965. Developmental sequence in small groups. *Psychological Bulletin* 63: 384–99.

24: Group Orienting and Monitoring

Ford, P., and J. Blanchard. 1993. *Leadership and administration of outdoor pursuits.* 2nd ed. State College, PA: Venture Publishing.

Johnson, D. W., and F. P. Johnson. 2000. *Joining together: Group theory and group skills*. 7th ed. Boston: Allyn & Bacon.

Jordan, D. J. 1999. *Leadership in leisure services: Making a difference*. State College, PA: Venture Publishing.

Luckner, J. L., and R. S. Nadler. 1997. *Processing the experience: Strategies to enhance and generalize learning*. 2nd ed. Dubuque, IA: Kendall/Hunt.

North Carolina Outward Bound School. 1993. *The instructor handbook: North Carolina Outward Bound School*. Asheville, NC: North Carolina Outward Bound.

Schoel, J., D. Prouty, and P. Radcliffe. 1988. *Islands of healing: A guide to adventure-based counseling*. Hamilton, MA: Project Adventure.

25: Group Processing and Debriefing

Knapp, C. E. 1992. *Lasting lessons: A teacher's guide to reflecting on experience*. Charleston, WV: Clearinghouse on Rural Education and Small Schools.

Quinsland, L. K., and A. Van Ginkel. 1984. How to process experience. *Journal of Experiential Education* 7 (2): 8–13.

Rohnke, K., and S. Butler. 1995. *Quicksilver: Adventure games, initiative problems, trust activities and a guide to effective leadership*. Hamilton, MA: Project Adventure.

Schoel, J., and R. Maizell. 2002. *Exploring islands of healing: New perspectives on adventure-based counseling*. Hamilton, MA: Project Adventure.

Schoel, J., D. Prouty, and P. Radcliffe. 1988. *Islands of healing: A guide to adventure-based counseling*. Hamilton, MA: Project Adventure.

26: History of Outdoor Leadership

Cinnamon, J., and E. Raiola. 1991. Adventure skill and travel modes. In *The Wilderness Educator: The Wilderness Education Association Curriculum Guide,* ed. D. Cockrell. Merrillville, IN: ICS Books.

Cockrell, D., ed. 1991. *The wilderness educator: The Wilderness Education Association curriculum guide*. Merrillville, IN: ICS Books, Inc.

Environmental Protection Agency. 1988. *Report assessing environmental education in the United States and the implementation of the national Environmental Education Act of 1990*. EPA 171-R-001.

Miles, J. C., and S. Priest. 1990. *Adventure education*. State College, PA: Venture Publishing.

Miner, J. L., and J. R. Boldt. *Outward Bound USA: Crew not passengers*. 2nd ed. Seattle: The Mountaineers.

National Outdoor Leadership School. 1987. *State of the school*. Lander, WY: National Outdoor Leadership School.

———. 1991. *National Outdoor Leadership School 1991 catalog of courses*. Lander, WY: National Outdoor Leadership School.

———. 2004. Mission and values. www.nols.edu/about/values.shtml.

———. 2004. History. www.nols.edu/about/history/.

North Carolina Outward Bound. 1987. *Instructor's field manual: North Carolina Outward Bound School*. Morganton, NC: North Carolina Outward Bound School.

———. 1993. *The instructor's handbook: North Carolina Outward Bound School*. 7th ed. Asheville, NC: North Carolina Outward Bound School.

Outward Bound. 2004. Mission statement. www.outward-bound.org/about_sub1_mission.htm.

———. 2004. Outward Bound International annual reports. www.outward-bound.org/about_annual.htm.

Petzoldt, P. K. 1995. *Teton tales: And other Petzoldt anecdotes*. Merrillville, IN: ICS Books.

Priest, S. 1999. The semantics of adventure programming. In *Adventure Programming*, eds. J. C. Miles and S. Priest. State College, PA: Venture Publishing.

Raiola, E., and M. O'Keefe. 1999. Philosophy in practice: A history of adventure programming. In *Adventure Programming*, eds. J. C. Miles, and S. Priest. State College, PA: Venture Publishing.

Ringholz, R. C. 1997. *On belay!: The life of legendary mountaineer Paul Petzoldt*. Seattle: The Mountaineers.

Seldon, W. L. Get adventurous! Outward Bound. www.lynnseldon.com/article119.html.

Smith, J. W., R. E. Carlson, G. W. Donaldson, and H. B. Masters. 1972. *Outdoor education*. 2nd ed. Englewood Cliffs, NJ: Prentice Hall, Inc.

Wilderness Education Association. 1989. *The WEA affiliate handbook: For current and prospective affiliate members*. Saranac Lake, NY: Wilderness Education Association.

———. 2004. Welcome to WEA. www.weainfo.org/welcome.html.

27: Interpretation of the Natural and Cultural Environments

Ford, P., and J. Blanchard. 1993. *Leadership and administration of outdoor pursuits.* 2nd ed. State College, PA: Venture Publishing.

Gookin, J., and D. Wells, eds. 2002. *Environmental education notebook.* Lander, WY: National Outdoor Leadership School.

Ham, S. H. 1992. *Environmental interpretation: A practical guide for people with big ideas and small budgets.* Golden, CO: North American Press.

Knudson, D. M., T. T. Cable, and L. Beck. 1995. *Interpretation of cultural and natural resources.* State College, PA: Venture Publishing.

National Outdoor Leadership School. 1999. *Wilderness educator notebook.* Lander, WY: National Outdoor Leadership School.

Regnier, K., M. Gross, and R. Zimmerman. 1992. *The interpreter's guidebook: Techniques for programs and presentations.* Stevens Point, WI:. UW-SP Foundation Press.

Sharpe, G. W. 1976. *Interpreting the environment.* New York: John Wiley and Sons.

28: Knots: An Introduction

Ashley, C. 1944. *Ashley book of knots.* New York: Doubleday.

Bigon, M., and G. Regazzoni. 1981. *The Morrow guide to knots.* New York: William Morrow & Co.

Budworth, G. 2001. *The ultimate encyclopedia of knots and ropework.* London: Select Editions.

Cinnamon, J. 1994. *Climbing rock and ice: Learning the vertical dance.* Camden, ME: Ragged Mountain Press.

Cox, S., and K. Fulsaas, eds. 2003. *Mountaineering: The freedom of the hills.* 7th ed. Seattle: The Mountaineers.

Padgett, A., and B. Smith. 1996. *On rope: North American vertical rope techniques.* 2nd ed. Huntsville, AL: Vertical Section, National Speleological Society.

Raleigh, D., and M. Clelland. 2003. *Knots and ropes for climbers.* Mechanicsburg, PA: Stackpole Books.

29: Leadership

Adizes, I. 1991. *Mastering change: The power of mutual trust and respect.* Santa Monica, CA: Adizes Institute Publications.

Arnaud, D., and T. LeBon. 2000. Towards wise decision-making (ii): Decision-making and the emotions. *Practical Philosophy* 3:3 (March). www.decision-making.co.uk/Publications/DecisionMakingAndEmotions.htm.

Buell, L. 1983. *Outdoor leadership competency: A manual for self-assessment and staff evaluation.* Greenfield, MA: Environmental Awareness Publications.

Canadian Conservative Forum. n.d. Will Rogers quotations. www.conservative forum.org/authquot.asp?ID=60.

Clark, K. E., and M. B. Clark. 1990. *Measures of leadership.* West Orange, NJ: Leadership Library of America.

Cockrell, D., ed. 1991. *The wilderness educator: The Wilderness Education Association curriculum guide.* Merrillville, IN: ICS Books, Inc.

Daniels, A. 2002. The dangers of micromanagement. *Entrepreneur.com,* February 4. www.entrepreneur.com/Your_Business/YB_SegArticle/0,4621,296886,00.html.

Drury, J. K., and E. R. Holmlund. 1997. *The camper's guide to outdoor pursuits: Finding safe, nature-friendly and comfortable passage through wild places.* Champaign, IL: Sagamore Publishing.

Facione, P. A. 2004. *Critical thinking: What it is and why it counts.* California Academic Press. www.insightassessment.com/pdf_files/what&why2004.pdf.

Ford, P., and J. Blanchard. 1993. *Leadership and administration of outdoor pursuits.* 2nd ed. State College, PA: Venture Publishing.

Fulghum, R. 1990. *All I really need to know I learned in kindergarten.* New York: Ballantine Books, Inc.

Gookin, J., M. Doran, and R. Green, eds. 2001. *2001 NOLS leadership education tool-box.* Lander, WY: National Outdoor Leadership School.

Graham, J. 1997. *Outdoor leadership: Technique, common sense & self-confidence.* Seattle: The Mountaineers.

Guillot, W. M. 2004. Critical thinking for the military professional. *Air & Space Power Chronicles* (June 17). www.airpower.maxwell.af.mil/airchronicles/cc/guillot.html.

Harvey, M. 1999. *The National Outdoor Leadership School's wilderness guide: The classic handbook, revised and updated.* 2nd ed. New York: Simon & Schuster.

Hersey, P., and K. H. Blanchard. 1982. *Management of organizational behavior: Utilizing human resources.* 4th ed. Englewood Cliffs, NJ: Prentice Hall.

Infinite Innovations Ltd. 1999–2003. Definitions. www.brainstorming.co.uk/tutorials/definitions.html.

Keay, W. 1996. *Expedition guide.* 3rd ed. Wellingborough, Northamptonshire, UK: Sterling Press.

Kouzes, J. M., and B. Z. Posner. 1995. *The leadership challenge.* 3rd ed. San Francisco: Jossey-Bass Publishers.

Lunenburg, F. C., and A. C. Ornstein. 1991. *Educational administration concepts and practices.* Belmont, CA: Wadsworth Publishing Company.

Mehrabian, A. 1971. *Silent messages.* Belmont, CA: Wadsworth.

Mobilia, W., ed. 1999. *Education by design: Level 1 coaching kit.* Keene, NH: Antioch New England Graduate School.

National Outdoor Leadership School. 1999. *Wilderness educator notebook.* Lander, WY: National Outdoor Leadership School.

Palmer, P. 1998. *The courage to teach: Exploring the inner landscape of a teacher's life.* San Francisco: Jossey-Bass Publishers.

Petzoldt, P. 1984. *The new wilderness handbook.* 2nd ed. New York: W. W. Norton & Company.

Plous, S. 1993. *The psychology of judgment and decision making.* New York: McGraw-Hill.

Priest, S., and M. A. Gass. 1997. *Effective leadership in adventure programming.* Champaign, IL: Human Kinetics.

Resource Ministries International. 1999. Leadership credibility account. *GraceNotes* 6 (June). www.resourceministries.org/gracen6.htm.

Rosenbach, W. E., and R. L. Taylor, eds. 1984. *Contemporary issues in leadership.* Boulder, CO: Westview Press.

Silvester, S. 2003-4. Inspiring communication: Using more than words. 5.12 Solutions. www.512solutions.com/article2.html.

30: Navigation: Map Folding

Drury, J. K., and E. R. Holmlund. 1997. *The camper's guide to outdoor pursuits: Finding safe, nature-friendly and comfortable passage through wild places.* Champaign, IL: Sagamore Publishing.

31: Navigation: Map Interpretation

Braasch, G. 1973. Reading a map at a glance. *Backpacker* (Fall): 34.

Burns, B., M. Burns, and P. Hughes. 1999. *Wilderness navigation: Finding your way using map, compass, altimeter and GPS*. Seattle: The Mountaineers.

Drury, J. K., and E. R. Holmlund. 1997. *The camper's guide to outdoor pursuits: Finding safe, nature-friendly and comfortable passage through wild places*. Champaign, IL: Sagamore Publishing.

Ford, P., and J. Blanchard. 1993. *Leadership and administration of outdoor pursuits*. 2nd ed. State College, PA: Venture Publishing.

Groundspeak Inc. 2000–4. Geocaching: Benchmark hunting. www.geocaching .com/mark/.

Harvey, M. 1999. *The National Outdoor Leadership School's wilderness guide: The classic handbook, revised and updated*. 2nd ed. New York: Simon & Schuster.

Jacobson, C. 1988. *The basic essentials of map and compass*. Merrillville, IN: ICS Books, Inc.

Keay, W. 1996. *Expedition guide*. 3rd ed. Wellingborough, Northamptonshire, UK: Sterling Press.

Kjellstrom, B. 1976. *Be expert with map and compass: The orienteering handbook*. New York: Charles Scribner's Sons.

———. 1994. *Be expert with map and compass: The complete orienteering handbook*. New York: Macmillan.

National Outdoor Leadership School. 1999. *Wilderness educator notebook*. Lander, WY: National Outdoor Leadership School.

32: Navigation: An Introduction to the Compass

Burns, B., M. Burns, and P. Hughes. 1999. *Wilderness navigation: Finding your way using map, compass, altimeter and GPS*. Seattle: The Mountaineers.

Drury, J. K., and E. R. Holmlund. 1997. *The camper's guide to outdoor pursuits: Finding safe, nature-friendly and comfortable passage through wild places*. Champaign, IL: Sagamore Publishing.

Ford, P., and J. Blanchard. 1993. *Leadership and administration of outdoor pursuits*. 2nd ed. State College, PA: Venture Publishing.

Harvey, M. 1999. *The National Outdoor Leadership School's wilderness guide: The classic handbook, revised and updated.* 2nd ed. New York: Simon & Schuster.

Keay, W. 1996. *Expedition guide.* 3rd ed. Wellingborough, Northamptonshire, UK: Sterling Press.

Kjellstrom, B. 1976. *Be expert with map and compass: The orienteering handbook.* New York: Charles Scribner's Sons.

——. 1994. *Be expert with map and compass: The complete orienteering handbook.* New York: Macmillan.

National Outdoor Leadership School. 1999. *Wilderness educator notebook.* Lander, WY: National Outdoor Leadership School.

Warren, J. W. 1986. Map and compass fundamentals. *Adirondac* L 4 (May): 12–16.

33: Navigation: Combining the Map and Compass

Barnes, S. 2000. *Basic essentials: Global positioning systems.* Guilford, CT: The Globe Pequot Press.

Burns, B., M. Burns, and P. Hughes. 1999. *Wilderness navigation: Finding your way using map, compass, altimeter and GPS.* Seattle: The Mountaineers.

Drury, J. K., and E. R. Holmlund. 1997. *The camper's guide to outdoor pursuits: Finding safe, nature-friendly and comfortable passage through wild places.* Champaign, IL: Sagamore Publishing.

Ford, P., and J. Blanchard. 1993. *Leadership and administration of outdoor pursuits.* 2nd ed. State College, PA: Venture Publishing.

Harvey, M. 1999. *The National Outdoor Leadership School's wilderness guide: The classic handbook, revised and updated.* 2nd ed. New York: Simon & Schuster.

Keay, W. 1996. *Expedition guide.* 3rd ed. Wellingborough, Northamptonshire, UK: Sterling Press.

Kjellstrom, B. 1976. *Be expert with map and compass: The orienteering handbook.* New York: Charles Scribner's Sons.

——. 1994. *Be expert with map and compass: The complete orienteering handbook.* New York: Macmillan.

National Outdoor Leadership School. 1999. *Wilderness educator notebook.* Lander, WY: National Outdoor Leadership School.

Warren, J. W. 1986. Map and compass fundamentals. *Adirondac* L 4 (May): 12–16.

34: Navigation: Route Finding with Map and Compass

Barnes, S. 2000. *Basic essentials: Global positioning systems.* Guilford, CT: The Globe Pequot Press.

Burns, B., M. Burns, and P. Hughes. 1999. *Wilderness navigation: Finding your way using map, compass, altimeter and GPS.* Seattle: The Mountaineers.

Drury, J. K., and E. R. Holmlund. 1997. *The camper's guide to outdoor pursuits: Finding safe, nature-friendly and comfortable passage through wild places.* Champaign, IL: Sagamore Publishing.

Ford, P., and J. Blanchard. 1993. *Leadership and administration of outdoor pursuits.* 2nd ed. State College, PA: Venture Publishing.

Harvey, M. 1999. *The National Outdoor Leadership School's wilderness guide: The classic handbook, revised and updated.* 2nd ed. New York: Simon & Schuster.

Keay, W. 1996. *Expedition guide.* 3rd ed. Wellingborough, Northamptonshire, UK: Sterling Press.

Kjellstrom, B. 1976. *Be expert with map and compass: The orienteering handbook.* New York: Charles Scribner's Sons.

———. 1994. *Be expert with map and compass: The complete orienteering handbook.* New York: Macmillan.

National Outdoor Leadership School. 1999. *Wilderness educator notebook.* Lander, WY: National Outdoor Leadership School.

Warren, J. W. 1986. Map and compass fundamentals. *Adirondac* L 4 (May): 12–16.

35: Navigation: Triangulation with Map and Compass

Drury, J. K., and E. R. Holmlund. 1997. *The camper's guide to outdoor pursuits: Finding safe, nature-friendly and comfortable passage through wild places.* Champaign, IL: Sagamore Publishing.

Kjellstrom, B. 1976. *Be expert with map and compass: The orienteering handbook.* New York: Charles Scribner's Sons.

———. 1994. *Be expert with map and compass: The complete orienteering handbook.* New York: Macmillan.

National Outdoor Leadership School. 1999. *Wilderness educator notebook.* Lander, WY: National Outdoor Leadership School.

36: Navigation: An Introduction to GPS

Anon. 1998. *GPS 315/320 user manual.* San Dimas, CA: Magellan.

Barnes, S. 2005. *Basic essentials: Global positioning systems.* Guilford, CT: The Globe Pequot Press.

Burns, B., M. Burns, and P. Hughes. 1999. *Wilderness navigation: Finding your way using map, compass, altimeter and GPS.* Seattle: The Mountaineers.

Carnes, John. 2002. Map datums. MapTools. www.maptools.com/UsingUTM/mapdatum.html.

Centre for Topographic Information, Ottawa; Natural Resources Canada. 1999. Maps 101: Topographic Maps, the Basics. http://maps.NRCan.gc.ca/maps 101/utm.html.

Dana, P. H. 2000. Global positioning system overview. The Geographer's Craft, Department of Geography, University of Colorado at Boulder. www .colorado.edu/geography/gcraft/notes/gps/gps_f.html.

Eagle Electronics. 2002. Selective availability: What is the effect of SA on GPS navigation? (Last updated August 21.) www.eaglegps.com/support/faq/faq_sa.htm.

Garmin Ltd. 1996–2005. What is WAAS? www.garmin.com/aboutGPS/waas.html.

Grubbs, B. 1998. *Using GPS: Finding your way with the global positioning system.* Helena, MT: Falcon Press.

Hotchkiss, N. 1994. *A comprehensive guide to land navigation with GPS.* Herndon, VA: Alexis Publishing.

Interagency GPS Executive Board. 2003. U.S. policy statement regarding civil GPS availability (March 21). www.igeb.gov/sa.shtml.

Keay, W. 1996. *Expedition guide.* 3rd ed. Wellingborough, Northamptonshire, UK: Sterling Press.

Letham, L. 2003. *GPS made easy: Using global positioning systems in the outdoors.* 4th ed. Seattle: The Mountaineers.

Mehaffey, J., J. Yeazel, and D. DePriest. 1997–2004. Important features for a hiking GPS. gpsinformation.net. http://gpsinformation.us/main/gps hiking.htm.

37: Personal Hygiene

Drury, J. K., and E. R. Holmlund. 1997. *The camper's guide to outdoor pursuits: Finding safe, nature-friendly and comfortable passage through wild places.* Champaign, IL: Sagamore Publishing.

Jaret, P. 2003. What's in the water? *Backpacker* (December): 45–58.

MedicineNet, Inc. 1996–2005. Metronidazole. www.medicinenet.com/metronidazole/article.htm.

Meyer, K. 1994. *How to shit in the woods: An environmentally sound approach to a lost art.* 2nd ed. Berkeley, CA: Ten Speed Press.

National Outdoor Leadership School. 1999. *Wilderness educator notebook.* Lander, WY: National Outdoor Leadership School.

New York State Department of Health. 2004. Cryptosporidiosis (last revised, June). www.health.state.ny.us/nysdoh/communicable_diseases/en/crypto.htm.

Offshore Pharmacy. 1996–2004. Rulid. www.smart-drugs.com/Inserts/insert-Roxithromycin.htm.

Petzoldt, P. 1984. *The new wilderness handbook.* 2nd ed. New York: W. W. Norton & Company.

Schatz, C., and D. Seemon. 1994. *A basic guide to minimum impact camping.* Cambridge, MN: Adventure Publications, Inc.

Tilton, B., and R. Bennett. 1995. *Camping healthy: Hygiene for the outdoors.* Merrillville, IN: ICS Books.

———. 2002. *Don't get sick: The hidden dangers of camping and hiking.* 2nd ed. Seattle: The Mountaineers.

University of North Carolina at Chapel Hill student health service. 2003. Water purification. www.shs.unc.edu/library/articles/waterpurification.html.

Welch, T. R. 2004. A rational approach to backcountry water use. Presentation at 2004 Wilderness Education Association Annual Conference, Bloomington, IN.

Welch, T. P., and T. R. Welch. 1995. Giardiasis as a threat to backpackers in the United States: A survey of state health departments. *Wilderness and Environmental Medicine* 6: 162–66.

Williamson, J. E., and N. Hansen, ed. 2002. *Accidents happen: Lessons from 2001's mountaineering accident report* (excerpt). Seattle: The Mountaineers. www.dcsar.org/featuredbooks.html.

38: Rock Climbing: Leadership Considerations for Top Roping

Cinnamon, J. 1994. *Climbing rock and ice: Learning the vertical dance*. Camden, ME: Ragged Mountain Press.

Cox, S., and K. Fulsaas. eds. 2003. *Mountaineering: The freedom of the hills*. 7th ed. Seattle: The Mountaineers.

Dougherty, N. J., ed. 1998. *Outdoor recreation safety*. Champaign, IL: Human Kinetics.

Ford, P., and J. Blanchard. 1993. *Leadership and administration of outdoor pursuits*. 2nd ed. State College, PA: Venture Publishing.

Graydon, D., and K. Hanson, eds. 1997. *Mountaineering: The freedom of the hills*. 6th ed. Seattle, WA: The Mountaineers.

Long, J. 1998. *How to rock climb*. 3rd ed. Helena, MT: Falcon Press.

Powers, P., and M. Cheek, eds. 2000. *NOLS climbing instructor notebook*. Lander, WY: National Outdoor Leadership School.

39: Safety: Emergency Procedures

Auerbach, P. S., ed. 1995. *Wilderness medicine: Management of wilderness and environmental emergencies*. 3rd ed. St. Louis: Mosby, Inc.

——. 2001. *Wilderness medicine*. 4th ed. St. Louis: Mosby, Inc.

Auerbach, P. S., H. Donner, and E. Weiss. 2003. *Field guide to wilderness medicine*. 2nd ed. St. Louis: Mosby, Inc.

Forgey, W. 2000. *Wilderness medicine: Beyond first aid*. 5th ed. Guilford, CT: The Globe Pequot Press.

Morrissey, J. 2000. *Wilderness medical associates field guide*. 2nd ed. Bryant Pond, ME: Wilderness Medical Associates.

Schimelpfenig, T. 2000. *NOLS wilderness first aid*. Lander, WY: National Outdoor Leadership School.

40: Safety: Risk Management

Auerbach, P. S., ed. 1995. *Wilderness medicine: Management of wilderness and environmental emergencies*. 3rd ed. St. Louis: Mosby, Inc.

———. 2001. *Wilderness medicine*. 4th ed. St. Louis: Mosby, Inc.

Auerbach, P. S., H. Donner, and E. Weiss. 2003. *Field guide to wilderness medicine*. 2nd ed. St. Louis: Mosby, Inc.

Beyer, S. 2002. *Risk management in wilderness education*. Chicago, IL: Wilderness Drum, Inc.

Cline, P. B. 1999. Outline to creating a risk management plan. *Outdoor Network Newsletter* (10) 4.

Drury, J. K., and E. R. Holmlund. 1997. *The camper's guide to outdoor pursuits: Finding safe, nature-friendly and comfortable passage through wild places*. Champaign, IL: Sagamore Publishing.

Ford, P., and J. Blanchard. 1993. *Leadership and administration of outdoor pursuits*. 2nd ed. State College, PA: Venture Publishing.

Forgey, W. W. 1989. *The basic essentials of first aid for the outdoors*. Merrillville, IN: ICS Books, Inc.

Gass, M., ed. 1998. *Administrative practices of accredited adventure programs*. Needham Heights, MA: Association for Experiential education.

Gregg, C. 1998. Almost safe, and proud of it! Paper presented at NOLS Wilderness Risk Managers Conference, Lander, WY.

———. 1999. Analyze, manage, inform. Workshop given at the Association for Experiential Education International Conference, Rochester, NY.

Isaac, J., and P. Goth. 1991. *The Outward Bound wilderness first-aid handbook*. New York: Lyons & Burford.

Jensen, C. R. 1995. *Outdoor recreation in America*. 5th ed. Champaign, IL: Human Kinetics.

Johanson, K. M., ed. 1984. *Accepted peer practices in adventure programming*. Boulder, CO: Association for Experiential Education.

Miles, J. C., and S. Priest. 1990. *Adventure education*. State College, PA: Venture Publishing.

Morrissey, J. 2000. *Wilderness Medical Associates field guide*. Bryant Pond, ME: Wilderness Medical Associates.

National Outdoor Leadership School. 1999. *Wilderness educator notebook*. Lander, WY: National Outdoor Leadership School.

Schimelpfenig, T., and L. Lindsey. 1991. *NOLS wilderness first aid*. Lander, WY: National Outdoor Leadership School.

Tilton, B., and F. Hubbell. 1994. *Medicine for the backcountry.* 2nd ed. Merrillville, IN: ICS Books.

Van der Smissen, B. J. 1980. *Legal liability: Adventure activities.* Las Cruces, NM: Educational Resources Information Center.

——. 1997. *Creating a proper risk management plan.* Boulder, CO: The Outdoor Network.

41: Safety: Waterfront Safety in the Backcountry

American National Red Cross. 1977. *Canoeing.* Garden City, NY: Doubleday & Company, Inc.

——. 1979. *Lifesaving: Rescue and safety.* Garden City, NY: Doubleday & Company, Inc.

——. 1992. *Aquatic safety.* St. Louis: Mosby, Inc.

——. 1995. *Water rescue.* St. Louis: Mosby, Inc.

——. 1996. *Community water safety.* St. Louis: Mosby, Inc.

——. 1997. *Basic water rescue.* St. Louis: Mosby, Inc.

Forgey, W. W. 1985. *Hypothermia: Death by exposure.* Merrillville, IN: ICS Books.

Girl Scouts of Milwaukee Area, Inc. 2005. Waterfront activities and safety standards. www.girlscoutsmilwaukee.org/tr_safety.htm.

Priest, S., and T. Dixon. 1990. *Safety practices in adventure programming.* Boulder, CO: Association of Experiential Education.

42: Stove Operation

Drury, J. K., and E. R. Holmlund. 1997. *The camper's guide to outdoor pursuits: Finding safe, nature-friendly and comfortable passage through wild places.* Champaign, IL: Sagamore Publishing.

Hart, J. 1977. *Walking softly in the wilderness.* San Francisco: Sierra Club Books.

National Outdoor Leadership School. 1999. *Wilderness educator notebook.* Lander, WY: National Outdoor Leadership School.

Simer, P., and J. Sullivan. 1983. *The National Outdoor Leadership School's wilderness guide.* New York: Simon & Schuster.

43: Travel Technique: An Introduction to Travel

Drury, J. K., and E. R. Holmlund. 1997. *The camper's guide to outdoor pursuits: Finding safe, nature-friendly and comfortable passage through wild places.* Champaign, IL: Sagamore Publishing.

Ford, P., and J. Blanchard. 1993. *Leadership and administration of outdoor pursuits.* 2nd ed. State College, PA: Venture Publishing.

Hampton, B., D. Cole, and D. Casey. 1995. *Soft paths: How to enjoy the wilderness without harming it.* Harrisburg, PA: Stackpole Books.

Keay, W. 1996. *Expedition guide.* 3rd ed. Wellingborough, Northamptonshire, UK: Sterling Press.

National Outdoor Leadership School. 1997. *Leave no trace: Outdoor skills and ethics.* Lander, WY: National Outdoor Leadership School.

———. 1999. *Wilderness educator notebook.* Lander, WY: National Outdoor Leadership School.

Petzoldt, P. 1984. *The new wilderness handbook.* 2nd ed. New York: W. W. Norton & Company.

Schatz, C., and D. Seemon. 1994. *A basic guide to minimum impact camping.* Cambridge, MN: Adventure Publications, Inc.

Simer, P., and J. Sullivan. 1983. *The National Outdoor Leadership School's wilderness guide.* New York: Simon & Schuster.

44: Travel Technique: Hiking

Cox, S., and K. Fulsaas, eds. 2003. *Mountaineering: The freedom of the hills.* 7th ed. Seattle: The Mountaineers.

Curtis, R. 1998. *The backpacker's field manual: A comprehensive guide to mastering backcountry skills.* New York: Three Rivers Press.

Drury, J. K., and E. R. Holmlund. 1997. *The camper's guide to outdoor pursuits: Finding safe, nature-friendly and comfortable passage through wild places.* Champaign, IL: Sagamore Publishing.

Ford, P., and J. Blanchard. 1993. *Leadership and administration of outdoor pursuits.* 2nd ed. State College, PA: Venture Publishing.

Hart, J. 1977. *Walking softly in the wilderness.* San Francisco: Sierra Club Books.

Harvey, M. 1999. *The National Outdoor Leadership School's wilderness guide: The classic handbook, revised and updated.* 2nd ed. New York: Simon & Schuster.

Keay, W. 1996. *Expedition guide*. 3rd ed. Wellingborough, Northamptonshire, UK: Sterling Press.

National Outdoor Leadership School. 1997. *Leave no trace: Outdoor skills and ethics*. Lander, WY: National Outdoor Leadership School.

———. 1999. *Wilderness educator notebook*. Lander, WY: National Outdoor Leadership School.

Petzoldt, P. 1984. *The new wilderness handbook*. 2nd ed. New York: W. W. Norton & Company.

Simer, P., and J. Sullivan. 1983. *The National Outdoor Leadership School's wilderness guide*. New York: Simon & Schuster.

45: Travel Technique: Canoeing and Sea Kayaking

American Canoe Association. 1987. *Canoeing and kayaking: Instruction manual*. Newington, VA: American Canoe Association.

American Red Cross. 1977. *Canoeing*. Garden City, NY: Doubleday & Company, Inc.

———. 1979. *Lifesaving: Rescue and safety*. Garden City, NY: Doubleday & Company, Inc.

———. 1995. *Canoeing and kayaking*. St. Louis: Mosby, Inc.

Belknap, L., C. Walbridge, M. Thornton, and R. Bowers. 1998. Personal preparedness and responsibility safety code of American Whitewater. Retrieved from American Whitewater Online. www.americanwhitewater.org/archive/safety/safety.html#river%20signals.

Conlan, T. 1998. *NOLS sea kayaking instructor notebook*. Lander, WY: National Outdoor Leadership School.

Ford, P., and J. Blanchard. 1993. *Leadership and administration of outdoor pursuits*. 2nd ed. State College, PA: Venture Publishing.

Grant, G. 1997. *Canoeing: A trailside guide*. New York: W. W. Norton & Company.

Gullion, L. 1987. *Canoeing and kayaking instruction manual*. Birmingham, AL: Menasha Ridge Press.

Hutchinson, D. 1999. *Expedition kayaking*. 4th ed. Guilford, CT: The Globe Pequot Press.

Jacobson, C. 1989. *Canoeing wild rivers*. 2nd ed. Merrillville, IN: ICS Books, Inc.

———. 2000. *Canoeing and camping: Beyond the basics.* 2nd ed. Guilford, CT: The Globe Pequot Press.

———. 2000. *Expedition canoeing: A guide to canoeing wild rivers in North America.* 3rd ed. Guilford, CT: The Globe Pequot Press.

46: Trip Planning

Drury, J. K., and E. R. Holmlund. 1997. *The camper's guide to outdoor pursuits: Finding safe, nature-friendly and comfortable passage through wild places.* Champaign, IL: Sagamore Publishing.

Ford, P., and J. Blanchard. 1993. *Leadership and administration of outdoor pursuits.* 2nd ed. State College, PA: Venture Publishing.

Harvey, M. 1999. *The National Outdoor Leadership School's wilderness guide: The classic handbook, revised and updated.* 2nd ed. New York: Simon & Schuster.

National Outdoor Leadership School. 1999. *Wilderness educator notebook.* Lander, WY: National Outdoor Leadership School.

Wilderness Education Association. 2000. *Affiliate handbook.* 6th ed. Bloomington, IN: Wilderness Education Association.

Wilderness Recreation Leadership Program. 1984. *Winter practicum manual.* Saranac Lake, NY: North Country Community College.

———. 1985. *Winter practicum manual.* Saranac Lake, NY: North Country Community College.

———. 1986. *Winter practicum manual.* Saranac Lake, NY: North Country Community College.

47: Water Treatment

Backer, H. 1989. Field water disinfection. In *Management of wilderness and environmental emergencies,* eds. Auerbach and Geehr. St. Louis: C. V. Mosby.

Bloch, J. D., and G. L. Patzkowsky. 1985. Giardiasis. *Family Practice Recertification 7* (1): 106–19, 122.

Drury, J. K., and E. R. Holmlund. 1997. *The camper's guide to outdoor pursuits: Finding safe, nature-friendly and comfortable passage through wild places.* Champaign, IL: Sagamore Publishing.

Harvey, M. 1999. *The National Outdoor Leadership School's wilderness guide: The classic handbook, revised and updated.* 2nd ed. New York: Simon & Schuster.

Jaret, P. 2003. What's in the water? *Backpacker* (December): 45–58.

Kahn, F. H., and B. R. Visscher. 1977. Water disinfection in the wilderness: A simple method of iodination. *Summit* 23 (3): 11–14.

Keay, W. 1996. *Expedition guide.* 3rd ed. Wellingborough, Northamptonshire, UK: Sterling Press.

MedicineNet, Inc. 1996–2005. Metronidazole. www.medicinenet.com/metronidazole/article.htm.

New York State Department of Health. 2004. Cryptosporidiosis (last revised, June). www.health.state.ny.us/nysdoh/communicable_diseases/en/crypto.htm.

Offshore Pharmacy. 1996–2004. Rulid. www.smart-drugs.com/Inserts/insert-Roxithromycin.htm.

Schatz, C., and D. Seemon. 1994. *A basic guide to minimum impact camping.* Cambridge, MN: Adventure Publications, Inc.

Schimelpfenig, T., and L. Lindsey. 1991. *NOLS wilderness first aid.* Lander, WY: National Outdoor Leadership School.

Tilton, B., and R. Bennett. 2002. *Don't get sick: The hidden dangers of camping and hiking.* 2nd ed. Seattle: The Mountaineers.

University of North Carolina at Chapel Hill student health service. 2003. Water purification. www.shs.unc.edu/library/articles/waterpurification.html.

Welch, T. R. 1986. Letter to the editor. *Adirondac,* September 30.

———. 2004. A rational approach to backcountry water use. Presentation at 2004 Wilderness Education Association Annual Conference, Bloomington, IN.

Welch, T. P., and T. R. Welch. 1995. Giardiasis as a threat to backpackers in the United States: A survey of state health departments. *Wilderness and Environmental Medicine* 6: 162–66.

Williamson, J. E., and N. Hansen, ed. 2002. *Accidents happen: Lessons from 2001's mountaineering accident report* (excerpt). Seattle: The Mountaineers. www.dcsar.org/featuredbooks.html.

48: Weather

Boy Scouts of America. 1984. *Fieldbook*. 3rd ed. Irving, TX: Boy Scouts of America.

Department of Atmospheric Sciences, Texas A & M University. n.d. Weather, lore, jingles and proverbs. www.met.tamu.edu/class/Metr304/Dir-test/lore.html.

Fisher, R. M. 1955. *Talk about the weather*. New York: Birk & Co., Inc.

Hardy, R., P. Wright, J. Kington, and J. Gribbin. 1982. *The weather book*. Boston: Little, Brown and Company.

Harvey, M. 1999. *The National Outdoor Leadership School's wilderness guide: The classic handbook, revised and updated*. 2nd ed. New York: Simon & Schuster.

Hodgson, M. 1992. *Basic essentials of weather forecasting*. Merrillville, IN: ICS Books, Inc.

Kovachick, R. J., ed. n.d. *United States weather: Northeastern New York and New England edition* (pp. 27–29). Albany, NY: WTEN-10 and WCDC-19.

Lehr, P. E., R. W. Burnett, and H. S. Zim. 1964. *Weather: A guide to phenomena and forecasts* (pp. 16–20, 142–45). New York: Golden Press.

National Oceanic and Atmospheric Administration. 2004. National Weather Service marine forecasts: Coastal marine forecasts by zone. Last modified July 9. www.nws.noaa.gov/om/marine/zone/usamz.htm.

——. n.d. Great Lakes Online. www.glakesonline.nos.noaa.gov/.

——. n.d. Tides Online. www.tidesonline.nos.noaa.gov/.

National Oceanic and Atmospheric Administration National Climatic Data Center. 2004. Past weather. Last updated December 30. www.noaa.gov/pastweather.html.

National Oceanic and Atmospheric Administration National Weather Service Internet Services Team. 2004. www.nws.noaa.gov/.

National Water and Climate Center. n.d. Climate reports and data. www.wcc.nrcs.usda.gov/climate/.

National Weather Service Storm Prediction Center. 2004. Last updated December 23. www.spc.noaa.gov/.

Old Farmer's Almanac. 2005. Cricket chirps to temperature. Dublin, NH: Yankee Publishing, Inc. www.almanac.com/outdoors/crickets.php.

Petterssen, S. 1958. *Introduction to meteorology*. 2nd ed. New York: McGraw-Hill Books.

Schlanger, V. 2003. Last updated December 12. Weather basics: Short range forecasting by plants and animals. www.atmosphere.mpg.de/enid/5057ce0c8397 e666f5a77ee2a0017790,55a304092d09/1qx.html.

Simer, P., and J. Sullivan. 1983. *The National Outdoor Leadership School's wilderness guide.* New York: Simon & Schuster.

Spooner, T. 1944. *Man's heritage of the skies: The ways of weather and climate and how they reach into our daily lives.* (p. 9.) Pittsburgh: Westinghouse Electric & Manufacturing Company.

Western Regional Climate Center. n.d. National and regional climate centers. www.wrcc.dri.edu/rcc.html.

Wilson, J. 2001. SkyWatch: Signs of the weather. www.wilstar.com/skywatch.htm.

United States Weather Bureau. 1962. Cloud forms (poster).

Index

monitoring groups. *See* group
monitoring
mountaineering certification, 314
mountain/valley winds, 522–23, 530
multipitch climbing, 431
multipurpose trips, 285

N

National Outdoor Leadership School
(NOLS), 178–79, 310, 311–12, 314
natural and cultural interpretation.
See interpretation, of natural/
cultural environments
navigation (compass introduction),
383–89
compass parts, 385–86
direction and, 384
field bearing, 386–87, 393–95
function of compass, 386
instructional strategies, 388–89
outcomes, 383
See also navigation (map and
compass combined)
navigation (GPS systems), 407–17
coordinate systems, 412–14
coordinating with map/
compass, 415
instructional strategies, 415–17
latitude/longitude coordinates,
412–13
mechanics of GPS, 409
outcomes, 407
receiver features/functions, 410–12
system overview, 408–9
UTM (Universal Transverse
Mercator) system, 413–14
navigation (map and compass
combined), 391–95
declination, 392–95

GPS systems and. *See* navigation
(GPS systems)
instructional strategies, 395
map bearings, 392
orienting maps, 395
outcomes, 391
philosophy, 392
procedures, 392–95
Time Control Plan (TCP), 399–400,
476–78
triangulation, 403–5
See also navigation (route finding)
navigation (map folding), 371–73
demonstration, 371–72
instructional strategies, 373
map storage, 372–73
outcomes, 371
reason for folding, 372
navigation (map interpretation)
details, 377–81
directions, 377–78
elevation markings, 378–81
general background, 375–76
instructional strategies, 381–82
margin information, 376–77
outcomes, 375
symbols, 377–78, 380
See also navigation (map and
compass combined)
navigation (route finding), 397–401
altitude gain/loss, 399
comfort considerations, 398
establishing guideposts, 398–99
instructional strategies, 400–401
outcomes, 397
terrain considerations, 398
time/distance, 398–400
navigation (triangulation), 403–5
instructional strategies, 404–5

outcomes, 403
steps, 404
triangulation defined, 404
navigators, 493
nonverbal communication, 8, 197–99
nonviolent interventions, 132, 135–37
nonwoven fabrics, 105
note takers, 51
nutrition. *See* food (nutrition/rations/
planning/packaging)

O

objectives. *See* outcomes
observation skills/steps, 293–95
opinion/information givers, 277
opinion/information seekers, 278
organizational goals, 286
organizations. *See* leadership
organizations
orienting groups. *See* group orienting
outcomes, 19–20. *See also specific topics*
outdoor education, 308–9
outdoor ethics, 174–75. *See also*
environmental ethics
Outward Bound (OB), 309–11
overhand knot, 330
overhand loop knot, 333

P

pace, 473, 476
parking lot/trash bin (for questions),
47–48
peer feedback, 40
"people" groups, 120–21
personal hygiene, 419–28
aesthetic concerns, 425–26
brushing teeth, 426
challenge, 427
grooming hair, 426

importance of, 420
instructional strategies, 426
microbes causing illness, 420–23
outcomes, 419
preventing injury, 424–25
preventing spread of illness,
423–24, 516
product quality checklist, 428
washing hands, 423, 516
See also bathing/washing
Petzoldt, Paul, 123, 311, 312, 313
physical fitness, 478–79
planning trips. *See* trip planning
PMI (Plus, Minus, Interesting)
debrief, 38–39
Decision at High Mountain, 163
defined, 48
positive interdependence, 24, 48–49
Post-Traumatic Stress Disorder
(PTSD), 133
post-trip considerations, 503–4
pots/pans, 224
preventing
injuries, 424–25. *See also* safety (risk
management)
spread of illness, 423–24, 516
probes, 200
problem solvers, 278
problem-based teaching approach. *See*
SPEC approach
"process" groups, 122
processing groups. *See* group
processing/debriefing
"product" groups, 121
product quality checklist
described, 49
template, 56
See also challenges/product quality
checklists

prompts, 200
protozoa, 422–23, 511
psychomotor skills, 348
public relations, 504

Q

quality criteria, 25–28, 37–38
quality discussion/quality audience,
49–50
questions, parking lot/trash bin for,
47–48
quick-bread. *See* food (quick-bread
baking)

R

radiation, 99
rafting certification, 314
random groups, 43
rappelling, 431
rations. *See* food (nutrition/rations/
planning/packaging)
real life challenges, 35
recipes. *See* food (granola preparation);
food (quick-bread baking)
recorders, 51
recreational trips, 285
resources
organizations. *See* leadership
organizations
for planning trips, 503
respiration, 100–101
rest breaks, 473–74, 490
rhythmic breathing, 472–73
risk management. *See* safety (risk
management)
rock climbing, 429–38
certification, 314
ethics, 433–35
institutional climbing, 430

instructional strategies, 438
leadership considerations, 436–38
organizations supporting, 314, 430
outcomes, 429–30
preparation, 436
programming considerations,
436–37
rating systems, 433
safety, 436–38
specific training/experience, 430–31
terminology, 431
top-rope, 431, 435–38
types of, 431
roles
leadership, 52, 358–60
monitoring, 295
teacher, 4
See also group roles
ropes. *See* knots

S

safety
backpack packing, 72–73
blister prevention/care, 486
campsite selection, 83
cooking, 222–23
defined, 444
fire, 210, 214, 222–23
food, 222–23
preventing illness, 423–24
preventing injury, 424–25
rock climbing, 436–38
stove operation, 466–68
water, 490
safety (emergency procedures), 439–42
emergency procedures, 440–41
evacuation procedures, 441
instructional strategies, 442
outcomes, 439

water sports certification, 314

water travel. *See* travel technique (canoeing/sea kayaking)

water treatment, 509–17

  boiling, 513–14

  chemical treatment, 514–16

  chlorination, 515–16

  Cryptosporidium and, 422–23, 512–13, 514, 515, 516

  crystalline iodination, 514

  filtration, 514, 516

  Giardia lamblia and, 422–23, 511–13, 514, 515, 516

  infectious illness and, 510

  instructional strategies, 516–17

  iodine tablets, 515

  methods, 513–16

  microorganisms necessitating, 510–13

  outcomes, 509

  reason for, 510–13

  special filters/purifiers, 516

waterproof fabrics, 105, 106

weather, 519–34

  altimeter/barometers predicting, 520–21

  animals predicting, 531

  barometric pressure and, 520–21

  clouds, 524–29, 532

  deserts, 530

  dew, 529, 531–32

  difficulty of, 520

  extreme, 530

  fog, 527–29

  forecast agencies, 530

  heavenly bodies predicting, 533

  instructional strategies, 534

  leaves predicting, 532

  local conditions, 530

  lore about, 530–34

  mountain/valley winds, 522–23, 530

  outcomes, 519

  seasonal, 530

  smoke predicting, 533

  temperature, elevation and, 523–24

  trip planning and, 502

  wind, 522–23, 530

white-water canoeing/rafting certification, 314

Wilderness Education Association (WEA), 310, 312, 314

Wilderness Risk Managers Committee Incident Reporting Project, 450–56

wind, 522–23, 530

W.I.S.E. system, 108–9

wool fabric, 104

woven fabrics, 105

Y

yeast baking. *See* food (yeast baking)

yeast/fungi, 421–22

About the Authors

Jack K. Drury

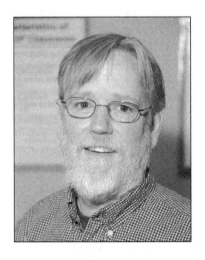

Jack has been working with learners of all ages and walks of life, ranging from youth at risk to longtime corporate executives. Jack is co-owner of Leading EDGE, a professional development organization of experienced educators who design and facilitate learning experiences for educators, businesses, nonprofit organizations, and government agencies. Jack was the founding director of the Wilderness Recreation Leadership Program and an associate professor at North Country Community College in Saranac Lake, New York. He has taught Wilderness Education Association (WEA) courses since 1979 and has been an Education By Design Institute coordinator affiliated with the Antioch New England Graduate School since 1992. He is past president of the WEA, a veteran of numerous National Outdoor Leadership School (NOLS) courses, and has been fortunate enough to lead and participate in ventures throughout North America, Central America, Europe, and Siberia during all the seasons.

Bruce F. Bonney

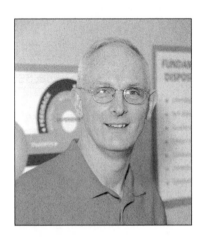

Bruce has played a leadership role in New York State in bringing change to the public school classroom by helping teachers and school systems take learning theory and turn it into real-life classroom and schoolwide practices. Bruce was a middle and high school social studies teacher for twenty-three years at Morrisville-Eaton Central School in upstate New York and was an associate of Education By Design at the Antioch New England Graduate School before cofounding Leading EDGE. He has presented at conferences and schools throughout the country and has played an instrumental role in introducing Education By Design to the United Kingdom.

Dene Berman

Dene Berman, Ph.D., a practicing psychologist, is clinical professor in the School of Professional Psychology at Wright State University in Dayton, Ohio. He has been involved with the wilderness therapy movement since the mid-1980s and is coauthor of *Wilderness Therapy: Foundations, Theory, and Practice* as well as numerous articles in professional journals. A Wilderness Education Association (WEA) instructor, Dene is on the board of trustees and is the current President of the WEA board.

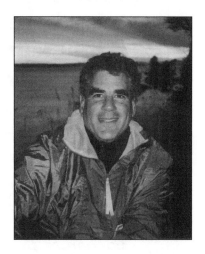

Mark C. Wagstaff

Mark is currently an associate professor of Recreation, Parks, and Tourism at Radford University, Virginia. Mark has been instructing for the Wilderness Education Association (WEA) since 1986 and served as executive director for three years. Mark's outdoor career includes instructing for the North Carolina Outward Bound School and professional white-water guiding throughout the United States and abroad.

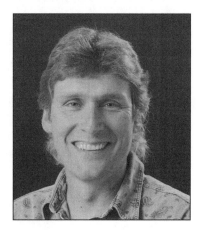

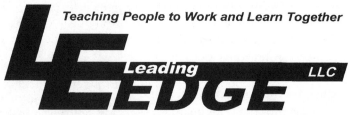

Wilderness Education Association

 Join The WEA Community!

The WEA is a non-profit membership organization that promotes wilderness education and preservation through wilderness leadership training within an affiliate network of colleges and outdoor programs.

WEA trains leaders, people who have good judgment and decision-making skills necessary to lead safe and environmentally-sound adventures. The WEA affiliate network is not limited to teaching outdoor skills or providing challenging adventures. WEA programs provide opportunities for learners to understand their own abilities and limitations, to make quality decisions, and to refrain from accepting responsibilities beyond their capabilities.

Member benefits include:
- **The WEA Journal.** The Journal is printed three times annually and includes, instructor profiles, national office updates, and messages from the President. Feature articles focus on field-based experiences.
- **Conference Discounts.** WEA members receive up to 20% off WEA conference registration fees.
- **Yahoo Groups.** Participate in lively industry discussion at wea@yahoogroups.com.
- **Professional Courtesy Discounts.** WEA Professional members, Instructors, and Certified Outdoor Leaders are eligible for discounts with a number of outdoor gear manufacturers

We rely on membership dues to carry out our important nonprofit work. The WEA works to train and certify outdoor leaders, develop new wilderness education curriculum, and form strategic alliances with wilderness land management agencies and other organizations.

The WEA mission: ***promoting the professionalism of outdoor leadership and to thereby improve the safety of outdoor trips and to enhance the conservation of the wild outdoors.***

WILDERNESS EDUCATION ASSOCIATION

900 East 7th Street - Bloomington IN, 47405
812.855.4095 voice - 812.855.8697 fax
E-mail: wea@indiana.edu - Web: www.weainfo.org

WHAT'S SO SPECIAL ABOUT UNSPOILED, NATURAL PLACES?

Beauty   Solitude   Wildness   Freedom   Quiet   Adventure
Serenity   Inspiration   Wonder   Excitement
Relaxation   Challenge

There's a lot to love about our treasured public lands, and the reasons are different for each of us. Whatever your reasons are, the national **Leave No Trace** education program will help you discover special outdoor places, enjoy them, and preserve them—today and for those who follow. By practicing and passing along these simple principles, you can help protect the special places you love from being loved to death.

THE PRINCIPLES OF LEAVE NO TRACE

- Plan ahead and prepare
- Travel and camp on durable surfaces
- Dispose of waste properly
- Leave what you find
- Minimize campfire impacts
- Respect wildlife
- Be considerate of other visitors

Leave No Trace is a national nonprofit organization dedicated to teaching responsible outdoor recreation skills and ethics to everyone who enjoys spending time outdoors.

To learn more or to become a member, please visit us at www.LNT.org or call (800) 332-4100.

Leave No Trace, P.O. Box 997, Boulder, CO 80306

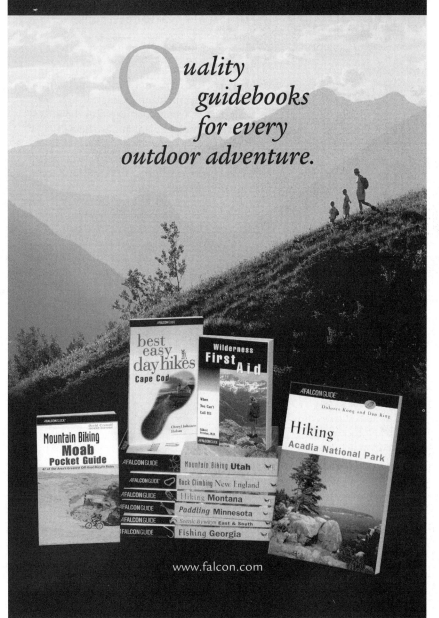

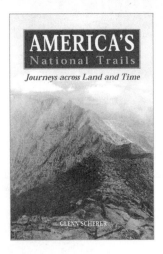
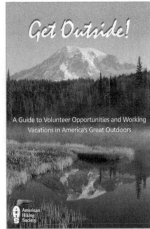
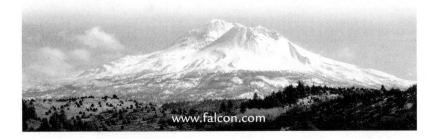